Certification and Core Review for

# Neonatal Intensive Care Nursing

## Fourth Edition

*Edited by*

**Robin L. Watson, RN, MN, CCRN**

Neonatal/Pediatric Clinical Nurse Specialist
Harbor-UCLA Medical Center
Torrance, California

AMERICAN
ASSOCIATION
*of* CRITICAL-CARE
NURSES

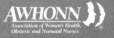

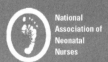

National
Association of
Neonatal
Nurses

**ELSEVIER**
SAUNDERS

3251 Riverport Lane
St. Louis, Missouri 63043

CERTIFICATION AND CORE REVIEW FOR
NEONATAL INTENSIVE CARE NURSING

ISBN: 978-1-4377-2633-6

---

**Notices**

Knowledge and best practice in this field are constantly changing. As new research and experience broaden our understanding, changes in research methods, professional practices, or medical treatment may become necessary.

Practitioners and researchers must always rely on their own experience and knowledge in evaluating and using any information, methods, compounds, or experiments described herein. In using such information or methods they should be mindful of their own safety and the safety of others, including parties for whom they have a professional responsibility.

With respect to any drug or pharmaceutical products identified, readers are advised to check the most current information provided (i) on procedures featured or (ii) by the manufacturer of each product to be administered, to verify the recommended dose or formula, the method and duration of administration, and contraindications. It is the responsibility of practitioners, relying on their own experience and knowledge of their patients, to make diagnoses, to determine dosages and the best treatment for each individual patient, and to take all appropriate safety precautions.

To the fullest extent of the law, neither the Publisher nor the authors, contributors, or editors, assume any liability for any injury and/or damage to persons or property as a matter of products liability, negligence or otherwise, or from any use or operation of any methods, products, instructions, or ideas contained in the material herein.

---

International Standard Book Number: 978-1-4377-2633-6

*Editor:* Maureen Iannuzzi
*Associate Developmental Editor:* Julia Curcio
*Publishing Services Manager:* Jeff Patterson
*Project Manager:* Megan Isenberg
*Design Direction:* Karen Pauls

Printed in the United States of America

Last digit is the print number:  9  8  7  6  5  4  3  2  1

Working together to grow
libraries in developing countries

www.elsevier.com | www.bookaid.org | www.sabre.org

ELSEVIER    BOOK AID International    Sabre Foundation

# Dedication

To those who walk with me—past, present, and future—who share in my laughter, who challenge me to climb higher, who guide me when I'm off course, who listen when I'm challenged, and who stand by me when I'm uncertain.

# Contributors

**Bobby B. Bellflower, DNSc, NNP-BC**
Option Coordinator
Neonatal Nurse Practitioner Program
College of Nursing
University of Tennessee Health Science Center
Memphis, Tennessee
Neonatal Nurse Practitioner
NICU
Pediatrix of Tennessee
Methodist Lebonheur Healthcare
Germantown, Tennessee
*Fluid and Electrolytes*

**Wanda Todd Bradshaw, RN, MSN, NNP-BC, PNP, CCRN**
Assistant Clinical Professor
Specialty Director-Neonatal
School of Nursing
Duke University
Durham, North Carolina
Neonatal & Pediatric Nurse Practitioner
Pediatrics: Neonatology
Duke University Health Care System
Durham, North Carolina
*Pharmacology*
*Pulmonary Disorders*

**Lucinda Brzozowski, RN, BSN, CCRN**
Neonatal Staff Nurse
ECMO Specialist
Intensive Care Nursery
Thomas Jefferson University Hospital
Philadelphia, Pennsylvania
*Neurologic Disorders*

**Robin Clifton-Koeppel, MS, RNC-NIC, CPNP, CNS**
Neonatal Clinical Nurse Specialist
Pediatric Nurse Practitioner
Neonatal Intensive Care Unit
Irvine Medical Center
University of California
Orange, California
*Nutrition Management*
*Patient Safety*

**Laura K. Cogswell, BSN, RNC**
Dartmouth Hitchcock Medical Center
Lebanon, New Hampshire
*Discharge Planning and Transition to Home Care*

**Beth Diehl-Svrjcek, RN, MS, CCRN, NNP, CCM, LNCC**
Neonatal Nurse Practitioner
Maryland Regional Neonatal Transport Program
Johns Hopkins Hospital
Baltimore, Maryland
*AACN Synergy Model for Patient Care*

**Janet Fogg, RNC-NIC, MSN**
Instructor
School of Nursing
The Pennsylvania State University
University Park, Pennsylvania
Staff Nurse
Neonatal Intensive Care Unit
The Milton S. Hershey Medical Center
Hershey, Pennsylvania
*Auditory and Ophthalmologic Disorders*
*Dermatologic Disorders*
*Perinatal Substance Abuse*

**Sharron Forest, DNP, NNP-BC**
Manager of Advanced Practice Nurses
Women and Children's Hospital
Lake Charles, Louisiana
*Immunologic Disorders and Infections*

**Debbie Fraser, MN, RNC-NIC**
Associate Professor
Centre for Nursing and Health Studies
Athabasca University
Athabasca, Alberta
Canada
Advanced Practice Nurse
Neonatal Intensive Care Unit
St. Boniface General Hospital
Winnipeg, Manitoba
Canada
Executive Editor
Neonatal Network
Santa Rosa, California
*Physical Assessment*

**Dodi Gauthier, M.Ed, RNC-OB, C-EFM**
Coordinator
Perinatal Education and Maternal Transport
Clinical Nurse, Labor and Delivery and High Risk OB
Santa Barbara Cottage Hospital
Santa Barbara, California
*Assessment of Fetal Well Being*
*Maternal-Fetal Complications*

**Sharyn Gibbins, NP, PhD**
Associate Professor
Nursing
University of Toronto
Toronto, Ontario
Canada
Professional Practice Lead
Professional Practice
Credit Valley Hospital
Mississauga, Ontario
Canada
*Pain Assessment and Management*

**Marie Hastings-Tolsma, PhD, CNM**
Associate Professor
Nurse Midwifery
College of Nursing
University of Colorado Denver
Aurora, Colorado
*Maternal-Fetal Complications*

**Ashley L. Hodges, PhD, WHNP-BC**
Assistant Professor
School of Nursing
University of Alabama at Birmingham
Birmingham, Alabama
*Legal Issues*

**Linda MacKenna Ikuta, MN, RN, CCNS, PHN**
Neonatal Clinical Nurse Specialist
Center for Nursing Excellence
Lucile Packard Children's Hospital at Stanford
    University Medical Center
Palo Alto, California
*Genetics and Congenital Anomalies*

**Beverly Inge-Walti, RNC-NIC, MSN, CPNP, CNS**
Clinical Nurse Specialist
Neonatal Intensive Care Unit
Children's Hospital of Orange County
Santa Margarita, California
*Ethical Issues*

**Anne M. Jorgensen, RNC, MS, NNP**
Assistant Professor of Pediatrics
Pediatrics
New York Medical College
Valhalla, New York
Assistant Director Neurodevelopmental Follow-up
    Center
Division of Neonatology
Good Samaritan Hospital
Suffern, New York
*Cardiovascular Disorders*

**Michelle LaBrecque, MSN, RN, CCRN**
Clinical Nurse Specialist
Neonatal Intensive Care Unit
Children's Hospital Boston
Boston, Massachusetts
*Gastrointestinal Disorders*

**Ellen Mack, MN, RNC**
Neonatal Clinical Nurse Specialist
Pediatrics/NICU
Cedars-Sinai Medical Center
Los Angeles, California
*Care of the Extremely Low Birth Weight Infant*

**Lisa Miklush, PhD, RNC, CNS**
Associate Professor
College of Graduate Nursing
Western University of Health Sciences
Pomona, California
*Research Issues*

**Janet Pettit  MSN, NNP-BC, CNS**
Neonatal Nurse Practitioner
Clinical Nurse Specialist
Neonatal Intensive Care Unit
Doctors Medical Center
Modesto, California
Assistant Nurse Manager
Maternal Child Health
Kaiser Permanente Medical Center
Modesto, California
*Renal and Genitourinary Disorders*

**Christine Retta, MSN, RNC, NNP-BC, CNS**
National Leader
National Risk Management and Patient Safety
Kaiser Permanente, Program Office
Oakland, California
*Adaptation to Extrauterine Life*
*Care of the Late Preterm Infant*

**Patricia Scheans, MSN, NNP-BC**
Neonatal Nurse Practitioner
Clinical Support for Neonatal Care
Legacy Health
Portland, Oregon
*Gestational Age Assessment*
*Developmental Support*

**Jennifer Stewart, RNC, MSN, CNS**
Clinical Nurse Specialist
Neonatal/Pediatric
Torrance Memorial Medical Center
Torrance, California
*Radiographic Evaluation*

**Laura S. Stokowski, RNC, MS**
Staff Nurse
Neonatal Intensive Care Unit
Inova Fairfax Hospital for Children
Fairfax Station, Virginia
*Metabolic and Endocrine Disorders*

**Shana Thompson, MSN, RNC, NNP-BC**
Clinical Instructor of Pediatrics
Boonshoft School of Medicine
Wright State University
Dayton, Ohio
Neonatal Nurse Practitioner
Regional Newborn Intensive Care Unit
The Children's Medical Center of Dayton
Dayton, Ohio
*Family Integration*

**Robin L. Watson, RN, MN, CNS, CCRN**
Clinical Nurse Specialist
Harbor-UCLA Medical Center
Torrance, California
*Cardiovascular Disorders*

**Linda Wynsma, RNC, MSN, CNS**
Neonatal/Pediatric Clinical Nurse Specialist
Long Beach, California
*Neonatal Resuscitation*
*Hematologic Disorders*

**Jenelle M. Zambrano, RN, MSN**
Neonatal Clinical Nurse Educator
Harbor-UCLA Medical Center
Torrance, California
*Gestational Age Assessment*
*Thermoregulation*

# Reviewers

Kelly Ballard, MSN, RNC-NIC, CNS, NNP-BC
Clinical Nurse Specialist, Neonatal/Pediatrics
Kern Medical Center
Bakersfield, California

Deanne Buschbach, RN, MSN, NNP, PNP
Duke University Medical Center
Cary, North Carolina

Dianne S. Charsha, RN, MSN, NNP-BC
Senior Vice President for Patient Care Services and
    Chief Nursing Officer
Cooper University Hospital
Camden, New Jersey

Christine Domonoske, PharmD
Children's Memorial Hermann Hospital
Houston, Texas

Linda L. Ehret, MSN, NNP-BC
Pediatrix Medical Group
Denver, Colorado

Susan A. Furdon, MS, RNC, NNP-BC
Albany Medical Center
Albany, New York

Carmen M. Hernandez, MSN, NNP-BC
Presbyterian St. Luke's Medical Center and The
    Rocky Mountain Hospital for Children
Denver, Colorado

Lisa Lima, MSN, PNP, CNS
Clinical Nurse Specialist
Neonatal Intensive Care Unit
St. John's Regional Medical Center
Oxnard, California

Annette S. Pacetti, RN, MSN, NNP-BC
Monroe Carell, Jr. Children's Hospital at Vanderbilt
Nashville, Tennessee

Sharyl L. Sadowski, MS, APN, NNP-BC
Neonatal Nurse Practitioner
Neonatal Outreach Educator
University of Illinois Perinatal Center
Chicago, Illinois

Julieanne Schiefelbein, DNP, M AppSc, MA (Ed),
    RNM, NNP-BC, PNP-BC, C-NPT
Primary Children's Medical Center
University of Utah, College of Nursing
Salt Lake City, Utah

Ann Petersen-Smith, PhD, RN, CPNP-AC
University of Colorado College of Nursing
Aurora, Colorado

Diane M. Szlachetka, APRN, NNP-BC
Baystate Medical Center
Springfield, Massachusetts

Mollie Frances Tripp, RN, MSN, NNP-BC
Clinical Assistant Professor
East Carolina University
Greenville, North Carolina

# Foreword

Three editions of the Core Curriculum for Neonatal Intensive Care Nursing and the Certification and Core Review for Neonatal Intensive Care Nursing confirm the successful collaboration of three preeminent nursing organizations: the American Association of Critical-Care Nurses; the Association of Women's Health, Obstetric and Neonatal Nurses; and the National Association of Neonatal Nurses. Their visionary leadership identified the need for essential resources that standardize the requisite knowledge for clinical practice in the rapidly evolving field of neonatal intensive care.

Once again, Editor Robin L. Watson, a master clinician and widely respected content expert, has assembled the energy, talent, and expertise of practicing nurses from these three associations to write and review study questions for neonatal nursing core content.

We applaud this singular example of how critical care nurses relentlessly and successfully foster true collaboration. With support from knowledgeable staff in each association, the editor and contributors have demonstrated the cooperation, collegiality, and quality that excellent care of critically ill infants and their families requires.

**Kristine Peterson, RN, MS, CCRN, CCNS**
Chief Executive Officer, American Association of Critical-Care Nurses

**Karen Peddicord, RNC, PhD**
Chief Executive Officer, Association of Women's Health, Obstetric and Neonatal Nurses

**Susan E. Reinarz, RN, MSN, NNP-BC**
President, National Association of Neonatal Nurses

# Preface

Care provided to critically ill newborns requires nurses who have specialized knowledge, skills, and experiences. Certification in neonatal nursing provides validation of these specialized competencies. Both the CCRN Certification Examination–Neonatal, offered by the AACN (American Association of Critical-Care Nurses) Certification Corporation, and the Neonatal Intensive Care Nursing certification examination, offered by the National Certification Corporation (NCC), are tools for assessing the acquisition of core knowledge essential to neonatal nursing practice.

This edition of the Certification and Core Review for Neonatal Intensive Care Nursing marks a new era for this resource. The accompanying Evolve Exam Review is an online, interactive version of this text. The participant can customize the Exam Review to simulate the CCRN–Neonatal or the RNC–NIC exam and choose between a study mode and a timed examination simulation. Using the access code found inside the front cover, visit http://evolve.elsevier.com/AACN/certification/ to take advantage of this helpful resource that comes free with the purchase of the Certification and Core Review for Neonatal Intensive Care Nursing, 4th edition.

The Certification and Core Review for Neonatal Intensive Care Nursing is designed as much to be a study guide and resource for nurses preparing to take a national certification examination in neonatal critical care nursing as it is a tool for nurses developing their critical thinking skills. I hope that experienced neonatal nurses will find the Certification and Core Review a refresher of their professional knowledge and that clinical nurse specialists and nurse educators who are responsible for assessing competency of neonatal nurses will refer to it as they design their own tools for assessing knowledge. The Certification and Core Review is an adjunct to the Core Curriculum for Neonatal Intensive Care Nursing and provides a mechanism for review and study of core content for neonatal intensive care nursing practice.

Content addressed in the Certification and Core Review is based on the AACN Certification Corporation's CCRN–Neonatal Test Plan and Testable Nursing Actions, as well as NCC's Test Content Outline–Neonatal Intensive Care Nursing. (Both can be found in the back of this text.) These resources guided the identification of subject matter and distribution of items for each content area. The structure of the Certification and Core Review is similar to that of the Core Curriculum; content is organized into four sections. The first section, General Assessment and Management, addresses clinical issues related to assessment of the fetus and physical and gestational age assessment of the newborn, adaptation of the fetus to extrauterine life, and general management practices basic to the care of critically ill newborns. "Care of the Late Preterm Infant" is a new chapter addressing the unique needs of these patients. The second section, Pathophysiology, is divided into two subsections. The first subsection, System-Specific Disorders, addresses patient care problems primarily affecting single body systems. The second subsection, Multisystem Considerations, addresses disorders that impact multiple organ systems. The third section, Professional Caring and Ethical Practice, highlights behaviors inherent to professional practice, such as the neonatal nurse's role in legal, ethical, and research issues. "AACN Synergy Model for Patient Care" is included again to illustrate how the synergy model is used as a basis for developing test questions.

All study items are multiple-choice with four options, giving readers practice at selecting a correct answer amidst three distractors. The answer to each item and explanations for the correct and incorrect answers can be found in Section IV. Rationales for the correct answers provide nurses with the knowledge required to prioritize, plan, and evaluate care. References supporting the correct answers and rationales are also provided. Questions are organized by topic area, so that individuals wanting to review a particular subject can easily find the content they need.

Study items address the various cognitive levels—knowledge, application, and analysis—providing readers the opportunity to recall, apply, and evaluate their knowledge of neonatal intensive care nursing. All phases of the nursing process are represented by the study items. Every effort was made to ensure that each question represents universal knowledge and reflects core content of neonatal intensive and critical care nursing practice. None of these questions has been or will be used on any certification examination. Because certification examinations are revised frequently, all nurses who are preparing for an examination are encouraged to contact the appropriate sponsoring agency to obtain the most up-to-date materials related to the areas of knowledge being tested on specific examinations. Information about CCRN certification can be found on the Web at www.certcorp.org; visit www.nccnet.org for NCC information.

Robin L. Watson

# Acknowledgments

The Certification and Core Review for Neonatal Intensive Care Nursing would not be possible without the dedication of the many contributors who graciously shared their time and expertise. With much gratitude, I thank each one of them for their commitment to this project. For returning contributors, this revision brought a new challenge of having to create rationales for incorrect answer options, as well as for the correct answers.

The reviewers provided insightful comments regarding content as well as test construction to ensure that the questions represent universal and core neonatal nursing knowledge. I sincerely appreciate the reviewers and the thoroughness of their work.

Julia Curcio, my developmental editor at Elsevier, kept the ball rolling and masterfully orchestrated my and the reviewer comments, revisions, and revisions to the revisions! Her patience and encouragement was such a gift and I sincerely thank her for her contribution to this work. My appreciation also goes to Maureen Iannuzzi and the entire editorial and publication staff at Elsevier.

My journey with the Certification and Core Review began in 1995, when I responded to a call for proposals for a study resource for the CCRN Neonatal exam. Six years later, the first edition of the "Core Review for Neonatal Intensive Care Nursing" was published. And there grew one of the most important relationships of my life … my bond with the American Association of Critical-Care Nurses. AACN has provided me with opportunity, challenge, support, and life-long friendships. I am so very grateful for all that AACN has given me, am proud to call them "family," and want to thank AACN for walking with me on this journey.

I honor my commitment to the neonatal intensive care nurses at Harbor-UCLA Medical Center to never forget my roots … I have not forgotten how scared I was that first shift I walked into the NICU as a new graduate almost 30 years ago. Today, I continue to be encouraged by them. Their questions challenge me, and their answers inspire me.

# Contents

# General Assessment and Management

## Chapter 1

# Assessment of Fetal Well-Being

1. A patient who is G2P2 at 33 weeks' gestation arrives at the triage unit complaining of regular uterine contractions. Her pregnancy history includes a preterm delivery at 34 weeks. Prior to examining her, the nurse performs electronic fetal monitoring and obtains a complete history. The patient reports no bleeding and no rupture of membranes. She has had no vaginal examinations or sexual activity for more than 24 hours. The biochemical marker useful in this situation for predicting preterm birth is:
   A. cervical ferritin.
   B. fetal fibronectin.
   C. corticotropin-releasing hormone.
   D. placental α-microglobulin-1.

2. A patient comes to the triage unit at 32 weeks' gestation concerned because she has been "leaking fluid" from her vagina for the past hour. She says she has felt no contractions and reports normal fetal activity. A bedside immunoassay called AmniSure is performed. This test identifies a glycoprotein abundant in amniotic fluid. This glycoprotein is called:
   A. prolactin.
   B. α-fetoprotein.
   C. fetal fibronectin.
   D. placenta α-microglobulin-1.

3. When electronic fetal monitoring is used, the *best* indicator of fetal oxygenation status during labor is:
   A. fetal heart rate baseline within the normal range.
   B. moderate fetal heart rate variability.
   C. absence of decelerations of the fetal heart rate.
   D. presence of accelerations in the fetal heart rate.

4. The biophysical profile (BPP) is currently the primary method for evaluating fetal well-being through the assessment of various activities that are controlled by the central nervous system and are sensitive to oxygenation. The five variables included in the BPP are:
   A. fetal tone, fetal breathing, fetal movement, non-stress test, and amniotic fluid volume.
   B. fetal movement, fetal tone, nonstress test, amniotic fluid index, and fetal position.
   C. fetal tone, fetal position, amniotic fluid volume, fetal heart rate, and fetal activity.
   D. fetal heart rate, fetal movement, nonstress test, amniotic fluid volume, and fetal tone.

5. An appropriate gestational length for glucose screening in women who are at low risk for developing gestational diabetes in pregnancy is:
   A. 20 to 21 weeks' gestation.
   B. 22 to 23 weeks' gestation.
   C. 24 to 28 weeks' gestation.
   D. 32 to 34 weeks' gestation.

6. When women give birth sitting upright, which of the following indicators show lower values in cord blood?
   A. pH
   B. $P_{CO_2}$
   C. $P_{O_2}$
   D. Base excess

7. Which test is most reliable in predicting fetal lung maturity in the infant of a diabetic mother?
   A. Fetal lung maturity test
   B. Phosphatidylglycerol level
   C. Lamellar body count
   D. Lecithin/sphingomyelin ratio

8. What is the physiologic cause of late decelerations?
   A. Fetal distress
   B. Sympathetic response to fetal activity
   C. Rapid fetal descent through the pelvis
   D. Transient interruption in fetal oxygenation

9. An intrauterine pressure catheter, once used to dilute meconium-stained amniotic fluid, perform amnioinfusion, or instill either normal saline or lactated Ringer solution into the uterus, is useful in the treatment of:
   A. polyhydramnios.
   B. late decelerations.
   C. variable decelerations.
   D. decreased fetal heart rate variability.

10. A patient is experiencing preterm labor at 33 weeks' gestation. She has a history of preterm labor and is currently showing regular contractions. To ensure that she receives her two doses of steroids to promote fetal lung maturity, a tocolytic medication is prescribed. This medication, a calcium channel blocker, has been marketed to treat hypertension, angina, and arrhythmia and does not commonly have adverse effects on the fetus or neonate. The medication is:
    A. magnesium sulfate.
    B. ketorolac (Toradol).
    C. terbutaline (Brethine).
    D. nifedipine (Procardia).

# Chapter 2

# Adaptation to Extrauterine Life

1. Which of the following pressure changes accurately represents normal postnatal adaptation to extrauterine life?
   A. Increase in pulmonary vascular resistance, increase in systemic vascular resistance
   B. Increase in pulmonary vascular resistance, decrease in systemic vascular resistance
   C. Decrease in pulmonary vascular resistance, increase in systemic vascular resistance
   D. Decrease in pulmonary vascular resistance, decrease in systemic vascular resistance

2. What is the name of the fetal shunt that is responsible for shunting blood between the aorta and pulmonary artery?
   A. Foramen ovale
   B. Ductus venosus
   C. Ductus arteriosus
   D. Blalock-Taussig shunt

3. The nurse in the labor, delivery, and recovery (LDR) department calls the nursery to request an immediate assessment of a term infant displaying signs and symptoms of respiratory distress following an uneventful vaginal delivery. Upon arrival to the LDR, the nursery nurse observes that the LDR nurse is providing bag-and-mask ventilation. The infant is dusky and has a scaphoid abdomen with an asymmetric-appearing chest with breath sounds greater on the right side. Based on this information, the infant most likely has what condition?

   A. Pneumothorax
   B. Diaphragmatic hernia
   C. Tracheoesophageal fistula
   D. Gastrointestinal obstruction

4. A 40⅔-week-gestation infant is delivered with vacuum assistance after a prolonged second stage of labor. The infant weighs 3.75 kg. This is the mother's first baby. The Apgar scores were 3, 5, and 8 at 1, 5, and 10 minutes, respectively. After stabilizing the infant following the delivery, the nurse conducts the head-to-toe assessment. Scalp edema is noted. When the head and neck areas are palpated, it is observed that swelling crosses the suture lines and feels boggy. The infant's overall tone is decreased. Based on these findings, what would be a probable diagnosis and care plan for this infant?
   A. Cephalohematoma; admit to the NICU for close observation.
   B. Subgaleal hemorrhage; admit to the NICU for close observation.
   C. Cephalohematoma; keep mother and baby together in the labor and delivery department.
   D. Caput succedaneum; keep mother and baby together in the labor and delivery department.

5. A 38-week-gestation infant is delivered by cesarean section due to a breech presentation. The Apgar score is 8 at 1 minute and 9 at 5 minutes. The mother received late prenatal care. The hepatitis B status of the mother is unknown. The plan

of care for this infant should include which one of the following options?

A. Administer monovalent hepatitis B vaccine before discharge from the hospital.

B. Draw maternal blood for determination of surface antigen status before performing any interventions.

C. Administer hepatitis B vaccine and 0.5 ml of hepatitis B immune globulin (HBIG) within 12 hours of birth.

D. Administer hepatitis B vaccine within 12 hours of birth. Determine mother's hepatitis B surface antigen (HBsAg) status as soon as possible and, if HBsAg positive, administer HBIG (no later than age 1 week).

6. A 37-week-gestation infant was delivered precipitously to a 33-year-old G4P3 mother. The mother's pregnancy was uneventful. The Apgar score was 7 at 1 minute and 9 at 5 minute. The infant was placed skin to skin on the mother's chest immediately after birth. The infant is now 1 hour old, and the nurse has just completed the first assessment. The infant has mild peripheral cyanosis of the hands and feet. The axillary temperature is 36.4° C (97.6° F). The head is rounded. Petechiae are noted on the face. Breath sounds are slightly coarse and equal with occasional expiratory grunting noted. Respiratory rate is 50 to 60 breaths/minute with an occasional increase to 70. Heart rate is 144 beats/minute. Tone is normal with flexion of arms and legs. Abdomen is soft and nondistended with bowel sounds present. Based on these assessment findings, follow-up care should include which of the following interventions?

A. Transfer the infant to the special care nursery/neonatal intensive care nursery.

B. Contact the pediatric provider to assess the respiratory status and peripheral cyanosis of this infant.

C. Keep the infant with the mother. Have the mother attempt to breast-feed and continue to monitor vital signs as per protocol.

D. Closely observe this infant under an open warmer. Delay feeding this infant due to the slight increase in respiratory rate and occasional grunting.

7. A term infant is now 24 hours old. The infant underwent a normal spontaneous vaginal delivery. Rupture of membranes occurred 12 hours prior to delivery. Results of the prenatal group B streptococcus screen were negative. Maternal temperature prior to delivery was normal. The amniotic fluid had light meconium staining. The infant was vigorous at birth and did not require resuscitation other than drying and clearing of the airway. The Apgar score was 8 at 1 minute and 9 at 5 minutes. The infant has been rooming in with the mother. The nurse on the mother/baby unit completed her shift assessment of the infant with the following findings: color slightly pale with decreased perfusion and pulses in the lower extremities compared with the upper extremities; slightly lethargic; respiratory rate 70 to 80 breaths/minute; no grunting, flaring, or retractions; last effective breast-feed was 6 hours ago. Based on the assessment findings, the nurse should carry out which of the following interventions?

A. Keep the baby with the mother, check glucose level, monitor temperature and respiratory rate, and observe for other signs of sepsis.

B. Notify the physician; transfer the infant to the nursery for observation and place under a radiant warmer with a possible diagnosis of coarctation of the aorta.

C. Keep the baby with the mother; obtain a lactation consultation; and place baby skin to skin on the mother's chest, knowing that these findings represent a normal transition.

D. Notify the physician; transfer the infant to the nursery for observation and place under a radiant warmer with a possible diagnosis of persistent pulmonary hypertension due to meconium aspiration.

8. Which hormone activates nonshivering thermogenesis?

A. Insulin
B. Vasopressin
C. Epinephrine
D. Norepinephrine

9. During fetal life, the lungs are fluid-filled. At the time of delivery, air fills the alveolar space and pulmonary vasodilation occurs. Adequate amounts of surfactant are needed to maintain adequate ventilation. The air-liquid interface is where the exchange of oxygen and carbon dioxide occur. Which of the following statements correctly describes the role of surfactant?

A. Surfactant decreases lung compliance.

B. Surfactant is responsible for clearing the lungs of secretions.

C. Surfactant increases the surface tension to prevent alveolar collapse.

D. Surfactant decreases surface tension to maintain end-expiratory pressure in the lungs.

10. A large-for-gestational-age infant is delivered to a G4P2 mother. There is no maternal history of diabetes. The term infant weights 4.5 kg. The glucose level is initially screened at 45 minutes of age with a result of 33 mg/dl. The baby is alert and active, and responds appropriately to stimuli. As the nurse caring for this infant, what would be your first intervention?

A. As long as the baby remains asymptomatic, recheck the glucose in 1 hour.
B. Attempt to feed the baby 10 ml of glucose water; recheck glucose level in 2 hours.
C. Begin an infusion of dextrose 10% in water at 80 ml/kg/day; recheck glucose level in 1 hour.
D. Attempt to have the mother breast-feed the infant immediately; recheck glucose level in 1 hour.

11. Where is the optimal place to measure preductal oxygen saturation?
A. Left foot
B. Left hand
C. Right foot
D. Right hand

## Chapter 3

# Neonatal Resuscitation

1. Although the Apgar score is useful for describing the status of the newborn after delivery, it is not used for decision making during resuscitation. The primary reason is that the Apgar score is:
A. a subjective scoring tool.
B. not assessed until 1 minute of age.
C. influenced by the ethnicity of the patient.
D. influenced by interventions and gestational age.

2. Following the birth of an infant through "pea soup" meconium, what would be the appropriate first steps if the infant appears vigorous?
A. Place the infant on the mother's chest and dry the infant.
B. Intubate and suction the trachea because of the pea soup meconium.
C. Place the infant on the radiant warmer, dry, stimulate, and clear the airway.
D. Place the infant on the radiant warmer and begin positive pressure ventilation.

3. An infant is born at 39 weeks' gestation. He is cyanotic, is grunting, and has a barrel chest and scaphoid abdomen. Upon auscultation, the nurse hears bowel sounds in the left side of his chest. Breath sounds are diminished. Based on this assessment, this infant is most likely to have:
A. a left pneumothorax.
B. a tracheoesophageal fistula.
C. meconium aspiration syndrome.
D. a congenital diaphragmatic hernia.

4. If the intestines have herniated up into the chest cavity, what is the most effective intervention to treat respiratory distress?
A. High-flow nasal cannula
B. Bag-and-mask ventilation
C. Intubation and endotracheal tube ventilation
D. Continuous positive airway pressure

**Questions 5 and 6 refer to following scenario:** An infant is delivered via crash cesarean section after a motor vehicle accident. The infant weighs approximately 3 kg. Following 30 seconds of positive pressure ventilations and chest compressions, the heart rate is 40 beats/minute.

5. An umbilical venous catheter is placed and epinephrine is given. What are the actions of epinephrine?
A. Increases heart rate, decreases contractility
B. Decreases cerebral perfusion, increases contractility
C. Causes vasoconstriction of the peripheral vessels and coronary arteries
D. Causes vasoconstriction of the peripheral vessels, increases contractility

6. Following the resuscitation, the physician orders that the infant be transferred to the NICU for observation. With an oxygen saturation of 98% on room air, the infant is noted to be pale. The blood pressure is 34/22 mm Hg with a mean of 28 mm Hg. Her tone is diminished. Her blood glucose level is 50 mg/dl. The first action at this time would be to:
A. give 30 ml O-negative blood.
B. start dextrose 10% in water ($D_{10}W$) at 10 ml/hour.
C. give 30 ml normal saline.
D. give a push of 6 ml $D_{10}W$.

**Questions 7 and 8 refer to the following scenario:** A woman has been seeing a perinatologist throughout the second trimester of her pregnancy because of a history of a stillbirth delivery due to hydrops fetalis. The cause of the hydrops fetalis is not known.

7. What prenatal test will be most helpful in anticipating the condition of the infant at delivery?
   A. Amniocentesis
   B. Kleihauer-Betke test
   C. High-resolution ultrasonography
   D. Glycosylated hemoglobin test

8. When preparing for the delivery of a hydropic infant, the team should be prepared to immediately carry out what priority action?
   A. Pericardiocentesis
   B. Provision of respiratory support
   C. Bilateral tube thoracotomy
   D. Placement of an umbilical arterial line

9. A term infant is born via normal spontaneous vaginal delivery. He is noted to be cyanotic when quiet but pinks up when he is crying. What is the most likely diagnosis for this infant?
   A. Choanal atresia
   B. Pierre Robin syndrome
   C. Congenital cardiac disease
   D. Respiratory distress syndrome

10. Despite continuous positive pressure ventilation via an endotracheal tube, a 1300-g, 31-week-gestation premature infant is persistently cyanotic. Breath sounds can be heard over both the lung fields and the stomach. No chest rise is visible. Which statement best describes the placement of the endotracheal tube?
    A. The endotracheal tube is on the carina.
    B. The endotracheal tube is in the esophagus.
    C. The endotracheal tube is in the correct position.
    D. The endotracheal tube is in the right mainstem bronchus.

---

## Chapter 4

# Physical Assessment

1. When beginning the assessment of a newborn infant, which of the following should be performed last?
   A. Checking the hips
   B. Testing the reflexes
   C. Palpating the pulses
   D. Examining the spine

2. Prior to delivery, a mother received a number of doses of magnesium sulfate to treat her preeclampsia. Which of the following would be an expected finding in her newborn infant?
   A. Anemia and hypotension
   B. Exaggerated deep tendon reflexes
   C. Hypernatremia and hypoglycemia
   D. Hypotonia and respiratory depression

3. A full-term male infant is born by vaginal delivery with vacuum extraction. His Apgar score is 7 at 1 minute and 8 at 5 minutes. He is pink and active. The nurse notices that he has a fluctuant swelling over the back of the head. Bruising around the ears is also noted. The most likely cause is:
   A. skull fracture.
   B. cephalohematoma.
   C. subdural hematoma.
   D. subgaleal hemorrhage.

4. A newborn infant born at 37 weeks' gestation is at the 5th percentile for weight and the 30th percentile for length and head circumference. The infant is at an increased risk of:
   A. anemia.
   B. hypoglycemia.
   C. chronic lung disease.
   D. respiratory distress syndrome.

5. A female infant is born by cesarean section without difficulty. She is admitted to the NICU with a weight of 1.5 kg at 34 weeks' gestation. On examination the nurse notes that the head and length are proportional to the body weight. These findings are most likely associated with:
   A. large size for gestational age.
   B. appropriate size for gestational age.
   C. symmetric intrauterine growth restriction.
   D. asymmetric intrauterine growth restriction.

6. A 4.2-kg, 41-week-gestation infant is admitted to the NICU because of tachypnea, grunting, and cyanosis. He was delivered vaginally with forceps, and his Apgar score was 4 at 1 minute and 7 at 5 minutes. On admission he requires an inspired oxygen fraction (Fio$_2$) of 0.50 to achieve an oxygen saturation of 94%. Despite attempts to wean to

room air, the infant has an increasing oxygen requirement. A chest radiograph is ordered that reveals patchy infiltrates with expansion of the chest to the tenth rib. This infant most likely has:
A. meconium aspiration.
B. respiratory distress syndrome.
C. cyanotic congenital heart disease.
D. transient tachypnea of the newborn.

7. When examining a term infant of appropriate size for gestational age, the nurse finds several anomalies that include heart murmur, malformed ears, a short neck with excessive skin, Brushfield spots, a large tongue, and simian creases. The nurse also notices that the infant is hypotonic when the Ballard assessment is performed. These findings are most likely related to:
A. trisomy 18.
B. Down syndrome (trisomy 21).
C. Turner syndrome.
D. Klinefelter syndrome.

8. A term male infant is born by vaginal delivery to a 35-year-old primigravida mother. Following delivery, the infant is noted to have dramatic cyanosis and severe respiratory distress. He is transferred to the NICU for further evaluation. Physical findings include poor perfusion, diminished breath sounds, sunken abdomen, and loud heart sounds on the right side of the chest. The most likely diagnosis is:
A. pneumothorax.
B. congenital diaphragmatic hernia.
C. congenital cyanotic heart disease.
D. severe respiratory distress syndrome.

9. An infant born at 34 weeks' gestation is noted to have respiratory distress. A radiograph shows hazy lung fields, ascites, and pleural effusions. A review of the history is most likely to reveal maternal:
A. alcohol ingestion.
B. HELLP syndrome (*h*emolysis, *e*levated *l*iver function, and *l*ow *p*latelets).
C. parvovirus infection.
D. group B streptococcus colonization.

10. Cyanosis at birth is most likely to be present in an infant with:
A. atrial septal defect.
B. patent ductus arteriosus.
C. ventricular septal defect.
D. transposition of the great vessels.

11. During the initial physical examination of a newborn infant, the nurse palpates the pulses while assessing cardiac function. The nurse compares both brachial pulses for timing and intensity, and then compares both femoral pulses. A significant difference is noted when the brachial and femoral pulses are compared. What is the most likely diagnosis for this infant?
A. Coarctation of the aorta
B. Patent ductus arteriosus
C. Ventricular septal defect
D. Persistent pulmonary hypertension of the newborn

12. An infant is noted to have a moist erythematous rash in the groin area. Small white pustules are present. The most likely diagnosis is:
A. herpes infection.
B. *Candida* infection.
C. scalded skin syndrome.
D. erythema toxicum.

13. Dermal sinuses are most commonly found on which area of the spinal cord?
A. Sacral
B. Lumbar
C. Cervical
D. Thoracic

14. Following prolonged pushing, a term female infant is delivered by vaginal delivery. Her head is elongated, and she is noted to have bruising on the back of her head. The crown of the head is spongy to the touch with edema that does not cross the suture lines. This is likely a:
A. skull fracture.
B. cephalohematoma.
C. caput succedaneum.
D. subdural hematoma.

15. When assessing the perfusion of an infant in the NICU, the nurse notices a line of demarcation down the infant's midline. One half of the infant appears pale, whereas the other side appears red. The most likely cause of this finding is:
A. cold stress.
B. hypovolemia.
C. overstimulation.
D. autonomic nervous system imbalance.

16. To auscultate a suspected tricuspid stenosis, the examiner should position the stethoscope over which of the following landmarks?
A. Second intercostal space, left sternal angle
B. Second intercostal space, right sternal angle
C. Fourth intercostal space, left sternal angle
D. Fifth intercostal space, midclavicular line

17. A nurse in the NICU is caring for a 28-week-gestation, 3-day-old infant receiving total parenteral nutrition. The nurse notices that the baby has

developed hypotonia, temperature instability, hypotension, and hyperglycemia. Based on these findings, the nurse suspects that this infant has which of the following conditions?
A. Sepsis
B. Pneumothorax
C. Patent ductus arteriosus
D. Intraventricular hemorrhage

18. An infant is born by vaginal delivery with forceps. There is moderate shoulder dystocia. The infant is noted to have an asymmetric Moro reflex and diminished movement in his right arm. What is the most likely cause?
A. Bell palsy
B. Fractured clavicle
C. Phrenic nerve paralysis
D. Fractured cervical spine

19. A Ballard assessment is done to determine:
A. gestational age.
B. narcotic exposure.
C. developmental care needs.
D. intrauterine growth patterns.

20. On examination of a newborn infant, the nurse notices several hyperpigmented skin lesions. Three small light brown flat spots are noted over the body. These are most likely:
A. salmon patches.
B. mongolian spots.
C. café au lait spots.
D. congenital melanocytic nevi.

21. A 2-day-old full-term male infant has a history of low Apgar scores, poor urine output, and hypertonicity. Which of the following would the infant likely demonstrate if he developed subtle seizures?
A. Repetitive jerking of the legs
B. Lip smacking and eye deviations
C. Tremulous movements that cease with flexion
D. Exaggerated startle reflex with occasional jerky movements

22. A nurse is caring for a 42-week gestational age infant in the NICU. The infant was delivered by emergency cesarean section because of an atypical fetal tracing. The Apgar score was 1 at 1 minute, 3 at 5 minutes, and 6 at 10 minutes. At 8 hours of age, the nurse notices that the infant begins pedaling movements and has lip smacking; she suspects seizures. The nurse immediately notifies the physician, who orders stat measurement of electrolyte levels. The results are Na, 133 mEq/L; K, 3.2 mEq/L; Cl, 101 mEq/L; glucose, 52 mg/dl;

and Ca, 7.5 mg/dl. Which of the following is the most likely cause of the seizures?
A. Hyponatremia
B. Hypoxic ischemia
C. Subdural hemorrhage
D. Intraventricular hemorrhage

23. The best method of evaluating postural tone in the newborn is to:
A. place the newborn supine and turn the head side to side.
B. stimulate the palmar surface of the newborn's hand with a finger.
C. hold the newborn upright and allow the soles of the feet to touch a flat surface.
D. grasp the newborn's hands and pull slowly from the supine to sitting position.

24. Following surfactant administration, a 30-week gestational age infant demonstrates severe respiratory distress despite adequate ventilatory pressures. Breath sounds are diminished on the right side, and the oxygen saturation is 72%. What is the most likely cause of the respiratory distress?
A. Pneumothorax
B. Pulmonary hypoplasia
C. An endotracheal tube that is too deep
D. Congenital cystic adenomatoid malformation

25. Following delivery, a 39-week gestational age female infant presents with frothy oral secretions and was noted to choke when attempting to breast-feed. Polyhydramnios was noted at delivery. The most likely cause of these findings is:
A. pyloric stenosis.
B. gastroesophageal reflux.
C. atresia of the duodenum.
D. tracheoesophageal fistula.

26. During labor, a fetus at 35 weeks' gestation is noted to have sustained sinus bradycardia with a heart rate of 72 to 84 beats/minute. Following an emergency cesarean section, the infant is pink with good respiratory efforts and good tone. The heart rate remains 82 to 88 beats/minute. Which of the following maternal conditions explains this heart rate pattern?
A. Diabetes
B. Preeclampsia
C. Chorioamnionitis
D. Systemic lupus erythematosus

27. Talipes equinovarus is defined as:
A. hyperextension of the knee.
B. webbing or fusion of two or more digits.
C. external rotation of the lower extremities.
D. medial turning and inversion of the sole of the foot with deformity of the hindfoot.

28. On examination of a full-term newborn male infant, the nurse notices that the scrotum is large and nontender, and appears to be "full." The nurse can successfully palpate both testes in the scrotum. This is most likely which of the following?
    A. Hydrocele
    B. Hypospadias
    C. Cryptorchidism
    D. Testicular torsion

29. At birth, a 4.3-kg infant is noted to have an asymmetric startle reflex. His wrist is noted to be flexed and adducted. There is a history of shoulder dystocia at birth. The nurse suspects the infant of having:
    A. Erb palsy.
    B. Bell palsy.
    C. neonatal stroke.
    D. fracture of the radius.

30. Risk factors for developmental dysplasia of the hip include:
    A. male sex.
    B. polyhydramnios.
    C. frank breech position.
    D. Black race.

31. A large anterior fontanelle is a finding in which of the following conditions?
    A. Craniosynostosis
    B. Turner syndrome
    C. Maternal diabetes
    D. Congenital hypothyroidism

32. A 2-day-old term infant is noted to have bile-stained emesis. The abdomen is soft and nondistended, and bowel sounds are faint. The infant has been passing meconium stools. The most urgent condition to rule out in this infant is:
    A. volvulus.
    B. pyloric stenosis.
    C. duodenal atresia.
    D. Hirschsprung disease.

33. When performing a physical examination on a female newborn infant, the nurse finds the following physical characteristics: widely spaced nipples, pedal edema, and redundant skin at the back of the neck. These findings are most consistent with:
    A. trisomy 13.
    B. Turner syndrome.
    C. DiGeorge syndrome.
    D. Down syndrome (trisomy 21).

34. A 1-day-old term female infant with a history of sneezing and tachypnea is noted to be jittery. The infant feeds poorly and vomits a large amount

following the feeding. These findings are likely related to in utero exposure to:
    A. heroin.
    B. alcohol.
    C. cocaine.
    D. selective serotonin reuptake inhibitors.

35. Low-set ears are associated with various syndromes and chromosomal abnormalities. Which of the following is the correct position of the ears?
    A. The bridge of the nose is even with the tragus.
    B. The ear is above an imaginary line drawn from the top of the eyebrow to the helix.
    C. The entire ear is above an imaginary line drawn from the outer canthus toward the mastoid process.
    D. The insertion of the ear is above a line drawn from the inner to the outer canthus of the eye.

36. A 2-day-old infant develops a petechial rash over his scalp, face, and trunk. Which of the following is most likely to be a contributing factor to this rash?
    A. Low platelet count
    B. Low hematocrit
    C. Low hemoglobin level
    D. Low white blood cell count

37. A 6-day-old infant born by spontaneous vaginal delivery at 34 weeks' gestation develops a cluster of three fluid-filled vesicles at the site of the scalp clip insertion. The most likely cause of this skin condition is an infection due to:
    A. *Candida*.
    B. *Klebsiella*.
    C. herpes simplex.
    D. *Staphylococcus aureus*.

38. An expected finding in an infant with Sturge-Webber syndrome is a port-wine stain over the infant's:
    A. neck.
    B. chest.
    C. buttocks.
    D. eyes and nose.

39. Rocker-bottom feet and overlapping clenched fingers are characteristic findings in infants with:
    A. trisomy 18.
    B. Down syndrome (trisomy 21).
    C. DiGeorge syndrome.
    D. osteogenesis imperfecta.

40. Which of the following is an expected finding in congenital cytomegalovirus infection?
    A. Macrosomia
    B. Microphthalmia
    C. Chorioretinitis
    D. Pleural effusions

41. Which of the following congenital malformations is most likely to have other associated malformations?
    A. Gastroschisis
    B. Omphalocele
    C. Pyloric stenosis
    D. Hirschsprung disease

42. The nurse caring for a 2-day old infant notices a scattered rash on an infant's face and trunk. The lesions are pustular with a reddened base. The nurse notes that some of the lesions seen earlier have faded and new ones have appeared. The infant is afebrile and feeding well. The rash is most likely to represent:
    A. milia.
    B. erythema toxicum.
    C. neonatal candidiasis.
    D. transient neonatal pustular melanosis.

## Chapter 5

# Gestational Age Assessment

1. Low birth weight is classified as birth weight less than:
   A. 500 g.
   B. 1000 g.
   C. 1500 g.
   D. 2500 g.

2. Length measurement entails measuring the infant:
   A. hip to hip.
   B. head to toe.
   C. crown to heel.
   D. shoulder to shoulder.

3. Large for gestational age is birth weight:
   A. at the 50th percentile.
   B. less than the 10th percentile.
   C. greater than the 90th percentile.
   D. between the 10th and 90th percentiles.

4. Small for gestational age is birth weight:
   A. at the 50th percentile.
   B. less than the 10th percentile.
   C. greater than the 90th percentile.
   D. between the 10th and 90th percentiles.

5. Appropriate weight for gestational age is birth weight:
   A. at the 50th percentile.
   B. less than the 10th percentile.
   C. greater than the 90th percentile.
   D. between the 10th and 90th percentiles.

6. Head circumference indicates brain:
   A. growth.
   B. function.
   C. anatomy.
   D. physiology.

7. An infant is born at 36 weeks' gestation. This infant is considered to be:
   A. term.
   B. postterm.
   C. late preterm.
   D. extremely preterm.

8. When assessing a premature infant born at 27 weeks' gestation, the nurse would expect to find:
   A. no lanugo.
   B. sparse lanugo.
   C. lanugo with balding areas.
   D. lanugo covering the entire body.

9. When assessing an infant with intrauterine growth restriction, the nurse can anticipate finding that the infant's:
   A. skin is covered in vernix.
   B. head is disproportionately large for the infant's trunk.
   C. umbilical cord is thickened with abundant Wharton jelly.
   D. anterior fontanelles are small with overlapping cranial sutures.

10. A physical assessment performed on a newborn infant notes that the skin of the infant is wrinkling, the areolae are raised with 10-mm buds, and the pinna springs back from being folded. Based on these physical assessment findings, this infant is considered to be:
    A. term.
    B. preterm.
    C. late preterm.
    D. very postterm.

11. Following the initial assessment of the newborn infant, the infant's weight, length, and head

circumference are plotted out on a growth chart. The growth chart shows that the infant's weight is at the 15th percentile, length is at the 20th percentile, and head circumference is at the 30th percentile. These results indicate that the infant is:

A. small for gestational age.
B. large for gestational age.
C. appropriate for gestational age.
D. none of the above.

12. A 4000-g male infant has just been delivered via cesarean section due to fetal distress. The infant is born through thick meconium and requires endotracheal suctioning. At the initial assessment, the infant's skin is noted to be leathery, cracked, and wrinkled. The infant's scrotum is noted to be pendulous with the testes descended. The nurse assessing this infant can anticipate that this infant is:

A. preterm.
B. late preterm.
C. term.
D. postterm.

13. A gestational age examination has just been performed on a newborn infant. The infant was noted to be in flexed position. The assessment shows that the square window angle is 0 degrees, the popliteal angle is 45 degrees, and the scarf sign evaluation shows increased resistance to crossing the midline. The infant's skin is noted to be cracking with no veins visible. Creases over the entire sole of the plantar surface are noted. Based on these findings, which of the following gestational ages would this infant be likely to be?

A. 24 weeks' gestation
B. 32 weeks' gestation
C. 36 weeks' gestation
D. 40 weeks' gestation

14. The correct way to assess the scarf sign in an infant is to:

A. position the infant supine, flex the arms for 5 seconds, then fully extend the infant's arms by pulling the hands downward, then release.
B. position the infant supine, take the infant's hand and pull it across the infant's chest and around the neck as far posterior as possible toward the opposite shoulder, and observe the elbow position in relation to the midline of the infant's body.
C. flex the infant's hand on the forearm between the examiner's thumb and index finger, use enough pressure to get full flexion, and visually measure the angle between the hypothenar eminence and the ventral aspect of the forearm.
D. position the infant supine with the pelvis flat on a surface, hold the infant's thigh in knee-chest position with the left index finger and thumb, place the right index finger behind the infant's ankle and extend the leg gently, and measure the angle between the lower leg and thigh.

15. The correct way to assess the arm recoil of an infant is to:

A. position the infant supine, flex the arms for 5 seconds, then fully extend the infant's arms by pulling the hands downward, then release.
B. position the infant supine, take the infant's hand and pull it across the infant's chest and around the neck as far posterior as possible toward the opposite shoulder, and observe the elbow position to the midline of the infant's body.
C. flex the infant's hand on the forearm between the examiner's thumb and index finger, use enough pressure to get full flexion, and visually measure the angle between the hypothenar eminence and the ventral aspect of the forearm.
D. position the infant supine with the pelvis flat on a surface, hold the infant's thigh in knee-chest position with the left index finger and thumb, place the right index finger behind the infant's ankle and extend the leg gently, and measure the angle between the lower leg and thigh.

16. The correct way to perform the square window test is to:

A. position the infant supine, flex the arms for 5 seconds, then fully extend the infant's arms by pulling the hands downward, then release.
B. position the infant supine, take the infant's hand and pull it across the infant's chest and around the neck as far posterior as possible toward the opposite shoulder, and observe the elbow position relative to the midline of the infant's body.
C. flex the infant's hand on the forearm between the examiner's thumb and index finger, use enough pressure to get full flexion, and visually measure the angle between the hypothenar eminence and the ventral aspect of the forearm.
D. position the infant supine with the pelvis flat on a surface, hold the infant's thigh in knee-chest position with the left index finger and thumb, place the right index finger behind the infant's ankle and extend the leg gently, and measure the angle between the lower leg and thigh.

17. A newborn's mother asks why the nurse is performing a gestational age assessment when she had ultrasonography to determine her due date. The best explanation to give her is that:

A. ultrasonographic estimates are often inaccurate by 3 to 4 weeks.

B. only dating based on the mother's last menstrual period is considered accurate.

C. the newborn's care is based on the gestational age and size-date plotting.

D. gestational age assessment determines the baby's future neurodevelopmental outcome.

18. After performing size-date plotting for an infant, the nurse shows the mother the growth chart. The mother asks why this is important. Which of the following is the best teaching point to explain at this moment?

A. Babies who plot between the 10th and the 90th percentiles have grown in utero as expected.

B. Babies who plot between the 10th and the 90th percentiles often have more problems than other babies.

C. Babies who plot above the 90th percentile are bigger and therefore always are healthier than other babies.

D. Babies who plot below the 10th percentile have grown larger than expected and can have problems with blood glucose level.

19. The mother of an infant born at 28 weeks' gestation tells the nurse that she is very worried because her baby's ears do not look normal. Which of the following is the best explanation to give her?

A. All very preterm babies end up with deformed ears due to their prematurity.

B. A preterm baby's ears are not formed yet, and this is what leads to deafness in preterm infants.

C. As a baby matures, the pinnae of the ears will mature and the cartilage will eventually firm up.

D. Growth and development stop at birth, so preterm infants have flatter ears than term babies, but their hearing is intact.

20. The nurse is performing a gestational age assessment on a premature infant. Observations will likely include which of the following?

A. Vernix in the axilla only

B. Very few visible veins on the abdomen

C. Palpable breast buds with raised and stippled areolae

D. Smooth plantar surfaces and large amounts of lanugo over the shoulders and back

21. Which of the following findings and related causes would a nurse likely see when size-date plotting is done for a 42⅗-week, postdate newborn?

A. All parameters less than the 10th percentile due to placental insufficiency

B. Weight greater than the 90th percentile but head circumference less than the 10th percentile due to hypoxic insult

C. Head circumference greater than the 90th percentile and length less than the 10th percentile due to intrauterine growth restriction

D. Weight less than the 10th percentile and head and length appropriate for gestational age due to placental insufficiency

22. Which of the following is a true statement about the neurologic portion of the gestational age examination?

A. Posture and flexion decrease with advancing gestational age and muscle mass.

B. The square window angle increases with advancing gestational age due to increasing muscle tone.

C. The values of neurologic indicators are not accurate in preterm infants of less than 30 weeks' gestation.

D. Gestational examination scoring can be altered by neurologic disorders and asphyxia injury and therefore may not be reliable.

23. Small-for-gestational-age infants are at risk for which of the following?

A. Anemia

B. Hyperthermia

C. Hypoglycemia

D. Brachial plexus palsy

24. A 40-week, 2000-g infant is admitted to the NICU. The nurse should assess for:

A. birth trauma.

B. polycythemia.

C. hyperglycemia.

D. respiratory distress syndrome.

25. Which of the following problems is a full-term large-for-gestational-age infant at highest risk for developing?

A. Hypothermia

B. Hyponatremia

C. Hypokalemia

D. Hypoglycemia

26. Which statement best describes intrauterine growth and development?

A. Subcutaneous fat and skin thickness decrease as gestational age increases.

B. Lanugo develops continuously as the fetus matures and is most prevalent close to term.

C. Nipple development progresses with advancing age, whereas breast tissue decreases with advancing age.

D. Female genitalia develop with advancing age, and by term, the labia majora and minora completely cover the clitoris.

27. An extremely low birth weight infant born at less than 25 weeks' gestation can be scored using the New Ballard Score gestational age examination. Which of the following findings is expected in an infant born at less than 25 weeks' gestation?
    A. Eyes are open.
    B. Lanugo is abundant.
    C. Skin is dry and paperlike.
    D. Plantar creases are absent and foot length is 45 mm.

28. A postterm infant of up to 44 weeks' gestation can be scored using the New Ballard Score gestational age examination. Which statement best describes the examination of these infants?
    A. Skin has superficial peeling, the ears are stiff, and the labia majora do not cover the clitoris.
    B. Skin is cracked and wrinkled, plantar creases cover the entire foot sole, and lanugo is mostly absent.
    C. Skin has few visible veins, the ears are well curved with ready recoil, and lanugo is thinning.
    D. Plantar creases extend to two-thirds of the feet, the ears are firm with instant recoil, and breast areolae are stippled.

29. Which of the following is an accepted method of accurately assessing gestational age?
    A. Birth weight
    B. Ultrasonography performed after 24 weeks' gestation
    C. Calculation of dates based on date of implantation spotting
    D. Examination of the anterior capsule of the vascular lens of the eye

30. The principal basis for gestational age determination by physical assessment is that development is predictable, so that specific characteristics are common to all infants of a given gestational age. Which statement best describes gestational age assessment tools?
    A. There are no limitations; the findings of gestational age examination are not altered by intrauterine events.
    B. There are no limitations; the findings of gestational age examination are always accurate to within 1 week of gestation time.
    C. There are limitations; the findings of the gestational age examination can be affected by maternal medications, breech positioning, and asphyxia.
    D. There are limitations; there is very high interrater reliability for the current tools.

31. General considerations for accurate use of a gestational age assessment tool, such as the Dubowitz score or New Ballard Score, include which of the following?
    A. Perform the examination with 1 week of life for best accuracy.
    B. Perform the examination within 48 hours of life for best accuracy.
    C. Gestational age assessment is most accurate when performed on infants in a deep sleep state.
    D. The combined score of the physical and neurologic components has a lower correlation than either component used separately.

32. A 4.5-kg infant born at 38 weeks' gestation is most at risk for which of the following?
    A. Erb palsy
    B. Hypothermia
    C. Congenital anomalies
    D. Respiratory distress syndrome

## Chapter 6

# Thermoregulation

1. Conduction is:
   A. heat transfer via air currents.
   B. heat transfer via direct contact.
   C. heat loss by conversion of liquid into vapor.
   D. transfer of radiant energy without direct contact through absorption and emission of infrared rays.

2. Convection is:
   A. heat transfer via air currents.

   B. heat transfer via direct contact.
   C. heat loss by conversion of liquid into vapor.
   D. transfer of radiant energy without direct contact through absorption and emission of infrared rays.

3. Evaporation is:
   A. heat transfer via air currents.
   B. heat transfer via direct contact.
   C. heat loss by conversion of liquid into vapor.

D. transfer of radiant energy without direct contact through absorption and emission of infrared rays.

4. Radiation is:
   A. heat transfer via air currents.
   B. heat transfer via direct contact.
   C. heat loss by conversion of liquid into vapor.
   D. transfer of radiant energy without direct contact through absorption and emission of infrared rays.

5. Thermoregulation is:
   A. a balance of heat loss, heat gain, and heat production.
   B. a state in which the temperature of the body is out of the expected normal range.
   C. the inability to maintain core temperature above that of the environment.
   D. a physiologic response to changes in ambient temperature in an attempt to maintain normal core temperature.

6. Thermal instability is:
   A. a balance of heat loss, heat gain, and heat production.
   B. a state in which the temperature of the body is out of the expected normal range.
   C. the inability to maintain core temperature above that of the environment.
   D. a physiologic response to changes in ambient temperature in an attempt to maintain normal core temperature.

7. Infants are at risk of hyperthermia because infants have:
   A. a large body surface area.
   B. limited glycogen stores.
   C. limited brown fat stores.
   D. limited ability to dissipate heat.

8. Maintaining a neutral thermal environment is important because it:
   A. limits the neonate in maintaining normothermia.
   B. promotes minimal consumption of oxygen and glucose.
   C. increases the neonate's metabolic rate.
   D. enables the neonate to maximize glucose consumption.

9. Which of the following puts an infant at risk for experiencing hypothermia?
   A. Increased muscle tone
   B. Increased glycogen stores
   C. Increased brown fat stores
   D. Increased body surface area

10. Which of the following puts an infant at risk for experiencing hyperthermia?
    A. Infection
    B. Prematurity
    C. Increased ability to dissipate heat
    D. Decreased ability to metabolize drugs

11. A premature infant has just been delivered vaginally because of prolonged premature rupture of the membranes. The nurse thoroughly dries the infant, places the infant on a warming mattress, and puts a knit cap on the infant. Which of these interventions reduces conductive heat loss?
    A. Thoroughly drying the infant
    B. Placing the infant on a warming mattress
    C. Putting a knit cap on the infant
    D. None of the above

12. A premature infant has just been delivered via cesarean section. The infant is dried thoroughly and placed on a warming mattress, and a knit cap is placed on the infant. Which of these interventions reduces convective heat loss?
    A. Thoroughly drying the infant
    B. Placing the infant on a warming mattress
    C. Putting a knit cap on the infant
    D. None of the above

13. A neonate has just been born at 24 weeks' gestation. The nurse determines that the use of a polyethylene bag is appropriate for this patient. When should the polyethylene bag be applied to the infant?
    A. After drying the infant
    B. Prior to drying the infant
    C. Once the infant is intubated
    D. Once respiratory distress is noted

14. A mother has just given birth via normal spontaneous vaginal delivery. The nurse thoroughly dries the infant and places the infant directly on the mother's skin for skin-to-skin (kangaroo) care. The action of placing the infant on the mother's skin reduces:
    A. radiant heat loss.
    B. convective heat loss.
    C. conductive heat loss.
    D. evaporative heat loss.

15. The body responds to cold stress by:
    A. increasing glycogen stores.
    B. storing brown adipose tissue.
    C. vasoconstricting peripherally.
    D. decreasing oxygen consumption.

16. Which of the following increases the risk that the neonate will experience hyperthermia?
    A. A dislodged skin temperature probe
    B. A skin temperature probe covered by an insulated probe cover

C. The placement of the skin temperature probe away from brown adipose tissue areas

D. Continuous monitoring of the skin temperature of a neonate using a servocontrolled incubator

17. Upon initial assessment of a preterm infant, the nurse finds that the infant is tachypneic, tachycardic, and irritable, shows signs of dehydration, and looks flushed. When checking the recent chemistry values for the infant, the nurse finds that the infant's serum sodium concentration is 152 mEq/L. These findings are consistent with the infant being:
    A. hypothermic.
    B. poikilothermic.
    C. hyperthermic.
    D. normothermic.

18. A premature neonate has just been born at 24 weeks' gestation with a birth weight of 525 g. Which of the following statements demonstrates that the nurse attending the delivery of this neonate understands how to use a polyethylene wrap?
    A. "I need to make sure that the baby is dried thoroughly before I apply the polyethylene wrap."
    B. "I need to make sure that I cover the baby's head and body with the polyethylene wrap before I dry the baby."
    C. "I need to make sure that I apply the polyethylene wrap once the baby gets to the nursery from the delivery room."
    D. "I need to make sure that I remove the polyethylene wrap once the baby is in a warm environment in the nursery."

19. At the delivery of a term infant born via cesarean section, the infant is thoroughly dried, wrapped in an unwarmed blanket, and transferred to the nursery without a cap via an open crib. In the nursery, the infant is placed under an operating prewarmed radiant warmer, which is located by the unit's drafty windows. The initial temperature of the infant indicates that the infant is hypothermic. The low temperature most likely resulted from:
    A. conductive, convective, and radiant heat loss.
    B. convective, radiant, and evaporative heat loss.
    C. conductive, radiant, and evaporative heat loss.
    D. conductive, convective, and evaporative heat loss.

20. During the assessment of a premature infant, the nurse notes that the infant is in an incubator and on a phototherapy blanket. The infant is positioned appropriately with the aid of positioning devices that promote flexion, alignment, containment, and security. The nurse takes the initial temperature of the infant and finds the infant to be hyperthermic. It would be appropriate for the nurse first to:
    A. leave the infant as is.
    B. turn off the incubator.
    C. remove the positioning devices.
    D. turn off the phototherapy for a while until the temperature decreases.

21. A term infant has just been admitted to the nursery and has been placed under a radiant warmer, which was prewarmed prior to the admission. Which of the following statements made by the admitting nurse demonstrates correct understanding of how to operate the radiant warmer?
    A. "It's important to make sure the radiant warmer alarms are off when it's in use."
    B. "Once the radiant warmer has finished prewarming, be sure to turn it off before using it."
    C. "Once I put the temperature probe on the patient, I need to make sure that I switch the radiant warmer mode from manual to servocontrolled."
    D. "I need to make sure that I switch the radiant warmer mode from servocontrolled to manual once I put the temperature probe on the patient."

Chapter 7

# Fluid and Electrolytes

1. The main ion that constitutes more than 90% of the total amount of solutes in the extracellular space is:
    A. chloride.
    B. magnesium.
    C. potassium.
    D. sodium.

2. Which of the following would cause hyponatremia in the neonate?

A. Antenatal steroid administration
B. Placental dysfunction
C. Maternal diabetes that has not been adequately controlled
D. Excessive administration of oxytocin or hypotonic intravenous fluid to the mother

3. Fluid requirements need to be determined accurately by evaluating the factors that influence insensible water loss (IWL). One factor that may decrease IWL is:
   A. increasing gestational age.
   B. high minute ventilation.
   C. use of a radiant warmer.
   D. low relative ambient humidity.

4. A 26-week gestational age infant with a birth weight of 800 g is 2 days old and currently weighs 660 g. Total fluids are 110 ml/kg/day. Urine output is 2.8 ml/kg/hr. Core temperature is 36.8° C (98.2° F), incubator temperature is 37° C (98.6° F), and humidity is 45%. The most appropriate action is to:
   A. increase humidity and fluids.
   B. change the incubator and increase fluids.
   C. decrease fluids and increase humidity.
   D. do nothing, because this is a normal weight loss.

5. When calculating medication doses for the premature infant, one should consider which of the following normal postnatal developments that could affect dosage?
   A. Renal blood flow decreases as renal vascular resistance rises.
   B. Renal blood flow increases as renal vascular resistance falls.
   C. Premature infants concentrate urine well, which decreases the excretion of medications.
   D. Preterm infants cannot dilute urine, which may cause decreased excretion of medications.

6. A 1200-g infant has oliguria and new-onset apnea. The infant has a history of being administered diuretics. Electrolyte levels are obtained. The results are Na 121 mEq/L, K 3.2 mEq/L, Cl 87 mEq/L, and $CO_2$ 32 mEq/L. The most appropriate action is to:
   A. discontinue the diuretic and allow Na to correct itself.
   B. provide NaCl supplementation to complete full correction in 24 hours.
   C. provide NaCl and KCl supplementation to correct hyponatremia over 24 to 48 hours.
   D. discontinue diuretic therapy and provide KCl and NaCl supplementation to correct hyponatremia and hypokalemia over 48 to 72 hours.

7. A 5-week-old 1100-g infant has oliguria and new-onset apnea. The infant has a history of being administered diuretics. Electrolyte levels are Na 115 mEq/L, K 3.8 mEq/L, Cl 86 mEq/L, $HCO_3$ 30 mEq/L, and creatinine 1.6 mg/dl. The infant is at highest risk for:
   A. seizures.
   B. severe dehydration.
   C. cardiopulmonary arrest.
   D. syndrome of inappropriate antidiuretic hormone.

8. A 4-day-old full-term infant, after being at home for 2 days, comes to the NICU with a high-pitched cry, lethargy, irritability, and apnea. The history reveals that the infant has been eating well, breast-feeding 10 to 12 times per day with two wet diapers per day. There is no history of fever or vomiting. These symptoms are most likely secondary to:
   A. excessive insensible water losses.
   B. sodium intake that is less than sodium losses.
   C. overhydration secondary to frequent feedings.
   D. dehydration from inadequate breast-feeding or breast milk.

9. A full-term infant with a history of atrial flutter has been receiving digoxin for the past 5 days. There have been no further episodes of flutter. The infant becomes apneic, and the monitor shows heart block. A specimen for electrolyte determination is sent stat. Which of the following is anticipated?
   A. Hypokalemia
   B. Hyperkalemia
   C. Hyponatremia
   D. Hypernatremia

10. A premature infant of 25 weeks' gestation experienced a traumatic delivery. The infant has generalized bruising and is requiring maximal support. The anticipated pathophysiologic effects with regard to potassium would be:
    A. a shift of potassium out of the cells due to metabolic alkalosis.
    B. higher potassium clearance due to increased glomerular filtration rate.
    C. endogenous release of potassium due to tissue destruction, hypoperfusion, hemorrhage, and bruising.
    D. intensification of the normal postnatal shift of potassium from the extracellular compartment to the intracellular compartment.

11. The primary intervention to decrease hyperbilirubinemia and minimize potassium increase in an extremely low birth weight infant with generalized bruising is to:
    A. obtain an electrocardiogram to detect cardiac dysrhythmias.

B. obtain the potassium level and total and direct bilirubin levels at delivery.

C. observe the infant and evaluate based on clinical presentation and assessment.

D. start phototherapy upon admission and obtain a potassium level and total and direct bilirubin levels at 8 to 12 hours of life.

12. A 665-g, 26-week gestational age infant in stable condition has a heart rate of 180. The following laboratory values were obtained on a sample from an umbilical catheter, through which dextrose 10% in water is infusing without additives:

Na 149 mEq/L
K 8.1 mEq/L
Cl 119 mEq/L
$CO_2$ 17 mEq/L
Ca 7.5 mEq/L
Blood urea nitrogen 30 mg/dl
Creatinine 1.3 mg/dl

The most appropriate intervention would be to notify the physician and prepare to administer a glucose and insulin infusion and calcium gluconate because:

A. glucose, insulin, and calcium facilitate the excretion of potassium.

B. glucose, insulin, and calcium gluconate bind to potassium and thereby reduce the serum ionized levels.

C. glucose and insulin temporarily shift potassium into the cells, whereas calcium lowers the cell membrane potential.

D. glucose and insulin will pull calcium from the cells, and supplemental calcium gluconate will further increase serum calcium levels.

13. A full-term, large-for-gestational-age infant comes to the NICU with jitteriness, seizure activity, a high-pitched cry, and stridor. This presentation is consistent with which of the following diagnoses?

A. Hypokalemia

B. Hyperkalemia

C. Hypocalcemia

D. Hypercalcemia

14. A 4.9-kg infant has a serum calcium level of 6.5 mg/dl. The physician writes an order to administer calcium gluconate. The person administering the corrective calcium should know that:

A. calcium gluconate should be given rapidly over 5 minutes.

B. calcium chloride is the drug of choice to correct hypocalcemia.

C. calcium gluconate does not require cardiac monitoring during administration.

D. calcium gluconate can cause intestinal necrosis and liver necrosis when administered via umbilical catheters.

15. A 36-week gestational age, 3.6-kg infant has hypoplastic left heart syndrome. The infant is acyanotic at birth, and a prostaglandin drip is started. The infant's calcium levels are consistently low with a continuous calcium drip of 500 mg/kg/day. The syndrome associated most frequently with hypocalcemia is:

A. trisomy 13.

B. trisomy 18.

C. trisomy 21 (Down syndrome).

D. DiGeorge syndrome.

16. An 865-g, 28-week gestational age infant is receiving dextrose 7.5% at 70 ml/kg/day. The glucose load is a(n):

A. sufficient quantity of glucose at 3.5 ml/hour, 5 mg/kg/minute of glucose.

B. sufficient quantity of glucose at 2.5 ml/hour, 3.6 mg/kg/minute of glucose.

C. insufficient quantity of glucose at 3.5 ml/hour, 5 mg/kg/minute of glucose.

D. insufficient quantity of glucose at 2.5 ml/hour, 3.6 mg/kg/minute of glucose.

17. Which of the following describes the body water composition of a fetus early in gestation?

A. Water makes up 75% of the body weight with the majority in the intracellular fluid compartment.

B. Water makes up 95% of the body weight with the majority in the intracellular fluid compartment.

C. Water makes up 95% of the body weight with the majority in the extracellular fluid compartment.

D. Water makes up 75% of the body weight with the majority in the extracellular fluid compartment.

18. A 3-day-old preterm infant weighing 965 g has a urine output of 160 ml/24 hours. Which of the following statements regarding this situation is accurate?

A. It is normal in the diuretic phase to have an output of 3 ml/kg/hour.

B. It is normal in the diuretic phase to have an output of 6.9 ml/kg/hour.

C. It is normal in the postdiuretic phase to have an output of 6.9 ml/kg/hour.

D. It is normal in the prediuretic phase to have an output of 6.9 ml/kg/hour.

19. A 1.265-kg preterm infant is ingesting 50 ml/kg/day of 24-kcal formula. In addition, the infant is receiving total fluids of 100 ml/kg/day of total parenteral nutrition, dextrose 15%. The total kilocalories per kilogram per day is:

A. 130.

B. 120.

C. 110.

D. 100.

20. A full-term 4.9-kg infant of a diabetic mother shows tremors, irritability, and hyperreflexia. The infant's calcium level is 4.5 mg/dl. Multiple calcium boluses have been administered, but the repeat calcium level is 5.5 mg/dl. The next consideration is to:

A. prepare to administer a calcium chloride bolus.

B. obtain the magnesium level and prepare to administer magnesium.

C. obtain the sodium level and prepare to administer a normal saline solution.

D. obtain the potassium level and prepare to administer a potassium correction.

21. A 30-day-old premature infant born at 24 weeks' gestation has a chest radiograph that indicates undermineralized bones. Serum calcium, phosphorus, and alkaline phosphatase levels are obtained. What results would be expected?

A. Low calcium, high phosphorus, high alkaline phosphatase, and low 1,25-dihydroxyvitamin D levels

B. High calcium, high phosphorus, high alkaline phosphatase, and normal 1,25-dihydroxyvitamin D levels

C. Normal calcium, low phosphorus, high alkaline phosphatase, and high 1,25-dihydroxyvitamin D levels

D. Low calcium, low phosphorus, high alkaline phosphatase, and high 1,25-dihydroxyvitamin D levels

# Chapter 8

# Nutrition Management

1. During a mother's first visit to the NICU, she mentions that she would like to breast-feed. She asks the nurse how soon she should start expressing her milk. The best response is:

A. as soon as she feels ready.

B. within the first 6 to 8 hours after delivery.

C. within the next few days when her baby is beginning enteral feedings.

D. tomorrow is best as she is just newly delivered and requires recovery time.

2. A mother of a preterm infant is undecided about breast-feeding. In discussing the issue with her, which of the following should the nurse emphasize?

A. Breast milk is high in protein.

B. Infants fed breast milk have fewer infections.

C. It makes no difference for preterm infants whether they are breast-fed or bottle-fed.

D. Breast milk provides the preterm infant all the nutrients for adequate growth.

3. A mother expresses interest in providing breast milk to her preterm infant and in exclusively breast-feeding at discharge. To optimize her success, the nurse should:

A. introduce the bottle first, to ensure the infant has an efficient suck.

B. ensure that the mother gets adequate rest periods away from her infant.

C. provide opportunities to have the mother hold the infant skin to skin.

D. tell the mother to avoid using a nipple shield during breast-feeding, because this inhibits adequate latch.

4. For adequate growth and development, a healthy full-term infant requires how many kilocalories per kilogram per day?

A. 50 to 60

B. 70 to 80

C. 100 to 120

D. 150 to 180

5. The presence of reducing substance in the stool is indicative of which of the following conditions?

A. Hepatobiliary disease

B. Necrotizing enterocolitis

C. Slow gastrointestinal motility

D. Possible carbohydrate malabsorption

6. A major limiting factor in providing enteral feedings to the premature newborn is:

A. small gastric capacity.

B. gastroesophageal reflux.

C. immature gastrointestinal motility.

D. limited absorption of nutrients from the gastrointestinal tract.

7. Infants at risk for developing osteopenia of prematurity include those with a history of:

A. near term delivery, prolonged nothing-by-mouth (NPO) status, and poor nutritional state.
B. severe prematurity, prolonged NPO status, and poor nutritional state.
C. poor nutritional state, prolonged NPO status, and use of fortified breast milk.
D. severe prematurity, TPN exposure for one week, and use of commercial formula.

8. Which of the following is a significant risk factor for the development of total parenteral nutrition (TPN)–associated cholestasis?
A. Presence of illness
B. Use of formula for enteral feeds
C. Long duration of TPN exposure
D. Use of TPN with protein, 3-4 grams/kg/day

9. Early minimal feeding of the premature newborn is associated with which of the following conditions?
A. Intestinal perforation
B. Apnea and bradycardia
C. Earlier attainment of full enteral feedings
D. Increased incidence of necrotizing enterocolitis

10. Carnitine supplementation may be helpful in the preterm infant who is receiving nothing by mouth for which of the following reasons?
A. Carnitine supplementation reduces the severity of respiratory distress.
B. Carnitine supplementation decreases the incidence of feeding intolerance.
C. Carnitine supplementation is associated with decreased incidence of necrotizing enterocolitis.
D. Preterm infants have low carnitine stores and may be missing the necessary enzymes in carnitine synthesis.

11. A side effect of intravenous lipid administration is:
A. hypophospholipidemia.
B. alteration in leukocyte function.
C. increased pulmonary diffusion of gases.
D. increased binding of bilirubin to albumin.

12. Preterm infant formulas differ from full-term infant formulas in that preterm formulas have:
A. a soy base and increased fat and protein content.
B. increased calories and decreased minerals to lower osmolarity.
C. increased calcium and phosphorus and decreased carnitine content.
D. increased medium-chain triglycerides, reduced amount of lactose, and increased protein content.

13. Soy-based formulas are indicated for infants with which of the following conditions?

A. Bloody stools
B. Frequent emesis
C. Lactase deficiency
D. Birth weight less than 1800 g

14. A mother who just delivered a preterm newborn asks the nurse which breast pumping technique is optimal: pumping one breast at a time or pumping both breasts simultaneously. The best answer is which of the following?
A. Pumping one breast at a time increases milk production.
B. Pumping both breasts simultaneously will take less time.
C. Either pumping technique will produce equal amounts of milk.
D. Pumping both breasts simultaneously produces high milk volumes.

15. The primary reason for slow postnatal growth in very low birthweight infants fed fortified human milk is:
A. low fat intake.
B. restricted intake.
C. low protein intake.
D. poor intestinal absorption of nutrients.

16. While feeding a preterm infant, the nurse notices that the infant appears to have disorganized behavior and begins to fatigue. The nurse's next action is to:
A. continue to feed, because this response improves over time.
B. discontinue the feeding and offer the bottle again at a later time.
C. pull the bottle out of the mouth, rub the back, and wait for recovery.
D. leave the nipple in the mouth but tip the bottle to stop the flow of the feeding.

17. The early use of total parenteral nutrition (initiation within the first 24 hours after birth) is associated with:
A. increased sepsis rates.
B. improved weight gain.
C. reduced albumin synthesis.
D. clinically significant elevated blood urea nitrogen levels.

18. When added to human milk, human milk fortifier increases the:
A. iron content of the milk.
B. incidence of feeding intolerance.
C. risk of necrotizing enterocolitis.
D. protein, calcium, phosphorous, fat, and calories of the milk.

19. Giving enteral feeds as a bolus does which of the following?

A. Lengthens the time to establish full feedings
B. Reduces the time to establish full feedings
C. Increases the incidence of feeding intolerance
D. Increases the incidence of necrotizing enterocolitis

20. A feeding residual indicates:
  A. nothing; feeds can be continued.
  B. a need for further evaluation of the infant.
  C. feeding intolerance; the feeds should be withheld.

D. the development of early necrotizing enterocolitis.

21. Nonnutritive sucking in the preterm infant is associated with:
  A. fatigue during nipple feedings.
  B. poor breast-feeding performance.
  C. reduced bradycardia events during nipple feedings.
  D. improved feeding behavior and reduced length of hospital stay.

# Chapter 9

# Developmental Support

1. A nurse is teaching a mother to feed her preterm baby by keeping the nipple in the infant's mouth and regularly tilting the bottle slightly to stop the flow of pumped mother's milk. This method of shortened sucking bursts that lets the infant pause, swallow, and breathe is referred to as:
  A. paced feeding.
  B. synactive feeding.
  C. infant-led feeding.
  D. interactive feeding.

2. Repetitive noxious stimuli to the mouth such as suctioning can result in which developmental disorder?
  A. Oral aversion
  B. Feeding strike
  C. Feeding opposition
  D. Feeding intolerance

3. Which is true of noise exposure for premature infants in NICUs?
  A. A safe range to decrease physiologic stress is 100 to 110 dB.
  B. The human voice does not generally exceed the recommended decibel level.
  C. Noise levels higher than 50 dB are associated with autonomic instability.
  D. Being inside an incubator sufficiently protects the infant from excessive decibel levels.

4. Effects and benefits of kangaroo (skin-on-skin) care have been reported with as few as 10 minutes of kangaroo care. Which statement best describes the research findings on kangaroo care?
  A. Kangaroo care has positive effects on breast-feeding, sleep, and infection rates.

B. Kangaroo care dose is best described as one sleep cycle—approximately 2 hours.
  C. Kangaroo care increases anxiety in parents due to worry about monitoring of their baby.
  D. Kangaroo care is embraced uniformly by all staff members, and there are no barriers to its use.

5. Contraindications to kangaroo care include:
  A. paternal hair on chest.
  B. mechanical ventilation.
  C. maternal preeclampsia requiring magnesium sulfate therapy.
  D. infection of the skin of the chest of the kangaroo care provider.

6. Repeated exposure to painful stimuli has short- and long-term consequences. Which explanation best describes pain exposure in neonates?
  A. There are no appropriate pain assessment tools for preterm infants.
  B. Short-term effects of pain exposure include increases in oxygenation and heart rate.
  C. Long-term effects of pain exposure include increased somatic complaints and structural changes in the brain.
  D. The use of sucrose to reduce painful responses is mostly anecdotal and without supporting evidence.

7. Maturational hypotonia can lead to acquired positioning malformations in preterm infants, which include abnormal head molding, hip adduction and external rotation, and:
  A. arching posture.
  B. fixed neck flexion.

C. wrist and ankle torsion.

D. scapular abduction and shoulder extension.

8. Best practices for a developmentally supportive NICU environment include:
   A. windows that allow daylight in, use of auditory alarms, and cue-based nursing care.
   B. continuous fluorescent lighting, placement of pagers on vibrate mode, and provision of nonnutritive sucking.
   C. day-night cycling of light, avoidance of overhead paging, and rigid timing of nursing care.
   D. use of a procedure light, use of acoustical tile, and assessment of stress signals when providing nursing care.

9. Feeding success has implications for mother-infant bonding, as well as length of NICU hospitalization. Interventions that facilitate feeding success include:
   A. paced feeding, kangaroo care prior to feedings, and provision of nonnutritive sucking.
   B. continuous drip feedings, appropriate type of nipple, and increasing environmental stimuli at feeding time.
   C. appropriate temperature of feedings, vigorous patting to encourage adequate burping, and use of high-flow nipple.
   D. clustering of care, playing of music in the incubator for 6 to 12 hours a day, and use of a rocking mattress.

10. A 30-week gestation infant who is not in physiologically stable condition will be undergoing a painful procedure. Which of the following techniques can be taught to parents so that they can help to provide developmental support to their baby to reduce pain response behaviors?
    A. Singing to the baby during the procedure
    B. Rapid stroking along the long axis of the extremities
    C. Using their hands to provide flexed containment of the extremities
    D. Using a soft blanket to maintain gentle extension of the extremities

11. Although survival of preterm infants has steadily improved, the incidence of disability remains high. Which of the following best describes neurodevelopmental outcomes in preterm infants?
    A. The incidence of major sequelae in the youngest preterms ranges from 20% to 25%.
    B. Although motor and behavioral outcomes can be affected, intelligence quotient is never affected.
    C. Studies have failed to show a correlation between skin-to-skin care and outcomes.

D. Over the last three decades, depending on year of birth, gestational age, and birth weight, the incidence of major disability has ranged from 60% to 70%.

12. A parent begins tapping on the incubator to wake up a sleeping infant for a visit. The most appropriate intervention at this time is to:
    A. suggest the parent wait until the infant is awake.
    B. assist the parent with a state-appropriate activity.
    C. encourage the parent's interactions with the infant.
    D. gently discourage the parent by stating, "The baby doesn't like that."

13. An appropriate nursing intervention to provide developmental support to an infant during gavage feeding is to:
    A. feed on a strictly routine schedule.
    B. provide nonnutritive sucking before, during, and after the procedure.
    C. use a bright light to allow visualization of the correct placement of the tube.
    D. restrain the infant's body in an extended, supine posture with a soft fabric restraint to prevent the tube from being dislodged.

14. Signs of sensory overstimulation in neonates include finger and toe splaying, gaze aversion, and hiccups. The most appropriate nursing intervention to provide neurodevelopmental support to an infant exhibiting one or more of these behaviors during nursing care is to:
    A. swaddle the baby and provide a time-out for rest and recovery.
    B. dim the lights to decrease stimulation and continue with the care.
    C. play music during care to provide auditory distraction and calm the infant.
    D. hurry and finish the care being provided to shorten the noxious exposure.

15. The father of an infant in the NICU is worried because his baby's incubator is covered and is concerned that no one will notice if the baby's condition deteriorates or the baby needs attention. Which is the best explanation to provide?
    A. Looking at the fabric cover of the incubator stimulates the infant's retina to mature.
    B. Bright light is detrimental to the developing brain because it is too stimulating.
    C. NICU monitors detect adverse events and track the time of the event.
    D. Constant darkness will help the baby adjust to normal sleep patterns after discharge from the NICU.

16. Which of the following is true regarding nonnutritive sucking (NNS)?
    A. NNS can lead to oral aversion.
    B. NNS can be used as a sign of readiness for nipple feeding.
    C. NNS is thought to impair sucking skills if overutilized prior to initiating bottle feeding.
    D. NNS is synergistic with a sweet taste on the tip of the tongue in decreasing pain responses.

17. Which of the following is true of kangaroo care?
    A. Olfactory sensations occur with the rise and fall of the parent's chest.
    B. Documentation of length of kangaroo care time is not needed, because it is universally well tolerated.
    C. The practice of standing transfer may increase stress during movement from the incubator to the parent's chest.
    D. Skin-to-skin contact provides tactile stimulation, promotes physiologic stability, and improves maternal milk production.

18. Which of the following best describes neurodevelopmentally supportive positioning?
    A. Muscle tone and reflex development proceeds from upper to lower extremities.
    B. Intentional movement by newborns enhances neuromuscular development and stability.
    C. Pushing against boundaries should be avoided to prevent pressure on the developing joints.
    D. Any position that allows movement will increases physiologic stress and should be avoided.

19. Which of the following is true of newborn sleep states?
    A. Oxygen consumption is lowest during rapid eye movement sleep.

    B. The best state for interaction with parents is the active alert state.
    C. Early dominant states are light sleep, quiet sleep, and active alertness.
    D. Less time is spent in the quiet alert state as the infant matures.

20. Sensory integrative dysfunction occurs when the brain is not organizing the flow of sensory impulses in a manner that provides precise information to the individual. Which statement best describes this malfunction in neurodevelopment?
    A. Painful stimuli are adapted to and do not cause sensory integrative dysfunction.
    B. All preterm infants uniformly display problems associated with sensory integration.
    C. The symptoms of sensory integrative dysfunction are not expressed in higher-level functioning.
    D. The long-term problems associated with sensory integrative dysfunction include reduction in self-control, capacity for abstract thought, and self-esteem.

21. Which statement about the development of the human brain is the most accurate?
    A. The newborn brain is largely formed by term and is completely developed by 2 years of age.
    B. Developmental outcome is influenced almost entirely by genetic history, and environmental events have a minimal effect.
    C. The brain is a chain of communicating cells, and every touch, movement, and emotion affects its wiring and development.
    D. The brain of a preterm infant (24 weeks' gestation) has many cortical sulci, and these involutions can be harmed by inappropriate stimulation, excessive noise, and repetitive painful stimuli.

# Chapter 10

# Radiographic Evaluation

1. A chest radiograph described as showing normal pulmonary vascularity and right atrial hypertrophy, which rotates the heart and is evident as an upturned and prominent cardiac apex that creates a "boot-shaped" heart, is diagnostic of:
   A. tricuspid atresia.
   B. Ebstein anomaly.
   C. tetralogy of Fallot.
   D. total anomalous pulmonary venous return.

2. A chest radiograph described as showing hyperlucency between the chest wall and lung in the right thorax with a mediastinal shift from right to left is diagnostic of:
   A. pneumothorax.
   B. pneumopericardium.
   C. pneumomediastinum.
   D. pulmonary interstitial emphysema.

3. An abdominal radiograph described as showing hyperlucency within the liver, bowel dilation, and bowel wall thickening with a "bubbly" pattern is diagnostic of:
   A. duodenal atresia.
   B. meconium ileus.
   C. midgut malrotation.
   D. necrotizing enterocolitis.

4. A radiographic exposure performed by passing the x-ray beam from the anterior to the posterior aspect with the radiograph cassette flat against the infant's back and the infant positioned on his or her side is referred to as a(n):
   A. anteroposterior view.
   B. posteroanterior view.
   C. lateral decubitus view.
   D. cross-table lateral view.

5. A 24-week gestation infant was admitted to the NICU. An umbilical arterial and venous catheter was inserted. A chest and abdominal radiograph showed the umbilical venous catheter tip to be located at T6. The catheter is:
   A. in the appropriate position.
   B. too low and should be advanced 1 cm.
   C. too high and should be pulled back to T10.
   D. too high and should be pulled back to T8.

6. A 26-week gestation infant is intubated and placed on conventional mechanical ventilation. The infant's oxygen requirements have increased from 43% to 57% in the last hour. A chest radiograph has been obtained in which the infant's head is turned slightly to the right with the chin pointing down. The endotracheal tube is noted to be at T4. The primary intervention is to:
   A. suction the infant's airway.
   B. turn the infant's head to the left.
   C. pull back the tube to T2.
   D. repeat the chest radiograph with the infant's chin in the midline position.

7. A full-term infant is transferred to the NICU from the labor and delivery unit at 2 hours of life. The infant has severe retractions, tachypnea, and an oxygen saturation of 85%. A chest radiograph is obtained and shows bilateral asymmetry with areas of atelectasis and a patchy appearance, and hyperaeration with flattened hemidiaphragms. The clinical diagnosis and initial intervention would be:
   A. pulmonary interstitial emphysema; intubate.
   B. meconium aspiration syndrome; provide oxygen.
   C. pneumonia; obtain blood specimens for culture and initiate antibiotic therapy.
   D. transient tachypnea of the newborn; provide oxygen and begin feedings.

8. The nurse placed a peripherally-inserted central catheter in the patient's right arm. On the follow-up chest radiograph, the catheter tip is seen to be located at T7. This catheter is:
   A. in the appropriate position and does not need to be removed.
   B. too deep and needs to be pulled back to T1.
   C. too deep and needs to be pulled back to T3.
   D. not in the appropriate position and should be advanced to T10.

9. A term infant is admitted to the NICU because of respiratory distress and has unequal breath sounds and a barrel chest. The chest radiograph shows air-filled loops in the left thorax. The clinical diagnosis and initial intervention would be:
   A. pneumothorax; provide oxygen.
   B. pyloric stenosis; prepare for surgery.
   C. congenital diaphragmatic hernia; intubate.
   D. midgut volvulus; decompress the bowel with an orogastric tube connected to low intermittent suction.

10. On evaluation of a chest and abdominal radiograph, the tip of an umbilical arterial catheter is seen to be located at L1. The primary intervention is to:
    A. assess the infant for hypoglycemia.
    B. assess the infant for gluteal necrosis.
    C. pull back the catheter to L2.
    D. advance the catheter to just above T12.

# Chapter 11

# Pharmacology

1. An infant has liver disease and is receiving a drug that is highly metabolized by the liver. To achieve the desired pharmacodynamic response to the drug, the nurse would expect the drug's dose to be:
   A. higher than the standard dose.
   B. lower than the standard dose.
   C. the same as the standard dose.
   D. the same as the standard dose, but given more frequently.

2. An infant needs to rapidly achieve a therapeutic plasma drug concentration of a medication. Rather than wait for a plateau level (steady state) to be achieved, the care provider will order a:
   A. loading dose.
   B. maintenance dose.
   C. medication with no first-pass effect.
   D. medication with rapid cell entry properties.

3. β-Lactam antibiotics, such as penicillins and cephalosporins, cause bacterial cell death by:
   A. blocking the production of folic acid.
   B. activating the patient's immune system.
   C. inhibiting intracellular protein synthesis.
   D. disrupting the cell walls of the microorganism.

4. Which statement is true regarding the mechanism of action of antiseizure medications?
   A. They potentiate the effect of the inhibitory neurotransmitter glutamate.
   B. They stabilize neuronal cell membranes and suppress neuronal discharges.
   C. They reduce the excitatory neurotransmitter γ-aminobutyric acid (GABA).
   D. They reduce neuronal electrical discharges by opening sodium and calcium channels.

5. Methylxanthines, such as caffeine (Cafcit) and theophylline (Elixophyllin), are used in the treatment of apnea of prematurity. The infant receiving caffeine should be monitored for:
   A. hypocalcemia.
   B. hypersomnolence.
   C. feeding intolerance.
   D. temperature instability.

6. An intubated infant is given intravenous fentanyl (Sublimaze) postoperatively for pain control. Suddenly, the infant exhibits desaturation followed by decreasing heart rate. The infant remains intubated without an air leak. Which of the following is a possible cause of this infant's deteriorating condition?
   A. Hypertension
   B. Vagal response
   C. Anesthetic gases
   D. Chest wall rigidity

7. Digoxin (Lanoxin), a digitalis glycoside, exhibits which of the following actions?
   A. It increases plasma renin and aldosterone levels.
   B. It increases intracellular calcium, which produces a positive inotropic action.
   C. It has a positive dromotropic action, increasing sinoatrial and atrioventricular nodal conduction.
   D. It exhibits a positive chronotropic action secondary to increased vagal nerve tone.

8. A side effect of anticholinergic ophthalmic medications used in neonates undergoing an examination for retinopathy of prematurity is:
   A. bradycardia.
   B. somnolence.
   C. respiratory distress.
   D. increased gastrointestinal transit time.

9. The potassium-sparing diuretic spironolactone (Aldactone) is not useful in emergency situations such as florid pulmonary edema because:
   A. there is risk of an allergic reaction to the drug.
   B. the onset of action is approximately 60 hours.
   C. the intravenous form of the drug is highly caustic to veins.
   D. more than one dose results in hypokalemia and cardiac dysrhythmias.

10. The factor that most determines drug distribution is:
    A. half-life.
    B. drug interactions.
    C. plateau (steady-state) drug level.
    D. vascular perfusion of the tissue or organ.

11. Drugs with higher molecular weights are metabolized in the liver, excreted into bile, and delivered to the intestines. Prior to evacuation from the body, the drug may be reabsorbed into the portal venous system. This process is known as:

    A. metabolism.
    B. first-pass effect.
    C. hepatic clearance.
    D. enterohepatic cycling.

## Chapter 12

# Care of the Extremely Low Birth Weight Infant

**Questions 1 and 2 refer to the following scenario:**
The nurse is expecting the delivery of a female infant at 24 weeks' postconceptional age, with an estimated fetal weight of 800 g.

1. Which of the following elements of the delivery room setup is most specifically geared toward the extremely low birth weight infant?
   A. Nasal continuous positive airway pressure device
   B. Polyethylene wrap
   C. Meconium aspirator
   D. 3.5-mm endotracheal tube

2. At delivery, the infant is noted to be apneic. The attending physician intubates and orders the nurse to deliver positive pressure ventilation with an inspired oxygen fraction ($Fio_2$) of 0.40 while the respiratory therapist applies the oxygen saturation monitor. Based on the patient-specific data, which of the following is the most accurate interpretation of this order?
   A. This is an inappropriate order, because blended oxygen is not available in the delivery room.
   B. This is an appropriate order, because even brief hyperoxia can result in negative sequelae in the extremely low birth weight infant.
   C. This is an inappropriate order, because apneic infants all require resuscitation with 100% oxygen until their condition is stabilized.
   D. This is an inappropriate order, because apneic infants must be resuscitated with 100% oxygen until pulse oximetry indicates that their oxygen saturation is greater than 98%.

3. Care planning for an extremely low birth weight (ELBW) infant includes minimizing painful procedures, minimizing suctioning, positioning the head midline, minimizing postural changes, and maintaining the hips below the head. As a group, these interventions are intended to prevent which one of the following complications more common in the ELBW infant than in other newborn populations?
   A. Pneumothorax
   B. Thermal instability
   C. Intraventricular hemorrhage
   D. Iatrogenic musculoskeletal deformities

**Questions 4 and 5 refer to the following scenario:**
An infant born at 24 weeks' gestation is now 27 hours old. Since admission, the infant has received thermal support via double-walled unhumidified incubator on servocontrol and intravenous fluid consisting of dextrose 5% in water at 100 ml/kg/day. Current findings include dry, flaking, and wrinkled skin; thermal lability that requires very high incubator air temperatures; serum sodium level of 150 mEq/dl; weight 710 g; and urinary output 1.5 ml/kg/hour.

4. The RN's assessment of this infant suggests which of the following as most likely related to each of these findings?
   A. Dehydration due to diuresis
   B. Dehydration due to insufficient fluid intake
   C. Dehydration due to transdermal fluid losses
   D. Dehydration due to high incubator temperatures

5. Which of the following, if instituted within the first few hours of life, is the best proactive intervention with the fewest negative side effects to prevent the dehydration seen in this case?
   A. Use of relative humidity higher than 70%
   B. Initial intravenous fluid intake of 200 ml/kg/day
   C. Use of a heated mattress to prevent the need for higher air temperatures
   D. Addition of sodium to the intravenous solution to improve renal retention of fluids

# Chapter 13

# Care of the Late Preterm Infant

1. Late preterm infants (LPIs) are at risk for rehospitalization. Common causes of rehospitalization include sepsis, hyperbilirubinemia, failure to thrive, and feeding difficulties. What is another common cause of rehospitalization of the LPI?
   A. Abdominal distention
   B. Necrotizing enterocolitis
   C. Respiratory syncytial virus infection
   D. Persistent patent ductus arteriosus

2. A 36⅔-week gestational age infant of a diabetic mother was delivered vaginally, weighing 3.75 kg. Spontaneous rupture of membranes occurred 2 hours prior to delivery. Fluid was clear and nonodorous. Fetal electrocardiographic monitoring revealed a normal tracing. Immediately after birth, the infant displayed the following symptoms: tachypnea, grunting, retractions, and cyanosis. Continuous positive airway pressure was provided with supplemental oxygen at 50%. Initial arterial blood gas values revealed a respiratory acidosis with hypoxia. Which of the following differential diagnoses most likely correlates with this infant's presentation?
   A. Pneumonia
   B. Bronchopulmonary dysplasia
   C. Respiratory distress syndrome
   D. Transient tachypnea of the newborn

3. Late preterm infants are at a higher risk for developing which of the following conditions?
   A. Hyperthermia
   B. Hyperglycemia
   C. Hyperbilirubinemia
   D. Persistent pulmonary hypertension

4. A 35⅔-week gestational age infant has been cared for on the mother/baby unit. Comprehensive discharge teaching needs to specifically address the late preterm infant. Which care topics are specific for the LPI and should be included in the discharge teaching plan?
   A. Assessment for hyperthermia and cord care
   B. Hearing screen, bathing, and method for taking temperature rectally
   C. Follow-up with a primary care provider 1 week after discharge, hearing screen, and cord care
   D. Car seat evaluation, evaluation by a lactation consultant, and signs and symptoms of dehydration

5. A 35½-week gestational age infant who is 6 hours old is brought to the nursery because the temperature is 35.1° C (95.2° F). The nurse places the baby under a radiant warmer to rapidly rewarm the infant so that it can be returned to the mother for feeding. One-half hour later, the nurse reassesses the baby and notices that the baby is suddenly showing episodes of apnea, a heart rate of 170 beats/minute, and hypotension. What is most likely the cause of these changes in vital signs?
   A. Sepsis
   B. Hypothermia
   C. Vasodilation
   D. Hypoglycemia

# PATHOPHYSIOLOGY
## SYSTEM-SPECIFIC DISORDERS

### Chapter 14

# Cardiovascular Disorders

**Questions 1 and 2 refer to the following scenario:**
A 2-day-old female infant is noted to have hepatomegaly, tachycardia, and tachypnea. The mucous membranes are pink. A gallop rhythm is present. Brachial pulses are 3+ bilaterally, femoral pulses are 1+ bilaterally. The blood pressure is 62/45 mm Hg in the right upper arm and 40/28 mm Hg in the right thigh.

1. The nurse notifies the licensed practitioner because this infant most likely has:
   A. cardiomyopathy.
   B. patent ductus arteriosus.
   C. coarctation of the aorta.
   D. persistent pulmonary hypertension of the newborn.

2. The infant also is noted to have a webbed neck, epicanthal folds, and lymphedema of the hands and feet. A genetics consult is indicated to evaluate this infant for which of the following?
   A. Trisomy 21 (Down syndrome)
   B. Turner syndrome
   C. Klinefelter syndrome
   D. Beckwith-Wiedemann syndrome

3. The effectiveness of prostaglandin $E_1$ therapy for a patient with hypoplastic left heart syndrome is *best* demonstrated by:
   A. increased oxygen saturation measured by pulse oximetry.
   B. decreased heart rate.
   C. decreased murmur intensity.
   D. improved peripheral perfusion.

4. For an infant with tricuspid atresia, prostaglandin $E_1$ is started at 0.05 mcg/kg/minute. Which of the following should the nurse monitor to assess effectiveness of the prostaglandin $E_1$ therapy?

   A. Oxygen saturation measured by pulse oximetry.
   B. Heart rate
   C. Blood pressure
   D. Capillary refill

5. Digoxin is used in the long-term management of supraventricular tachycardia because of which effect?
   A. It improves contractility.
   B. It constricts the splanchnic circulation.
   C. It slows conduction through the atrioventricular node.
   D. It prolongs the refractory period in myocardial tissue.

6. When assessing an infant with hypoplastic left heart syndrome, the nurse should anticipate:
   A. diminished pulses.
   B. diastolic murmur.
   C. profound cyanosis.
   D. excessive urine output.

7. The care plan for an infant receiving indomethacin should include monitoring for which of the following?
   A. Leukopenia
   B. Hypertension
   C. Thrombocytosis
   D. Decreased urine output

8. The main goal of preoperative management of an infant with hypoplastic left heart syndrome is to:
   A. close the ductus arteriosus.
   B. maintain blood pressure as high as possible.
   C. maintain oxygen saturation levels above 90%.
   D. provide a balance of the systemic and pulmonary circulations.

9. A 26-week gestation infant has been oliguric for 14 hours. The electrocardiogram (ECG) shows peaked T waves and a widened QRS complex. Serum laboratory values are Na 128 mEq/L, K 6.9 mEq/L, Cl 85 mEq/L, Ca 6.8 mg/dl, glucose 30 mg/dl. What is the most likely cause of the infant's ECG abnormalities?
   A. Hyperkalemia
   B. Hyponatremia
   C. Hypoglycemia
   D. Hypocalcemia

10. The rationale for performing a balloon septostomy in transposition of the great vessels is to increase:
    A. cardiac output.
    B. pulmonary blood flow.
    C. right ventricular outflow tract blood flow.
    D. mixing of oxygenated and deoxygenated blood at the atrial level.

11. Supplemental oxygen should be used with caution in infants with single-ventricle anatomy because:
    A. it can lead to retinopathy of prematurity.
    B. increased $Po_2$ will prevent the ductus arteriosus from closing.
    C. oxygen is of little use in raising the oxygen saturation levels in infants with cyanotic heart lesions.
    D. it can lead to pulmonary vasodilation and increased pulmonary blood flow at the expense of systemic perfusion.

12. The plan of care for an infant of a diabetic mother should include monitoring the infant for signs and symptoms of decreased cardiac output due to hypoglycemia because hypoglycemia:
    A. decreases preload.
    B. increases afterload.
    C. decreases heart rate.
    D. decreases cardiac contractility.

13. Which of the following statements about cyanosis is correct?
    A. Anemia increases the visibility of cyanosis.
    B. A cyanotic heart lesion is always associated with cyanosis.
    C. Cyanosis can occur in a healthy infant with polycythemia.
    D. Cyanosis does not occur if pulmonary blood flow is increased.

**Questions 14 through 16 refer to the following scenario:** A 2-week-old, 4-kg neonate with Ebstein anomaly demonstrates the rhythm illustrated in the electrocardiogram shown here. The infant is alert, color is slightly pale, and capillary refill is 2 seconds.

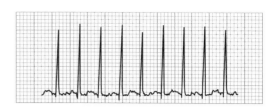

14. Which of the following best describes this rhythm?
    A. Sinus tachycardia
    B. Normal sinus rhythm
    C. Ventricular tachycardia
    D. Supraventricular tachycardia

After conversion, a 12-lead electrocardiogram is obtained. Lead $V_2$ is shown here.

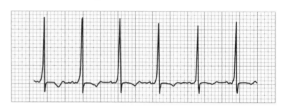

15. The abnormality in this tracing is best described as:
    A. complete atrioventricular block.
    B. first-degree heart block.
    C. premature atrial contractions.
    D. Wolff-Parkinson-White syndrome.

16. Which long-term drug treatment should the nurse expect for this condition?
    A. Digoxin
    B. Atropine
    C. Adenosine
    D. Propranolol

17. Which of the following would be most beneficial to the infant with pulmonary atresia?
    A. Digoxin
    B. Furosemide
    C. Propranolol
    D. Prostaglandin $E_1$

18. A 2-day-old, full-term infant has become moderately ill after a normal postnatal course. Capillary refill is 3 seconds and peripheral pulses are adequate. The cardiac monitor shows a heart rate of 280 beats/minute with a narrow QRS complex. Vagal maneuvers have been unsuccessful. Two doses of adenosine are administered with no resulting change on the electrocardiogram. The next therapeutic intervention of choice is:
    A. transesophageal pacing.
    B. defibrillation at 2 J/kg.
    C. administration of atropine at 0.02 mg/kg.
    D. synchronized cardioversion at 0.5 to 1.0 J/kg.

19. Zero referencing is important because it:
    A. calibrates the monitor.
    B. calibrates the transducer.
    C. negates the effect of atmospheric and hydro-static pressure on physiologic measurements.
    D. ensures that all components of the hemodynamic monitoring system are functioning accurately.

20. When an umbilical artery catheter monitoring system is zero balanced and leveled, which component must be leveled with the infant's phlebostatic axis?
    A. Transducer
    B. Intraflow/fast flush device
    C. Air-fluid interface of the zeroing stopcock
    D. Stopcock connecting the catheter to the fluid tubing

21. A serum digoxin level is ordered. The nurse should obtain the sample:
    A. 1 hour after a dose.
    B. 6 hours after a dose.
    C. just before giving a dose.
    D. immediately after giving a dose.

22. What is the primary mechanism by which cardiac output is increased in neonates?
    A. Increase in preload
    B. Decrease in afterload
    C. Increase in heart rate
    D. Increase in cardiac contractility

23. A 2-week-old infant with tetralogy of Fallot suddenly becomes agitated, hyperpneic, and very cyanotic. The nurse auscultates the infant's heart sounds and notes that the systolic murmur, which is usually very loud, is now very quiet. Administration of which of the following would be least helpful?
    A. Oxygen
    B. Morphine
    C. Sodium bicarbonate
    D. Sodium nitroprusside

24. Right ventricular preload is assessed in the clinical setting by evaluating which pressure?
    A. Central venous pressure
    B. Arterial systolic pressure
    C. Arterial diastolic pressure
    D. Pulmonary artery systolic pressure

25. Which of the following best describes the transitional events immediately following birth in the healthy newborn infant?
    A. Pulmonary vascular resistance increases and systemic vascular resistance decreases.
    B. Pulmonary vascular resistance decreases and systemic vascular resistance decreases.
    C. Pulmonary vascular resistance decreases and systemic vascular resistance increases.
    D. Pulmonary vascular resistance increases and systemic vascular resistance increases.

26. What is the purpose of the ductus arteriosus in the fetus?
    A. It allows mixing of blood at the atrial level.
    B. It shunts blood from the left to the right ventricle.
    C. It shunts blood from the pulmonary artery to the aorta.
    D. It shunts blood from the umbilical vein to the inferior vena cava.

27. An infant with a suspected congenital heart defect is being evaluated in the NICU. As part of the education provided to the parents, the nurse explains that echocardiography is a useful diagnostic tool because it:
    A. measures the electrical activity of the heart.
    B. evaluates adequacy of myocardial perfusion.
    C. measures intracardiac pressures and oxygen saturation.
    D. visualizes heart structures and measures heart function.

28. An umbilical artery catheter was placed 1 hour ago. The nurse notes that the toes on the infant's right foot are bluish. The nurse's first intervention should be to:
    A. administer oxygen.
    B. massage the right foot vigorously.
    C. remove the umbilical artery catheter.
    D. apply a warm compress to the left foot.

29. The nurse notices that the umbilical artery waveform is dampened. Which of the following troubleshooting strategies would be least helpful in assessing line function and/or resolving the problem?
    A. Checking for kinks in the line
    B. Checking the tightness of all connections
    C. Attempting to aspirate blood, and then flushing
    D. Adding extension tubing to the line

30. What are two important goals in the management of an infant with congestive heart failure?
    A. Minimize heart rate; maximize blood pressure.
    B. Optimize cardiac function; minimize cardiac demands.
    C. Decrease systemic vascular resistance; increase preload.
    D. Decrease cardiac output; increase oxygen consumption.

**Questions 31 and 32 refer to the following scenario:**
A 4-week-old infant with an atrioventricular canal defect is admitted to the NICU. Vital signs are heart

rate 180 beats/minute, respiratory rate 50 breaths/minute, blood pressure 60/45 mm Hg, oxygen saturation 95%. Assessment findings include the following: color is pale, capillary refill is 3 seconds, extremities are cool to the touch, grade III-VI murmur is present, rales are heart bilaterally, liver is 4 cm below the right costal margin.

31. Which of the following conditions does the nurse suspect?
    A. Sepsis
    B. Pneumonia
    C. Dehydration
    D. Congestive heart failure

32. Pharmacologic management of this infant may include which of the following?
    A. Adenosine
    B. Dobutamine
    C. Ibuprofen
    D. Prostaglandin $E_1$

33. In the case of which of the following congenital heart defects should the nurse expect the infant to have cyanosis?
    A. Aortic stenosis
    B. Pulmonary atresia
    C. Atrial septal defect
    D. Ventricular septal defect

34. A 2-day-old 1000-g, 30-week gestation infant previously in stable condition develops an active precordium, widened pulse pressure, bounding pulses, and a murmur heard best at the left upper sternal border. The nurse suspects that this infant has which of the following conditions?
    A. Sepsis
    B. Pneumonia
    C. Patent ductus arteriosus
    D. Intraventricular hemorrhage

35. An intubated neonate has an intravenous line in the right antecubital fossa infusing dextrose 10% in water, an umbilical artery catheter infusing half-normal saline, and a heparin lock in the left foot. When administering adenosine to this patient, the nurse should administer it:
    A. in the umbilical catheter over 1 to 2 seconds, followed by a normal saline flush.
    B. diluted with normal saline and given via the left foot heparin lock over 20 to 30 seconds.
    C. diluted with normal saline and given via the endotracheal tube over 2 to 3 seconds.
    D. in the right antecubital vein over 1 to 2 seconds, and followed by a normal saline flush.

36. Dobutamine improves cardiac output primarily by:
    A. decreasing preload.
    B. increasing heart rate.

    C. improving cardiac contractility.
    D. decreasing systemic vascular resistance.

37. Cardiac troponin levels are useful in the diagnosis of:
    A. myocarditis.
    B. tetralogy of Fallot.
    C. infective endocarditis.
    D. Wolff-Parkinson-White syndrome.

38. The nurse is admitting an infant born to a mother with systemic lupus erythematosus. The nurse should assess the infant for what cardiac arrhythmia?
    A. Sinus bradycardia
    B. Long QT syndrome
    C. Supraventricular tachycardia
    D. Complete congenital heart block

39. A 6-hour-old, full-term, 4.3-kg male infant is admitted from the well baby nursery to the NICU because of hypoglycemia. The maternal laboratory report reveals that that the mother's hemoglobin $A_{1c}$ level was 14% at 6 weeks' gestation. Which of the following cardiac disorders is most likely to be present in this infant?
    A. Aortic stenosis
    B. Ebstein anomaly
    C. Tetralogy of Fallot
    D. Ventricular septal defect

40. Which of the following drugs is known to cause congenital heart disease?
    A. Insulin
    B. Phenytoin
    C. Labetalol
    D. Tetracycline

41. The apical impulse represents:
    A. pulmonic valve closing.
    B. closure of the mitral and tricuspid valves.
    C. forward thrust of the left ventricle during systole.
    D. transient left-to-right flow through the ductus arteriosus.

42. A 28-week gestation infant is 6 days old. The infant has been on a ventilator since birth, and for the past 2 days, no weaning of pressures or oxygen has been possible. A patent ductus arteriosus (PDA) is suspected. The clinical signs and symptoms of a PDA include:
    A. cardiac arrhythmias.
    B. diaphoresis and poor feeding.
    C. weak peripheral pulses and hypertension.
    D. murmur at the upper left sternal edge, bounding peripheral pulses, and increased precordial cardiac impulse.

43. The clinical signs and symptoms of a patent ductus arteriosus most typically manifest:

A. at birth.
B. 1 to 2 days after birth.
C. 3 to 4 days after birth.
D. 7 to 10 days after birth.

44. What is the most common congenital heart defect?
    A. Pulmonic stenosis
    B. Atrial septal defect
    C. Coarctation of the aorta
    D. Ventricular septal defect

45. What is the most common cyanotic congenital heart defect?
    A. Pulmonary atresia
    B. Tetralogy of Fallot
    C. Hypoplastic left heart syndrome
    D. Transposition of the great arteries

46. A full-term female infant is admitted to the NICU. Her physical examination reveals the following dysmorphic craniofacial features: cleft palate, prominent nose with squared nasal root, narrow palpebral fissures, abundant scalp hair, vertical maxillary excess with a long face, and a low-set chin. Tetralogy of Fallot is seen on echocardiography. The infant's initial serum ionized calcium level is 2.4 mg/dl (0.6 mmol/L). Of the following, the infant is most likely to have:
    A. trisomy 21 (Down syndrome).
    B. Gilbert syndrome.
    C. DiGeorge syndrome.
    D. Cornelia de Lange syndrome.

47. Which of the following congenital heart defects is most often associated with Noonan syndrome?
    A. Ebstein anomaly
    B. Ventricular septal defect
    C. Valvular pulmonic stenosis
    D. Hypoplastic left heart syndrome

48. Of the following, which best describes the cardiac anatomy of transposition of the great arteries?
    A. There is a single arterial outflow from both ventricles in association with a ventricular septal defect.
    B. The descending aorta is narrowed adjacent to insertion of the ductus arteriosus.
    C. The pulmonary veins drain into the right atrium directly or through connection with the systemic veins.
    D. The aorta serves as the outflow of the right ventricle and the pulmonary artery serves as the left ventricular outflow.

49. A 6-hour-old term newborn is suspected of having hypoplastic left heart syndrome. Of the following, what is the most consistent clinical finding of this syndrome?

A. Severe cyanosis
B. Split second heart sound
C. Hyperdynamic precordial activity
D. Decreased amplitude of peripheral pulses

50. Cardiac output is compromised in supraventricular tachycardia primarily due to:
    A. increased preload.
    B. increased afterload.
    C. decreased cardiac contractility.
    D. decreased diastolic filling time.

51. Which metabolic disorder is associated with hypertrophic cardiomyopathy?
    A. Galactosemia
    B. Pompe disease
    C. Niemann-Pick disease type C
    D. Congenital adrenal hyperplasia

52. The immediate management priority for infants suspected to have hypoplastic left heart syndrome is administration of:
    A. sildenafil.
    B. lidocaine.
    C. indomethacin.
    D. prostaglandin $E_1$.

53. Reliability of noninvasive blood pressure measurements depends on use of the appropriate blood pressure cuff size. In the newborn, the correct cuff width should be what percentage of the circumference of the extremity?
    A. 20% to 30%
    B. 30% to 40%
    C. 40% to 50%
    D. 50% to 60%

**Questions 54 and 55 refer to the following scenario:**
A 28-week gestation male infant who weighed 975 g at birth is 6 weeks old. The infant's history includes respiratory distress syndrome requiring mechanical ventilation for the first 7 days of life and oxygen supplementation via nasal canula for 11 days, umbilical artery catheterization, apnea of prematurity, clinical sepsis, and hyperbilirubinemia. The infant is currently breathing room air, oxygen saturation is consistently over 93%, and the infant is tolerating full enteral feeds. Findings of his physical examination are unremarkable. The NICU nurse measures the infant's blood pressure in the right arm by the oscillometric method using the correct size cuff and while the infant is sleeping. The systolic blood pressure is 98 mm Hg and the diastolic pressure is 60 mm Hg. The nurse looks back at the flow sheet and notes that the infant's blood pressure has been elevated for the last three readings.

54. What is the most appropriate diagnostic test to confirm the cause of this infant's hypertension?
    A. Renal sonogram
    B. Thyroid studies
    C. Head ultrasonography
    D. Chest radiograph

55. Which of the following medications would most likely be used to treat this infant's hypertension?
    A. Digoxin
    B. Amiodarone
    C. Hydralazine
    D. Procainamide

## Chapter 15

# Pulmonary Disorders

1. The formation of respiratory bronchioles (i.e., acini) during the canalicular stage of fetal lung development is significant because it heralds:
   A. initiation of surfactant synthesis.
   B. creation of alveolar ducts and alveoli.
   C. rapid proliferation of pulmonary vasculature.
   D. primitive development of the gas exchange section of the lung.

2. Which of the following statements is the most accurate about what occurs during the terminal sac stage of fetal lung development?
   A. The adult component of alveoli is obtained.
   B. A decrease in pulmonary vascularization occurs.
   C. Surface-active phospholipid (lecithin) is first detected.
   D. A progressive increase in alveolar capillary surface area occurs that is necessary for gas exchange.

3. A newborn infant with respiratory difficulty is diagnosed with a congenital chylothorax. A thoracentesis followed by placement of a tube thoracotomy for continuous drainage is performed. The nurse must monitor this patient closely for:
   A. apnea.
   B. air leak.
   C. infection.
   D. subcutaneous emphysema.

4. Lung development is completed by what age?
   A. 38 to 40 weeks of gestation
   B. 12 to 15 months of age
   C. 6 to 8 years of age
   D. 16 to 18 years of age

5. Surfactant improves lung function by:
   A. increasing opening pressure.
   B. inhibiting alveolar fluid clearance.
   C. promoting structural maturation of the lung.

   D. reducing surface tension at the air-liquid interface in the alveolus.

6. Which of the following populations of infants at 36 weeks of gestation would be at increased risk for developing respiratory distress syndrome?
   A. Infants of heroin-addicted mothers
   B. Infants of mothers with hypertension
   C. Infants of class A/B/C diabetic mothers
   D. Infants with intrauterine growth restriction

7. Surfactant is produced in the lungs by:
   A. acini.
   B. type I pneumocytes.
   C. type II pneumocytes.
   D. surfactant protein A.

8. Early signs of respiratory disease in a neonate include:
   A. retractions.
   B. hypotension.
   C. acrocyanosis.
   D. respiratory rate of 30 to 40 breaths/minute.

9. Mechanically ventilated infants must be monitored for acid-base status. Prolonged, severe hypocapnia resulting in respiratory alkalosis places the infant at risk for:
   A. apnea.
   B. renal failure.
   C. periventricular leukomalacia.
   D. gastroesophageal reflux disease.

10. In the delivery room a 1200-g infant at 30 weeks' gestation shows grunting, nasal flaring, and chest wall retractions. Which of the following pulmonary pathophysiologic conditions is most likely occurring?
    A. Pulmonary air leak syndrome
    B. Respiratory distress syndrome
    C. Meconium aspiration syndrome
    D. Transient tachypnea of the newborn

11. Expiratory grunting represents the infant's attempt to:
    A. conserve energy.
    B. decrease upper airway resistance.
    C. overcome large airway obstruction.
    D. maintain a normal functional residual capacity.

12. To rule out group B streptococcal infection as an underlying cause of respiratory distress, which of the following studies would be most appropriate?
    A. Eye culture
    B. Blood cultures
    C. Cultures of nasopharyngeal secretions
    D. Cultures of axillary and rectal specimens

13. A radiographic picture of grainy lungs and prominent air bronchograms is characteristic of respiratory distress syndrome and indicates which of the following conditions?
    A. Pneumonia
    B. Pulmonary edema
    C. Pulmonary air leaks
    D. Aerated bronchioles superimposed over non-aerated alveoli

14. Results of an infant's arterial blood gas analysis are pH 7.25, $Paco_2$ 70, $HCO_3$ 21, base deficit –4, $Pao_2$ 50, and oxygen saturation 88%. These blood gas results are indicative of which acid-base condition?
    A. Metabolic acidosis
    B. Metabolic alkalosis
    C. Respiratory acidosis
    D. Respiratory alkalosis

15. An infant is being mechanically ventilated because of respiratory failure secondary to respiratory distress syndrome. Arterial blood gas results indicate a rising $Paco_2$. Breath sounds are coarse bilaterally, with bubbling of secretions observed in the endotracheal tube. The infant is extremely restless, with "seesaw" respirations. The ventilator is consistently sounding an alarm for high inspiratory pressure. The nurse's first action should be to:
    A. reposition the infant.
    B. administer an analgesic.
    C. silence the ventilator alarm.
    D. assess breath sounds, suction, and reassess breath sounds.

16. By 72 hours of life, a small preterm infant who has been treated with surfactant for respiratory distress syndrome develops a grade II-VI continuous murmur at the left upper sternal border. Bilateral rales are heard on auscultation of breath sounds. Bounding peripheral pulses with a widened pulse pressure are present. Urine output is less than 2 ml/kg/hour. Blood gas analyses reveal increasing hypoxemia, hypercarbia, and metabolic acidosis with subsequent need for increased ventilatory support. These findings are most consistent with which condition?
    A. Sepsis
    B. Air leak
    C. Pneumonia
    D. Patent ductus arteriosus

17. Medical management of an infant with respiratory distress complicated by patent ductus arteriosus would include which of the following?
    A. Volume expansion
    B. Indomethacin (Indocin)
    C. Acetaminophen (Tylenol)
    D. Prostaglandin $E_1$ (Alprostadil)

18. The clinical presentation of tachypnea, hypercarbia, tissue mottling, diminished capillary refill, and oliguria associated with patent ductus arteriosus in the preterm infant is the result of which of the following conditions?
    A. Systemic hypertension
    B. Pulmonary hypoperfusion
    C. Right-to-left shunting of blood
    D. Left-to-right shunting of blood

19. Which of the following is a complication associated with patent ductus arteriosus?
    A. Metabolic alkalosis
    B. Pulmonary air leak
    C. Pulmonary hypoplasia
    D. Pulmonary hemorrhage

20. Nursing management of a preterm infant with acute respiratory distress syndrome should be directed toward:
    A. liberalizing administration of fluids.
    B. handling frequently to provide developmental stimulation.
    C. maintaining the infant in a neutral thermal environment.
    D. decreasing inspired oxygen fraction ($Fio_2$) for oxygen saturation values of less than 88%.

21. When assessing an infant with respiratory distress syndrome, the nurse calculates the infant's urine output to be more than 5 ml/kg/hour for an 8-hour period. The nurse suspects that the increase in urine output is indicative of which of the following conditions?
    A. Renal failure
    B. Worsening pulmonary status
    C. Development of chronic lung disease
    D. Recovery phase of respiratory distress syndrome

22. A maternal history of chorioamnionitis, fever, premature rupture of membranes longer than 24 hours, prolonged labor with intact membranes, and excessive obstetric manipulations predisposes the infant to which of the following conditions?
    A. Congenital pneumonia
    B. Respiratory distress syndrome
    C. Meconium aspiration syndrome
    D. Transient tachypnea of the newborn

23. A 39-week large-for-gestational-age infant was delivered by cesarean section. The Apgar scores were 8 and 9 at 1 and 5 minutes, respectively, and initial vital signs were stable. At 2 hours of age, the infant exhibits increased work of breathing and a pulse oximetry reading of 88% on room air. Blow-by oxygen raises the oxygen saturation to 96%. An arterial blood gas analysis reveals the following: pH 7.36, $Paco_2$ 37, $HCO_3$ 24, and $Pao_2$ 65. Appropriate management for this infant would include which of the following interventions?
    A. Administration of surfactant
    B. Administration of inhaled nitric oxide
    C. Intubation and mechanical ventilation
    D. Provision of supplemental oxygen to maintain $Pao_2$ at 70 to 80

24. The initial chest radiograph for a large-for-gestational-term infant delivered by caesarean section reveals diffuse haziness with prominent perihilar streaking bilaterally and fluid in the fissures. This radiographic picture is consistent with which diagnosis?
    A. Respiratory distress syndrome
    B. Meconium aspiration syndrome
    C. Pulmonary interstitial emphysema
    D. Transient tachypnea of the newborn

25. The underlying clinical pathology of transient tachypnea of the newborn is respiratory distress resulting from which of the following conditions?
    A. Aspiration
    B. Retained lung fluids
    C. Pulmonary hypoplasia
    D. Progressive atelectasis

26. Which of the following would be included in the differential diagnosis of transient tachypnea of the newborn?
    A. Pneumonia
    B. Pneumothorax
    C. Pleural effusion
    D. Pulmonary interstitial emphysema

27. Severe asphyxia of the full-term infant in the early neonatal period may result in which of the following conditions?
    A. Pneumonia

B. Transient tachypnea of the newborn
    C. Left-to-right shunting through the foramen ovale
    D. Persistent pulmonary hypertension of the newborn

28. Central apnea is defined as:
    A. absence of airflow and respiratory effort.
    B. absence of airflow with continued respiratory effort.
    C. a condition with both neurologic and obstructive components.
    D. cyclic respirations of breathing for 10 to 15 seconds, followed by apnea for 5 to 10 seconds, that occur at least three times in succession.

29. The neonate's unique response to hypoxemia and carbon dioxide retention is characterized by:
    A. an initial decrease in respiratory effort.
    B. prolonged sustained increase in alveolar ventilation.
    C. a brief period of increased respiration followed by respiratory depression.
    D. an increase in minute ventilation above baseline until blood levels of oxygen and carbon dioxide normalize.

30. Which of the following nursing interventions may exacerbate apnea in preterm infants?
    A. Limiting loud noises
    B. Weighing on a cold scale
    C. Controlling environmental temperature
    D. Positioning with small rolls under the neck and shoulder

31. As the nurse prepares to administer a dose of caffeine to a preterm infant, the nurse determines that the infant is tachycardic, with a heart rate of 190 beats/minute. The infant is resting quietly in the incubator. The nurse should:
    A. administer the dose of caffeine.
    B. wait 5 minutes before administering the dose.
    C. withhold the dose and notify the physician or neonatal nurse practitioner.
    D. remeasure the heart rate and administer the dose if heart rate is less than 180 beats/minute.

32. An infant requires frequent arterial blood gas (ABG) monitoring, but obtaining ABG specimens is difficult in the infant. A transcutaneous oxygen and carbon dioxide monitor is ordered for this infant. The nurse knows that:
    A. no more ABG specimens will be needed.
    B. the umbilical arterial catheter can now be removed.
    C. use of this monitor will reduce the number of ABG specimens needed.

D. there is a direct correlation between the transcutaneous oxygen and carbon dioxide values and the ABG values.

33. Aspiration pneumonitis acquired at delivery manifests within the first hours to days of life. Which of the following pathogens is most commonly associated with aspiration pneumonitis?
    A. *Chlamydia trachomatis*
    B. Respiratory syncytial virus
    C. Group B β-hemolytic streptococci
    D. Fungi, especially *Candida* species

34. A 3.5-kg, postdate infant was born via cesarean section because of prolonged fetal bradycardia and thick meconium-stained fluid. At delivery the infant was limp, apneic, cyanotic, and bradycardic and required intubation. Suctioning of the trachea produced thick green material. On admission, the admitting nurse recognizes that this infant is at high risk for which of the following conditions?
    A. Pulmonary edema
    B. Nonspecific respiratory distress
    C. Meconium aspiration syndrome
    D. Transient tachypnea of the newborn

35. A newborn term infant with meconium aspiration syndrome is intubated and conventional ventilation is started. When the infant is 3 hours of age, the cardiorespiratory monitor sounds alarms for bradycardia and hypotension. The infant is extremely restless and cyanotic, with diminished breath sounds on the left side, poor peripheral pulses, asymmetric chest rise, and a mediastinal shift toward the right. The nurse should suspect the development of which of the following conditions?
    A. Pleural effusion
    B. Tension pneumothorax
    C. Pulmonary hemorrhage
    D. Pulmonary interstitial emphysema

36. A term infant is delivered vaginally following an uncomplicated labor and delivery. Immediately after birth, the infant becomes cyanotic with severe grunting, retracting, and nasal flaring. The infant is intubated and positive pressure ventilation is started. On physical examination, breath sounds are diminished on the left side with displacement of cardiac sounds toward the right. The abdomen is scaphoid in appearance. A chest radiograph reveals dilated loops of bowel in the thoracic space with right mediastinal shift. The nurse should prepare to assist with management of which of the following conditions?
    A. Pneumothorax
    B. Pneumomediastinum

C. Congenital diaphragmatic hernia
D. Cystic adenomatoid malformation

37. Factors that predispose an infant to bronchopulmonary dysplasia include which of the following?
    A. Hypovolemia
    B. Full-term birth
    C. Oxygen administration and mechanical ventilation
    D. Transient tachypnea of the newborn

38. Radiographic findings characteristic of severe bronchopulmonary dysplasia include which of the following?
    A. Pleural effusion
    B. Alveolar infiltrates
    C. Dark areas without parenchymal markings
    D. Cystic lung fields with hyperinflation and atelectasis

39. Which of the following would be the appropriate management for ventilator-induced respiratory alkalosis?
    A. Increase the ventilator rate
    B. Decrease minute ventilation
    C. Increase peak inspiratory pressure
    D. Decrease positive end-expiratory pressure

40. Which of the following statements about pulmonary physiology is accurate?
    A. Tidal volume is defined as the volume of air maximally inspired and maximally expired in one breath.
    B. Vital capacity is defined as the amount of air that moves into or out of the lungs with each normal respiration.
    C. Functional residual capacity is defined as the volume of gas that remains in the lungs after normal expiration.
    D. Physiologic dead space is defined as the volume of gas within the area of the pulmonary conducting airways that cannot engage in gas exchange.

41. Which of the following statements about the care of an infant with a chest tube is accurate?
    A. Repositioning of the patient should be minimized.
    B. Milking and stripping of the chest tube are routine interventions to ensure tube patency.
    C. Continuous bubbling in the water seal chamber is an indication that the chest tube is functioning effectively.
    D. Tube patency, fluctuation, and bubbling in the drainage system should be monitored and documented hourly.

42. A preterm infant being treated with mechanical ventilation for severe respiratory distress syndrome suddenly has hypotension, muffled heart sounds, and bradycardia. The chest radiograph reveals a "halo" surrounding the heart. The nurse should prepare to assist with management of which of the following conditions?
    A. Pneumothorax
    B. Pneumopericardium
    C. Pneumomediastinum
    D. Pulmonary interstitial emphysema

43. Why is inhaled nitric oxide useful in the treatment of persistent pulmonary hypertension?
    A. Inhaled nitric oxide supports cardiac function.
    B. Inhaled nitric oxide promotes bronchodilation.
    C. Inhaled nitric oxide decreases systemic arterial pressure.
    D. Inhaled nitric oxide is a potent selective pulmonary vasodilator.

44. The nurse anticipates that an infant will be scheduled for surgical reduction of a congenital diaphragmatic hernia:
    A. immediately after delivery.
    B. following surfactant therapy.
    C. after a trial period of treatment with inhaled nitric oxide.
    D. once pulmonary stabilization has been achieved.

45. Which of the following is a long-term complication associated with congenital diaphragmatic hernia repair?
    A. Chylothorax
    B. Potter syndrome
    C. Gastroesophageal reflux
    D. Necrotizing enterocolitis

46. In which phase of fetal lung development would the nurse expect distal pulmonary vasculature and capillary networks to develop?
    A. Canalicular
    B. Embryonic
    C. Pseudoglandular
    D. Alveolar expansion

47. Which of the following would cause an infant to exhibit signs and symptoms of decreased respiratory effort, lethargy, and bradycardia?
    A. Hyperglycemia
    B. Caffeine (Cafcit) administration
    C. Isoproterenol (Isuprel) administration
    D. Adenosine (Adenocard) administration

48. Initial blood gas analysis for an infant with respiratory distress syndrome reveals the following: pH 7.28, $Paco_2$ 65, $Pao_2$ 85, $HCO_3$ 22. The most appropriate management for this infant, who is being mechanically ventilated, is to:
    A. decrease the ventilator rate.
    B. decrease the inspiratory time.
    C. increase the peak inspiratory pressure.
    D. increase the positive end-expiratory pressure.

49. The chest radiograph for an infant who is being mechanically ventilated, taken 1 day after surfactant administration, reveals grossly hyperinflated lungs with coarse radiolucencies extending from the pleura to the hilum. This radiographic picture is most consistent with which of the following diagnoses?
    A. Respiratory distress syndrome
    B. Pulmonary interstitial emphysema
    C. Transient tachypnea of the newborn
    D. Persistent pulmonary hypertension of the newborn

50. While being mechanically ventilated, an infant becomes agitated and cyanotic. The infant's respirations are vigorous but asynchronous from those of the ventilator. The best initial response is to:
    A. obtain a chest radiograph.
    B. suction the endotracheal tube.
    C. administer pancuronium (Pavulon).
    D. change the mode of ventilation from synchronized intermittent mandatory ventilation to assist-control ventilation.

51. Surfactant secretion would most likely be stimulated by which of the following?
    A. Hypoventilation
    B. Lung hypoinflation
    C. Adenosine triphosphate
    D. β-Adrenergic receptor blocker

52. Which factor will cause a shift to the left in the oxygen-hemoglobin dissociation curve?
    A. Increase in pH
    B. Increase in $Paco_2$
    C. Increase in temperature
    D. Increase in diphosphoglycerate level

53. A full-term infant has apnea at 10 hours of life. The most likely cause is:
    A. sepsis.
    B. placement on the back to sleep.
    C. hyperglycemia.
    D. apnea of prematurity.

54. Which of the following is a pathologic condition characterized by right ventricular hypertrophy and right axis deviation on EKG, respiratory wheezing, hepatomegaly, and radiographic findings of cystic lesions with lung hyperinflation?

A. Bronchopulmonary dysplasia
B. Respiratory distress syndrome
C. Meconium aspiration syndrome
D. Pulmonary interstitial emphysema

55. An infant is admitted to the NICU from the delivery room exhibiting tachypnea, nasal flaring, cyanosis, and increased anteroposterior diameter of the chest. The amniotic fluid was characterized as thick "pea-stained" fluid. An initial arterial blood gas analysis determines that endotracheal intubation is warranted. Which of the following is most appropriate as an initial setting for this infant when synchronized intermittent mandatory ventilation is started?
A. Low rate
B. Low inspiratory time
C. Low peak inspiratory pressure
D. High positive end-expiratory pressure

56. Early signs of respiratory distress within the first 24 hours of life in a full-term neonate include:
A. hypotension.
B. acrocyanosis.
C. periodic breathing.
D. grunting, flaring, and retractions.

57. Hyponatremia associated with respiratory distress syndrome in a preterm infant with no documented weight loss within the first few days of life is indicative of:
A. total body sodium depletion.
B. excessive evaporative loss.
C. excessive total body water.
D. high-volume urinary output.

58. Which of the following nursing activities will optimize patient outcomes in the intubated extremely preterm infant with respiratory distress syndrome?
A. Multiple laboratory specimen draws via heel stick
B. Infusion of intravenous fluids at 150 ml/kg/day
C. Frequent and scheduled endotracheal suctioning
D. Placement of a transparent plastic covering over an infant who is on an open warmer bed

59. Which of the following statements is true regarding inhaled nitrogen oxide (iNO)?
A. iNO is inactivated after it combines with hemoglobin.
B. iNO is an effective pulmonary vasodilator with a half-life of 3 to 5 minutes.
C. iNO is initiated and maintained at 20 ppm until pulmonary vascular relaxation has occurred.
D. Once pulmonary vascular relaxation has been accomplished, it is safe to halt administration of iNO because the half-life is so short.

60. The administration of surfactant at the time of delivery is termed:
A. rescue therapy.
B. assisted ventilation.
C. prophylactic therapy.
D. chemical resuscitation.

61. The care provider has ordered indomethacin (Indocin) for an infant diagnosed with a patent ductus arteriosus. Which of the following would indicate to the nurse that it is safe to administer the medication?
A. Serum creatinine level of 2.0 mg/dl
B. Urine output of 0.5 ml/kg/hour
C. Platelet count of 110,000/mm$^3$
D. Radiographic evidence of necrotizing enterocolitis

62. The most common cause of stridor in the infant is:
A. choanal atresia.
B. laryngomalacia.
C. vocal cord paralysis.
D. congenital subglottic stenosis.

63. A 38-week gestation infant had apnea, hypotonia, cyanosis, and a heart rate of less than 100 beats/minute at delivery. When tactile stimulation and blow-by oxygen fail to induce spontaneous respiration, the nurse initiates positive pressure bag-and-mask ventilation, suspecting that the infant has which of the following conditions?
A. Idiopathic apnea
B. Obstructive apnea
C. Primary apnea associated with asphyxia
D. Secondary apnea associated with asphyxia

64. When an apnea monitor sounds an alarm 20 seconds after the cessation of breathing, the most appropriate immediate response is to:
A. assess breath sounds.
B. provide blow-by oxygen.
C. administer positive pressure ventilation with bag and mask.
D. provide gentle tactile stimulation of the chest and/or extremities.

65. Which of the following medications is used to treat apnea that is refractory to methylxanthine therapy?
A. Caffeine (Cafcit)
B. Doxapram (Dopram)
C. Theophylline (Theo-Dur, Slo-Bid)
D. Aminophylline (Phyllocontin, Truphylline)

66. A nursing intervention that helps alleviate apnea in preterm infants is:
A. performing endotracheal suction.
B. weighing on a cold scale.
C. controlling environmental temperature.
D. tapping on the outside of the isolette.

67. Which of the following is an advantage of caffeine (Cafcit) over theophylline (Theo-Dur, Slo-Bid) in the management of apnea of prematurity?
    A. Caffeine can be given only by mouth.
    B. Caffeine requires twice-a-day dosing.
    C. Caffeine is excreted more rapidly by the kidneys.
    D. Caffeine has a longer half-life, which result in smaller changes in its plasma concentration.

68. Continuous positive airway pressure ventilation would be indicated in an infant with which of following diagnoses?
    A. Cleft palate
    B. Choanal atresia
    C. Laryngomalacia
    D. Tracheoesophageal fistula

69. When the nurse is planning the care of the infant receiving continuous positive airway pressure ventilation at 8 cm $H_2O$, which of the following interventions should receive the *least* consideration?
    A. Monitoring $Paco_2$
    B. Monitoring and documenting urine output
    C. Monitoring vital signs and oxygen saturation via pulse oximetry
    D. Maintaining the nasogastric tube to gravity drainage

70. Inclusion criteria for the use of extracorporeal membrane oxygenation for the treatment of cardiorespiratory failure include:
    A. severe lung hypoplasia.
    B. gestational age of 32 weeks.
    C. bilateral grade IV intracranial hemorrhage.
    D. left congenital diaphragmatic hernia without liver herniation in a full-term infant.

71. Extrapulmonary causes of lower airway obstruction in the newborn include which of the following?
    A. Vascular ring
    B. Choanal atresia
    C. Bronchomalacia
    D. Pierre Robin sequence

72. Which of the following statements regarding extracorporeal membrane oxygenation (ECMO) is true?
    A. An oxygenation index of 40 for 4 hours is an inclusion criterion.
    B. A $Pao_2$ of 100 that is responsive to inhaled nitric oxide (iNO) is an inclusion criterion.
    C. A pH of 7.35 that is responsive to pharmacologic and ventilator management is an inclusion criterion.
    D. ECMO is rapidly replacing iNO for the therapeutic management of persistent pulmonary hypertension of the newborn.

73. Factors that predispose an infant to bronchopulmonary dysplasia include which of the following?
    A. Full-term birth
    B. Fluid restriction
    C. Mechanical ventilation
    D. Inspired oxygen concentration of 0.21

74. Factors that predispose infants with bronchopulmonary dysplasia to pulmonary edema include which of the following?
    A. Impaired lymphatic drainage
    B. Decreased capillary permeability
    C. Increased plasma oncotic pressure
    D. Decreased pulmonary vascular resistance

75. Diuretic therapy with furosemide (Lasix) has been shown to improve lung compliance in infants with bronchopulmonary dysplasia. Complications associated with its use include:
    A. ototoxicity.
    B. hyperkalemia.
    C. hyperchloremia.
    D. metabolic acidosis.

76. What are the caloric requirements for an infant with severe bronchopulmonary dysplasia?
    A. 80 to 100 kcal/kg/day
    B. 100 to 120 kcal/kg/day
    C. 120 to 140 kcal/kg/day
    D. 150 to 180 kcal/kg/day

77. Dexamethasone administration for the treatment of bronchopulmonary dysplasia has been associated with an increased incidence of which of the following?
    A. Pulmonary air leak
    B. Necrotizing enterocolitis
    C. Neurodevelopmental dysfunction
    D. Severe retinopathy of prematurity

78. An infant born at an estimated 25 weeks' gestation who is now 56 weeks corrected postconceptual age remains mechanically ventilated in synchronous intermittent mechanically ventilation mode. The chest radiograph is consistent with severe bronchopulmonary dysplasia. The ventilator settings most appropriate for this infant would include a(n):
    A. inspiratory time of 0.3 seconds.
    B. respiratory rate of 50 breaths/minute.
    C. inspired oxygen fraction ($Fio_2$) of 0.21 with a corresponding $Pao_2$ of 30.
    D. peak end-expiratory pressure of 4 cm $H_2O$.

79. An arterial blood gas analysis was obtained with the following results: pH 7.32, $Paco_2$ 67, $Pao_2$ 46, and base excess +2. What is the best interpretation of these results?
    A. Respiratory acidosis
    B. Hypoxemia and respiratory alkalosis

C. Partially compensated metabolic acidosis

D. Partially compensated respiratory acidosis and hypoxemia

80. Dexamethasone has been ordered by the nurse practitioner for an infant. The bedside nurse would expect which of the following for this infant?
    A. Urine output of 5 ml/kg/hour
    B. Increased ventilator support
    C. Mean arterial blood pressure of 40 mm Hg
    D. Biventricular atrophy on echocardiography

81. On physical examination of an infant, inspiratory and expiratory wheezing, intercostal retractions, and an oxygen saturation of 68% are noted. These signs would alert the nurse to the possibility of bronchospasm. The most appropriate intervention would be administration of which of the following medications?
    A. Caffeine (Cafcit)
    B. Furosemide (Lasix)
    C. Albuterol (Ventolin, Proventil)
    D. Theophylline (Theo-Dur, Slo-Bid)

82. An intubated infant's pulse oximeter sounds an alarm because oxygen saturation is 75%. The nurse suctions the infant's airway and pink-tinged secretions are obtained. The most appropriate action would be to:
    A. perform aggressive endotracheal suctioning.
    B. transfuse platelets to reach a platelet count of 200,000/mm$^3$.
    C. transfuse red blood cells to reach a hemoglobin level of 15 mg/dl.
    D. increase the peak end-expiratory pressure from 4 to 6 cm $H_2O$.

83. Extracorporeal membrane oxygenation is indicated for which of the following conditions?
    A. Bilateral pulmonary hypoplasia
    B. Bronchopulmonary dysplasia
    C. Transient tachypnea of the newborn
    D. Persistent pulmonary hypertension of the newborn

84. The most common cystic malformation of the lung resulting in obstructive air trapping is:
    A. bronchopulmonary dysplasia.
    B. congenital lobar emphysema.
    C. congenital diaphragmatic hernia.
    D. cystic adenomatoid malformation.

85. An infant has a prenatal history of polyhydramnios. On physical examination, the infant appears normal. At first feeding, he becomes dusky with respiratory distress, and suctioning of the nasopharynx/oropharynx is required. Further attempts to nipple-feed are met with the same results. The nurse expects the cause of this infant's respiratory distress to be:
    A. choanal atresia.
    B. pulmonary hypoplasia.
    C. congenital heart disease.
    D. esophageal atresia with tracheoesophageal fistula.

86. Which of the following statements about the oxygen-hemoglobin dissociation curve is accurate?
    A. The absence of cyanosis indicates a well-oxygenated infant.
    B. A right-shifted curve indicates increased affinity of hemoglobin for oxygen.
    C. The hemoglobin-oxygen dissociation curve reflects the affinity of hemoglobin for oxygen.
    D. Hemoglobin's affinity for oxygen is primarily influenced by serum glucose and electrolyte values.

87. Which of the following can cause a pulse oximeter to display inaccurate oxygen saturation values?
    A. Prematurity
    B. Use of vasodilating drugs
    C. Cyanotic heart disease
    D. Decreased peripheral perfusion

88. A newborn infant requires supplemental oxygen, and oxygen administration is initiated via oxygen hood. An appropriate nursing intervention would be to:
    A. switch the infant to a nasal cannula.
    B. do nothing, because no intervention is required.
    C. ensure sufficient gas flow to prevent carbon dioxide retention.
    D. obtain an order and change the patient to nasal continuous positive airway pressure ventilation.

89. Heliox, a mixture of helium and oxygen at a 4:1 ratio, has been demonstrated to have beneficial ventilatory effects in infants with:
    A. pneumothorax.
    B. intracranial hemorrhage.
    C. necrotizing enterocolitis.
    D. obstructive pulmonary disease.

90. Infants with micrognathia and glossoptosis require careful monitoring by the nurse for which of the following complications?
    A. Cor pulmonale
    B. Obstructive apnea
    C. Subglottic stenosis
    D. Reactive airway disease

# Chapter 16

# Gastrointestinal Disorders

1. The nurse is caring for an infant in whom esophageal atresia and tracheoesophageal fistula has been newly diagnosed. A priority in the care of this infant is:
   A. initiating enteral feeds.
   B. administering antibiotics.
   C. placing the infant on continuous positive airway pressure ventilation.
   D. gently passing a sump tube into the proximal esophageal pouch and connecting it to low continuous suction.

2. Infants with esophageal atresia and tracheoesophageal fistula have a high incidence of associated anomalies. What anomalies are commonly seen in these infants?
   A. Omphalocele, cardiomegaly, and macroglossia
   B. Vertebral anomalies, cardiac defects, and anal atresia
   C. Short stature, micrognathia, hearing loss, and low-set ears
   D. Cardiac defects, hypoplasia of the thymus, hypocalcemia, and microcephaly

3. The mother of an infant with esophageal atresia and a distal tracheoesophageal fistula (EA/TEF) is concerned about postoperative complications after a primary repair of the EA/TEF. Complications after primary repair surgery include:
   A. short bowel syndrome, intestinal dysfunction, and ileus.
   B. leakage or stricture at the anastomosis site, tracheomalacia, and pneumonia.
   C. leakage or stricture at the anastomosis site, renal dysfunction, and urosepsis.
   D. problems associated with increased intraabdominal pressure, including escalation of respiratory support requirements, hemodynamic compromise, and inferior vena cava compression.

**Questions 4 through 7 refer to the following scenario:**
A 39-week gestational age male infant born to a 35-year-old G2P2 mother via repeat cesarean section is now 2 days old. The infant was rooming with the mother until this afternoon, when the infant began bilious vomiting. The infant was then transferred to the NICU for evaluation of possible bowel obstruction. The infant is alert and in hemodynamically stable condition. Abdominal examination shows distention and tenderness. An abdominal radiograph reveals dilated loops of bowel. Specimens have been sent for blood cultures and a complete blood count, and antibiotic therapy has been started.

4. The immediate plan of care for this infant should include which of the following?
   A. Prepare the infant for an upper gastrointestinal tract contrast study.
   B. Obtain an abdominal radiograph and abdominal girth measurement.
   C. Initiate nothing-by-mouth status, insert a urinary catheter, and prepare to administer a glycerin suppository.
   D. Initiate nothing-by-mouth status, begin intravenous fluid therapy, and insert a Salem sump for gastric decompression.

5. An upper gastrointestinal tract contrast study confirms the diagnosis of malrotation and volvulus. The nurse understands that this is a surgical emergency due to the high risk for which of the following?
   A. Pneumonia
   B. Fluid and electrolyte imbalance
   C. Intestinal ischemic injury and infarction
   D. Disseminated intravascular coagulation

6. While being prepared for surgery, the infant becomes lethargic, hypotensive, and tachycardic. He is pale, and his perfusion is diminished. He has been intubated because of respiratory distress. The nurse should anticipate which of the following immediate interventions for this infant?
   A. Fluid resuscitation
   B. Blood transfusion
   C. Initiation of a dopamine infusion
   D. Delay of surgery until the infant's condition is stabilized

7. The infant undergoes a Ladd procedure, and it is now postoperative day 1. The infant is receiving a fentanyl infusion at 0.5 mcg/kg/hour and acetaminophen as needed, which he received 2 hours ago. The nurse notices that the infant is tachycardic and is grimacing. She assesses his pain as 6 out of 10 using the CRIES pain scale. The best intervention would be to:
   A. administer a midazolam bolus and evaluate its effectiveness within an hour.

B. administer a fentanyl bolus and evaluate its effectiveness within 15 minutes.

C. administer another dose of acetaminophen and evaluate its effectiveness within an hour.

D. increase the fentanyl infusion to 2 mcg/kg/hour and evaluate its effectiveness within 2 hours.

8. The father of a baby boy with an imperforate anus is worried about his son's bowel continence later in life. The nurse's explanation to the father is based on which of the following facts?
   A. It is impossible to predict bowel continence at such an early age.
   B. Females have a higher rate of associated bowel incontinence than males.
   C. If there is no associated urogenital fistula, bowel continence should be normal.
   D. There is a lower incidence of bowel incontinence with low defects than with high defects.

9. Hirschsprung disease should be suspected in any infant with which of the following?
   A. Acholic stools
   B. Projectile vomiting
   C. Oliguria in the first 24 hours after birth
   D. Failure to pass meconium spontaneously in the first 48 hours after birth

10. The nurse is caring for an infant in whom gastroesophageal reflux disease has been diagnosed. The nurse understands that the best conservative management for reflux is:
    A. postpyloric feeding via a nasojejunal tube.
    B. initiation of treatment with a prokinetic medication such as metoclopramide.
    C. initiation of treatment with a histamine-2 receptor antagonist such as ranitidine (Zantac).
    D. positioning the infant upright for 30 minutes after a meal with the head of the bed inclined to 30 degrees.

11. When providing medication teaching to the parents of an infant with severe gastrointestinal reflux, the nurse should be aware of which of the following about pantoprazole (Protonix)?
    A. Pantoprazole is a histamine-2 receptor antagonist.
    B. Pantoprazole should be administered 30 minutes after a meal.
    C. Pantoprazole use increases the risk of gastroenteritis and pneumonia.
    D. Pantoprazole is associated with an increased incidence of esophagitis.

12. An infant with symptoms of bowel obstruction has an abdominal radiograph which shows a "double bubble" pattern. What is the bowel obstruction that typically displays this radiographic pattern?

A. Duodenal atresia
B. Congenital diaphragmatic hernia
C. Malrotation with midgut volvulus
D. Esophageal atresia with tracheoesophageal fistula

13. An NICU orientee inquires about the differences between an omphalocele and a gastroschisis. As part of the response, the preceptor explains that:
    A. a prolonged ileus is a common complication of a gastroschisis.
    B. a gastroschisis is characterized by a higher incidence of associated anomalies.
    C. anticipated fluid losses are greater with an omphalocele than with a gastroschisis.
    D. an omphalocele is an abdominal wall defect that is usually to the right of the umbilicus with no sac covering the bowel.

**Questions 14 through 18 refer to the following scenario:** A 38-week gestational age female in whom a large gastroschisis was diagnosed prenatally has just been admitted to the NICU. She was delivered via planned cesarean section to a 28-year-old G1P1 mother after an uncomplicated pregnancy. Apgar scores were 6 and 7 at 5 and 10 minutes, respectively.

14. Which of the following should be given priority in the preoperative assessment?
    A. Examination for signs of sepsis
    B. Assessment of neurologic status and monitoring for seizure activity
    C. Assessment of temperature, blood pressure, fluid balance, and acid-base status
    D. Respiratory examination and assessment of need for exogenous surfactant therapy

15. The father of this infant asks the nurse why the lower two thirds of the infant's body were placed in a plastic bag in the delivery room. The nurse explains to the father that this was done to:
    A. decrease fluid and heat loss.
    B. protect the bowel from injury.
    C. decrease the risk of infection.
    D. cover the bowel to maintain the infant's privacy.

16. A staged reduction is planned given the size of the gastroschisis. The benefit of a staged reduction is that it:
    A. causes less surgical pain than a primary repair.
    B. carries less risk of infection than a primary repair.
    C. decreases stress on the respiratory and cardiovascular systems.
    D. improves bowel function, which allows for earlier initiation of feedings.

17. During the staged reduction, the infant is intubated and receives a moderate amount of ventilator support. A few hours after the final reduction and closure of the abdominal wall, the nurse notices a change in the infant's physical examination findings. The infant is hypotensive, capillary refill time is 4 to 5 seconds, the lower extremities are cool, and urine output has decreased. The nurse understands the likely cause of this change to be:
    A. sepsis.
    B. postoperative pain.
    C. intracranial hemorrhage.
    D. increased intraabdominal pressure.

18. The infant is given a fluid bolus of normal saline 20 mL/kg with a little improvement in the physical examination findings. An hour later the infant is hypotensive and anuric, and has the following arterial blood gas values: pH 7.15, $Pco_2$ 35, $Po_2$ 68, $HCO_3$ 16. The nurse pages the surgeon. Based on the nurse's understanding of postoperative care of the neonate with gastroschisis, the nurse should anticipate which of the following?
    A. Initiation of an epinephrine infusion
    B. Administration of a furosemide (Lasix) bolus
    C. Administration of a sodium bicarbonate bolus
    D. Surgical decompression to relieve intraabdominal pressure

19. Infants with duodenal atresia should be assessed for which associated condition?
    A. Trisomy 21
    B. Trisomy 18
    C. Turner syndrome
    D. Beckwith-Wiedemann syndrome

20. The nurse is called to the delivery of a 39-week gestational age male infant with a prenatal diagnosis of a left-sided congenital diaphragmatic hernia (CDH). A plan is made by the NICU team that calls for tracheal intubation to be performed by a skilled resuscitation team member immediately after delivery. The rationale for this plan is that:
    A. infants with CDH must immediately undergo surgical repair, which requires intubation.
    B. airway anomalies are often associated with CDH, so establishing a safe airway is the first priority.
    C. infants with CDH always have surfactant deficiency, and intubation is required to administer surfactant.
    D. positive pressure ventilation via face mask would cause distention of the bowel in the chest cavity and should be avoided.

21. Planning of the initial postnatal care of a neonate with congenital diaphragmatic hernia (CDH) should include assessment for which of the following conditions?

A. Bowel ischemia
B. Hepatic dysfunction
C. Pulmonary hypertension
D. Necrotizing enterocolitis

22. The single greatest risk factor for necrotizing enterocolitis is:
    A. infection.
    B. prematurity.
    C. enteral feedings.
    D. maternal substance abuse.

23. A 28-week gestational age female infant is now 8 days old. She is receiving continuous positive airway pressure ventilation and has occasional apnea and bradycardia episodes that are well controlled by caffeine therapy. She has been advancing on enteral feedings of breast milk. The nurse's morning assessment reveals abdominal distention, hypoactive bowel sounds, and increased residual aspirates. The infant's abdominal girth has increased 1 cm over the past 3 hours, and the nurse notices frank blood in her stool. An abdominal radiograph confirms the diagnosis of necrotizing enterocolitis. Which of the following is an indication for surgical intervention in this infant?
    A. Positive results on a blood culture
    B. Abdominal distention and lethargy
    C. The need for reintubation and mechanical ventilation
    D. Pneumoperitoneum seen on abdominal radiograph

24. An infant with necrotizing enterocolitis and intestinal perforation underwent bowel resection and an ileostomy was created. The infant had an extensive amount of bowel resected, including the ileum. As a result, the infant developed short bowel syndrome. A long-term nutritional concern for this infant is:
    A. constipation.
    B. malabsorption.
    C. deficiency of water-soluble vitamins.
    D. recurrence of necrotizing enterocolitis.

25. At the initial family meeting for an infant in whom a meconium ileus has been newly diagnosed, the physician recommends a genetic consultation for the infant. Based on the nurse's knowledge of meconium ileus, the nurse understands that a genetics consultation is needed because of the high association of meconium ileus with which of the following?
    A. Trisomy 18
    B. Cystic fibrosis
    C. DiGeorge syndrome
    D. Hirschsprung disease

# Chapter 17
# Metabolic and Endocrine Disorders

1. Which of the following infants is at lowest risk for hypoglycemia?
   A. A 32-week, small-for-gestational-age infant
   B. A 34-week, breast-feeding infant
   C. A 36-week, infant of a diabetic mother
   D. A 41-week, infant with clubfoot deformity

2. The nurse is about to administer a glucose bolus to a neonate with transient postnatal hypoglycemia. How can rebound hypoglycemia be prevented?
   A. By starting the baby on an insulin drip
   B. By repeating the bolus every 30 minutes
   C. By following the bolus with a continuous intravenous infusion or feedings
   D. By giving a bolus of glucagon simultaneously with the bolus of dextrose

3. What is the presumed cause of macrosomia in the infant of a diabetic mother?
   A. Fetal pancreatic beta cell hypoplasia
   B. Inherited predisposition for a larger body habitus
   C. Maternal insulin resistance, hyperglycemia, and hyperaminoacidemia
   D. Tendency for prolonged pregnancy and post-term delivery, resulting in more weight gain

4. A 36-week gestational age infant of a diabetic mother has a point-of-care blood glucose level of 23 mg/dl at 6 hours of age. The infant has breast-fed twice since birth. What is the best course of action under these circumstances?
   A. Draw a specimen for measurement of plasma glucose level and initiate treatment while awaiting the results.
   B. Send a blood sample to the laboratory for measurement of plasma glucose level and await the results.
   C. Have the mother breast-feed again and check the blood glucose level before the next feeding.
   D. Observe the baby for symptoms of hypoglycemia and feed or initiate intravenous therapy if symptoms occur.

5. An infant born at 24 weeks' gestation, now close to discharge, has an elevated alkaline phosphatase level. What nursing care measure is particularly important and should be taught to the infant's caregivers as well?

   A. Avoid kangaroo care.
   B. Handle the infant as carefully as possible.
   C. Switch the infant to a soy-based formula.
   D. Limit the infant's mobility as much as possible.

6. An infant with a low thyroxine level and an elevated thyroid-stimulating hormone level is presumed to have which condition until proven otherwise?
   A. Euthyroid sick syndrome
   B. Neonatal Graves disease
   C. Congenital hypothyroidism
   D. Thyroid-binding globulin deficiency

7. What is the most prevalent thyroid disorder in preterm and low birth weight infants?
   A. Thyroid dysgenesis
   B. Neonatal thyrotoxicosis
   C. Transient hypothyroxinemia
   D. Thyroid peroxidase deficiency

8. A 600-g neonate has a blood glucose level of 195 mg/dl. What physiologic consequence should the nurse be concerned about?
   A. Weight gain
   B. Ketonuria
   C. Hyperinsulinism
   D. Osmotic diuresis

9. Which of the following is associated with neonatal hypocalcemia?
   A. Perinatal asphyxia
   B. Hypophosphatemia
   C. Hypervitaminosis D
   D. Subcutaneous fat necrosis

10. The signs and symptoms of an inborn error of metabolism in a newborn infant are most likely to be mistaken for what other neonatal disorder?
    A. Sepsis
    B. Congenital heart defect
    C. Necrotizing enterocolitis
    D. Respiratory distress syndrome

11. Which of the following is the most important element of management when caring for a neonate with medium-chain acyl–coenzyme A dehydrogenase deficiency, a disorder of fatty acid oxidation?
    A. Prohibit breast-feeding.
    B. Feed with a phenylalanine-free formula.

C. Feed frequently and avoid prolonged periods of fasting.

D. Withhold all protein sources (formula, milk, and amino acid solutions).

12. A term infant is born with a large goiter. What nursing intervention is indicated?
    A. Have a defibrillator on standby for cardioversions.
    B. Delay sending the neonatal screen until the goiter has resolved.
    C. Position the infant with the head elevated and with slight extension.
    D. Allow nothing by mouth until after surgical correction of the goiter.

13. A 35-week gestational age infant is born to a mother who had been taking magnesium sulfate for pregnancy-induced hypertension. What should the nurse watch for?
    A. Lethargy and apnea
    B. Hypertension and fever
    C. Jitteriness and tachycardia
    D. Tachypnea and hypoglycemia

14. The XX virilization of the neonate, the most common cause of ambiguous genitalia, is a result of which of the following?

A. Pure gonadal dysgenesis
B. Partial androgen insensitivity
C. Congenital adrenal hyperplasia
D. Prenatal exposure to progestins

15. Which of the following findings on assessment of external genitalia should prompt further investigation for possible ambiguous genitalia?
    A. Hydrocele
    B. Physiologic phimosis
    C. Inguinal hernia in a female
    D. Blood-tinged vaginal mucus

16. The parents of a baby born with ambiguous genitalia are still awaiting test results to determine the sex of their infant. Which of the following interventions would be most helpful during this time?
    A. Telling them you are almost certain that the baby is a boy (or girl)
    B. Suggesting that they choose a name suitable for either a boy or a girl
    C. Arranging a meeting with a knowledgeable mental health professional
    D. Advising them to keep the baby's condition a secret from all but the immediate family

# Chapter 18

# Hematologic Disorders

1. A 32-week, small-for-gestational-age infant is born via primary cesarean section due to a nonreassuring fetal heart tracing. In addition to sending blood samples for TORCH (*t*oxoplasmosis, *o*ther infections, *r*ubella, *c*ytomegalovirus infection, and *h*erpes simplex) titers, the physician requests that immunoglobulin levels be determined. In the event of an in utero viral infection, which immunoglobulin level would be elevated in the period immediately after birth?
   A. Immunoglobulin G
   B. Immunoglobulin M
   C. Immunoglobulin A
   D. Immunoglobulin E

2. A 26-year-old primigravida was found to have pregnancy-induced hypertension at 22 weeks' gestation. After her infant was born at term, the infant was found to have a venous hematocrit of 68%.

What is the most likely reason for the polycythemia experienced by this infant?
   A. The infant has a higher level of erythropoietin in his body.
   B. The infant has been exposed to a maternal-fetal hemorrhage in utero.
   C. The infant has a higher percentage of hemoglobin F, which results in a higher hematocrit.
   D. The obstetrician stripped blood from the umbilical cord into the infant at the time of delivery.

3. Which of the following infants will show the greatest affinity for oxygen?
   A. A 28-week gestational age infant with a temperature of 36.5° C (97.8° F)
   B. A 30-week gestational age infant with a $Paco_2$ of 55
   C. A 35-week gestational age infant with a temperature of 38.0° C (100.4° F)

D. A 38-week gestational age infant with a $Paco_2$ of 40

4. Compared with adult red blood cells, newborn red blood cells:
   A. are more resilient.
   B. have a longer life span.
   C. have a decreased mean corpuscular volume.
   D. carry a larger amount of oxygen on the hemoglobin.

5. A 35-week gestational age infant was born in septic shock 36 hours ago. Cultures of blood specimens taken at birth grew out positive for *Escherichia coli*. The infant has been receiving mechanical ventilation since birth and has required dopamine (14 mcg/kg/minute) and dobutamine (5 mcg/kg/minute). A short while ago, the infant had a sudden pulmonary hemorrhage. Furthermore, he now has petechiae on his trunk. An examination of the maternal laboratory results shows that the platelet count is normal. Based on the history and clinical presentation of this infant, what disease process is occurring?
   A. Neonatal alloimmune thrombocytopenia
   B. Maternal systemic lupus erythematosus
   C. Disseminated intravascular coagulation
   D. Maternal idiopathic thrombocytopenic purpura

6. What are the expected laboratory results for a patient with disseminated intravascular coagulation?
   A. Normal platelet count, prolonged prothrombin time (PT), and prolonged partial thromboplastin time (PTT)
   B. Low platelet count, low fibrinogen level, and D-Dimer+
   C. Low platelet count, prolonged PT, and shortened PTT
   D. Normal platelet count, low fibrinogen level, and elevated level of fibrin split products

7. What blood transfusion product will most directly supply fibrinogen to an infant?
   A. Platelets
   B. Cryoprecipitate
   C. Fresh frozen plasma
   Ð. Packed red blood cells

**Questions 8 and 9 refer to the following scenario:**
A 32-week gestational age, 1700-g infant has an umbilical arterial line in place. Fifteen minutes after a radiograph of the infant is taken, the nurse notices a large pool of blood on the bed next to the infant. The estimated blood loss is 45 ml.

8. Which set of signs and symptoms is most likely to reflect the infant's condition in the first 30 to 60 minutes following this acute loss of blood?

|    | Hematocrit | Blood Pressure | Heart Rate | Multisystem |
|----|------------|----------------|------------|-------------|
| A. | Decreased | Hypotension | Tachycardia | Tachypnea, pallor |
| B. | Unchanged | Hypotension | Tachycardia | Pallor, capillary refill of 3 seconds, respiratory distress |
| C. | Unchanged | Hypotension | Bradycardia | Apnea, cyanosis |
| D. | Decreased | Unchanged | Unchanged | Hepatosplenomegaly |

9. What is the preferred first intervention for this baby?
   A. Placing the infant in the Trendelenburg position
   B. Administering a rapid infusion of isotonic saline
   C. Increasing the percentage of inspired oxygen to 100%
   D. Administering a transfusion of group O, Rh-negative whole blood

10. A 95-day-old infant (current weight, 2.2 kg; post-conceptual age, 36 weeks) is being cared for in the NICU. He has bronchopulmonary dysplasia and is receiving oxygen at 0.2 L/minute and 100% fraction of inspired oxygen ($Fio_2$) via nasal cannula. He is pale and lethargic and has had eight apneic episodes in the past 24 hours. His heart rate is 176 beats/minute. Complete blood cell count results include the following:
    White blood cell count: 15,000/mm³
    Hemoglobin: 7.5 g/dl
    Hematocrit: 23%
    Reticulocyte count: 1.8%
    Platelet count: 265,000/mm³
    Based on the clinical picture and laboratory results, what would the appropriate action be?
    A. Continue current care.
    B. Begin a course of supplemental iron with feeds.
    C. Transfuse the infant with 10 ml/kg packed red blood cells.
    D. Begin a course of recombinant human erythropoietin (Epogen).

11. A 4-day old, 28-week-gestation infant weighing 960 grams is on continuous positive airway pressure (CPAP) at +5 at a $Fio_2$ of 32%. He is given a transfusion of 10 cc packed red blood cells (PRBC) over 3 hours due to a hematocrit of 35. What signs would most likely indicate that the infant is having a transfusion reaction?
    A. Fever, tachycardia, and apnea
    B. Hypertension, erythema, and retractions
    C. Angioedema, bradycardia, and restlessness
    D. Diaphoresis, increasing jaundice, and tachypnea

**Questions 12 and 13 refer to the following scenario:**
A 36-week gestational age infant has been diagnosed with thrombocytopenia related to maternal idiopathic thrombocytopenic purpura. The infant's platelet count has been consistently below $25,000/mm^3$ for the last 4 days. The baby has received a platelet transfusion daily without significant results. The neonatologist orders intravenous immune globulin (IVIG) 0.5 mg/kg over 2 hours.

12. What is the mechanism of action of IVIG in this instance?
    A. It modulates complement activation.
    B. It decreases autoimmune hemolysis of the erythrocytes.
    C. It blocks the antibodies that destroy sensitized platelets.
    D. It increases mobilization of platelets from the platelet pool.

13. What physiologic signs would demonstrate an adverse immune reaction to the IVIG?
    A. Emesis, bradycardia, and pallor
    B. Tachycardia, wheezing, and skin flushing
    C. Hypertension, tachycardia, and skin flushing
    D. Hypotension, decreased urinary output, and mottling

14. A 38-week gestational age, 3100-g infant is admitted to the NICU. She is very pale, has a capillary refill of 4 seconds, and has a blood pressure of 43/26 mm Hg. She has a hemoglobin level of 4 g/dl. A positive result on which blood test would most likely indicate a prenatal hemorrhage?
    A. Apt test
    B. Direct Coombs test
    C. Indirect Coombs test
    D. Kleihauer-Betke test

15. According to the American Academy of Pediatrics, which infant is in the high-risk category for potential negative effects related to hyperbilirubinemia?
    A. A 36-week-gestation infant with temperature instability
    B. A 38-week-gestation infant with sepsis
    C. A 39-week-gestation infant with visible jaundice in the first 24 hours after birth
    D. A 40-week-gestation infant with ABO incompatibility and positive direct Coombs test result

16. A 5-day-old breast-feeding infant has been readmitted to the NICU for intensive phototherapy due to a total serum bilirubin level of 23 mg/dl. The infant is placed under fluorescent bulbs at room temperature. What potential side effect of phototherapy does the nurse need to be most concerned about at this point?

A. Dehydration
B. Loose stools
C. Hyperthermia
D. Bronze baby syndrome

17. A nurse is caring for a 30-week-old septic infant with an indirect bilirubin level of 23.8 mg/dl. The infant is intubated and receiving synchronized intermittent mechanical ventilation. Over the last 6 hours, the infant's pH has varied between 7.20 and 7.25 with a base deficit of –8. Which is the first priority before starting a double-volume exchange transfusion?
    A. Give a bolus of albumin.
    B. Correct the metabolic acidosis.
    C. Ensure that the infant is restrained.
    D. Ensure that emergency equipment is available at the bedside.

18. A 38-week-old small-for-gestational-age newborn has a venous hematocrit of 62%. The infant has shown some jitteriness and is not nipple-feeding well. The infant is not experiencing any respiratory difficulties, and the blood glucose level is 54 mg/dl. Urinary output is 2.1 ml/kg/hour. Anticipatory management at this time would include which of the following interventions?
    A. Continuing current care
    B. Performing a partial exchange transfusion with normal saline or 5% albumin
    C. Putting the infant on nothing-by-mouth status and beginning maintenance intravenous fluids at 80 ml/kg/day
    D. Closely monitoring the infant's respiratory status, glucose levels, and hydration while encouraging feeds

19. A 35-week gestational age breast-feeding infant is being discharged home from the hospital. Which of the following should the nurse tell the mother is an indication for contacting the pediatrician as soon as possible?
    A. The baby has four to six thoroughly wet diapers in 24 hours.
    B. The baby is still having meconium stools on day 3 of life.
    C. The baby is irritable and cries for a few hours each afternoon.
    D. The baby is sleepy and does not want to eat for more than 5 hours.

20. A 26-year-old G5P1 woman comes to the clinic with polyhydramnios at 32 weeks' gestation. Fetal ultrasonography shows cardiomegaly, hepatosplenomegaly, and ascites. Further questioning of the mother reveals that her firstborn was jaundiced at birth. She has not had prenatal care with any of her pregnancies. All of her other infants were stillborn

at 24 to 36 weeks' gestation. Blood tests show that she has O-negative blood type. What would be the most appropriate intervention at this time?
A. Delivery of the baby
B. Fetal thoracentesis
C. Intrauterine transfusion to minimize fetal anemia
D. Amniocentesis to assess the fetus's bilirubin level and reduce uterine volume to prevent premature delivery

<br>

## Chapter 19

# Neurologic Disorders

1. An appropriate size for gestational age term infant of a gravida 1 mother experienced a difficult delivery that required vacuum extraction. The nurse notes an expanding mobile scalp mass that crosses suture lines and extends into the neck, so the nurse will closely monitor the infant for:
A. shock.
B. seizures.
C. hydrocephalus.
D. craniosynostosis.

2. A term infant who is undergoing a workup for an inborn error of metabolism displays lip smacking and pedaling movements. The nurse suspects:
A. myoclonus.
B. hypercalcemia.
C. seizure activity.
D. readiness to feed.

3. Which of the following is the most common cause of neonatal seizures?
A. Hypercalcemia
B. Bacterial meningitis
C. Subarachnoid hemorrhage
D. Hypoxic-ischemic encephalopathy

4. A subgaleal shunt performs which function?
A. Connects the pulmonary artery to the subclavian artery
B. Connects the umbilical vein with the ductus venosus in utero
C. Allows cerebral spinal fluid to drain from the lateral ventricles to the third ventricle
D. Drains cerebrospinal fluid from the lateral ventricles to the loose connective tissue below the aponeurotic membrane

5. The best description of periventricular leukomalacia is a(n):
A. increased neutrophil count in the cerebrospinal fluid.
B. disease primarily affecting postterm infants.
C. insignificant finding on head ultrasonography.
D. loss of cerebral white matter secondary to ischemic injury.

6. Which is the correct statement about the difference between mild and moderate hypoxic-ischemic encephalopathy as defined in Sarnat staging?
A. The mildly affected infant has signs of autonomic depression.
B. The mildly affected infant has depressed deep tendon reflexes.
C. The more severely affected infant demonstrates hyperalertness.
D. The more severely affected infant displays hypotonia and stupor.

7. Which of the following is most specific for assessing seizures in the neonate?
A. Changes in vital signs
B. Low voltage baseline on bedside electroencephalogram
C. Abnormal movements followed by somnolence
D. Abnormal movements that cannot be stopped by gentle, passive flexion of the involved extremity

8. A term infant has just undergone surgical repair of a myelomeningocele. The most common complication for which the nurse should assess is:
A. seizure.
B. infection.
C. hydrocephalus.
D. skin breakdown.

9. When is it most beneficial to perform surveillance head ultrasonography for intraventricular/periventricular hemorrhage in the preterm infant?
A. At one week of life
B. By day 4 of life
C. Shortly after birth
D. After 30 weeks' postconceptual age

10. A 3-day-old, 25-week gestational age infant has a sudden drop in hematocrit. The nurse should first assess for:
    A. anemia of prematurity.
    B. severe intraventricular hemorrhage.
    C. bloody drainage from the nasogastric tube.
    D. blood loss from frequent laboratory blood draws.

11. The nurse is reinforcing teaching to parents about their infant's intraventricular hemorrhage (IVH). Which of the following is the most accurate statement to include in the parent teaching?
    A. Most infants with IVH have sequelae.
    B. Performance in school is usually not affected.
    C. Infants with IVH usually require ventriculo-peritoneal shunt placement.
    D. Outcomes are varied, so early interventions are important.

12. Brain growth is assessed most accurately by which of the following methods?
    A. Daily weight measurements
    B. Serial measurements of head circumference
    C. Weekly head ultrasonography
    D. Weekly Dubowitz assessments

13. The best positioning for an infant with congenital hydrocephalus is:
    A. in an infant seat or swing.
    B. supine with the head turned side to side.
    C. prone with the head elevated 45 degrees.
    D. with the head in the midline, elevated 30 degrees.

14. A primary goal in caring for the infant who has undergone surgical repair of a myelomeningocele is to:
    A. prevent hydrocephalus.
    B. promote early bottle- or breast-feeding.
    C. prevent soiling or tension at the incision site.
    D. promote regaining of lower extremity motor function.

15. The difference between grade III and grade IV intraventricular/periventricular hemorrhage is:
    A. decerebrate posturing.
    B. periventricular echogenicity.
    C. presence of ventricular dilation.
    D. bleeding into the parenchyma.

16. A late preterm infant is born via spontaneous vaginal delivery to a mother with no documented prenatal care. At 3 hours of age, the infant has fever and shows abnormal movement that raises suspicion of seizures. The nurse would expect treatment to include:
    A. acyclovir.

B. morphine.
C. immune globulin.
D. cerebral hypothermia.

17. Infants with hypoxic-ischemic encephalopathy who meet which of the following inclusion criteria may benefit from referral for hypothermia?
    A. $Po_2$ of 48, hypertonia
    B. $Pco_2$ of 55, irritability
    C. Base deficit of –9, hyperalertness
    D. Base deficit of –19, Apgar score of less than 5 at 5 minutes

18. Risk factors for intraventricular/periventricular hemorrhage in the preterm infant include:
    A. closure of a patent ductus arteriosus.
    B. central nervous system malformations.
    C. rapid volume expansion.
    D. advancing gestational age.

19. Rapid volume expansion is contraindicated in the neonate because:
    A. it may cause pulmonary edema.
    B. the kidneys rapidly excrete excess fluids.
    C. it may cause rupture of germinal matrix vessels.
    D. venous access devices in neonates are too small to accommodate rapid infusion.

20. Signs and symptoms of Erb palsy include:
    A. respiratory distress.
    B. drooping on one side of the face.
    C. holding of the affected hand next to the thorax in a claw position.
    D. decreased movement of the affected shoulder and upper arm.

21. Initial management of Erb palsy includes:
    A. performing surgical repair.
    B. administering a short course of antiviral medication.
    C. initiating physical therapy as soon as possible.
    D. limiting movement of the involved extremity until swelling and inflammation subside.

22. Eliciting gag, cough, and suck reflexes is an indirect assessment of the function of the:
    A. cranial nerves.
    B. cerebral cortex.
    C. peripheral nerves.
    D. autonomic nervous system.

23. Early-onset bacterial meningitis is characterized by:
    A. blueberry muffin rash.
    B. progression to shock in 24 hours.
    C. concomitant pulmonary hypertension.
    D. subtle, nonspecific signs and symptoms.

24. After phenobarbital, which class of medications is most often used to treat refractory seizures in the neonate?
    A. B vitamins
    B. Local anesthetics
    C. Benzodiazepines
    D. Neuromuscular blockers

25. To prevent secondary brain damage, hypothermia therapy for hypoxic-ischemic encephalopathy should be instituted:
    A. when the infant is less than 6 hours old.
    B. when the infant is less than 12 hours old.
    C. upon admission to intensive care.
    D. any time in the first day of life.

26. Which is the most accurate statement about neonatal cerebral metabolism?
    A. Hypoglycemia is well tolerated by the premature infant.
    B. The neonatal brain is dependent on glucose for substrate.
    C. Blood glucose levels of less than 30 mg/dl are associated with decreased cerebral blood flow.

    D. Blood glucose levels of more than 200 mg/dl are associated with increased cerebral blood flow.

27. Anencephalic infants do not strictly meet the criteria for brain death because:
    A. cerebral blood flow is present.
    B. brainstem function is present.
    C. parents must decide when brain death occurs.
    D. only the hospital ethics committee can determine brain death.

28. When administering neuromuscular blocking drugs like vecuronium, the nurse should be aware that:
    A. analgesia should be used concurrently, because sensation remains intact.
    B. medications that cause neuromuscular blockade also provide analgesia.
    C. neostigmine should be used concurrently to minimize cardiovascular effects.
    D. medications that cause neuromuscular blockade have anticholinergic effects.

# Chapter 20

# Renal and Genitourinary Disorders

1. Parents of a newborn with hypospadias should be instructed to:
   A. avoid having the infant circumcised.
   B. measure urine output daily.
   C. anticipate surgical correction at 4 weeks of age.
   D. provide daily antibiotics for prophylaxis against urinary tract infection.

2. A voiding cystourethrogram should be obtained following antimicrobial treatment of a urinary tract infection to detect:
   A. hypospadias.
   B. vesicoureteral reflux.
   C. renal vein thrombosis.
   D. polycystic kidney disease.

3. The medication most likely to cause ischemic and nephrotoxic renal injury is:
   A. dopamine.
   B. furosemide.
   C. indomethacin.
   D. aminophylline.

4. The most appropriate method for monitoring to detect complications associated with multicystic dysplastic kidney disease is:
   A. weekly voiding cystourethrogram studies.
   B. weekly urinalysis to monitor for glucosuria.
   C. daily weight measurement to ensure nutritional adequacy.
   D. frequent blood pressure measurement to monitor for hypertension.

5. A postrenal cause of acute renal failure is suggested by:
   A. hypotension.
   B. perinatal asphyxia.
   C. posterior urethral valves.
   D. anuria following indomethacin (Indocin) administration.

6. Hydronephrosis due to obstruction of urine flow in the newborn is most likely caused by:
   A. hypospadias.
   B. patent urachus.

C. urinary tract infection.

D. ureteropelvic junction obstruction.

7. Through its effect on the kidney, furosemide (Lasix) therapy is most likely to lead to the development of which of the following?
   A. Hypokalemia
   B. Hypoglycemia
   C. Hypernatremia
   D. Hyperchloremia

8. The most important intervention in caring for the infant with hypertension is to:
   A. monitor urine output and specific gravity.
   B. restrict oral intake to limit total daily fluid intake.
   C. assess weight daily to monitor for an inappropriate increase.
   D. measure resting blood pressure with an appropriately sized blood pressure cuff.

9. The most common sign or symptom of an incarcerated inguinal hernia in a neonate is:
   A. oliguria.
   B. vomiting.
   C. apnea and bradycardia.
   D. positive findings on transillumination of the scrotum.

10. An 8-day-old term female infant with virilized genitalia has a history of poor feeding, lethargy, diarrhea, hyponatremia, and dehydration. The most likely cause is:
    A. primary hyperthyroidism.
    B. intraventricular hemorrhage.
    C. congenital adrenal hyperplasia.
    D. low breast milk supply and intake.

11. Acute renal failure is diagnosed in a 3-day-old infant with a history of perinatal asphyxia. Which of the following sets of serum indices is most likely given this diagnosis?

|   | Creatinine | Sodium | Osmolality |
|---|---|---|---|
| A. | 1.2 mg/dl | 140 mEq/L | Increased |
| B. | 0.8 mg/dl | 145 mEq/L | Decreased |
| C. | 1.8 mg/dl | 125 mEq/L | Decreased |
| D. | 1.0 mg/dl | 150 mEq/L | Increased |

12. Hypotension following administration of enalapril maleate is most likely due to:
    A. volume depletion.
    B. electrolyte imbalance.
    C. undiagnosed congenital heart disease.
    D. too rapid an administration of the medication.

13. Which of the following statements best describes the disadvantage of peritoneal dialysis compared with hemodialysis in the infant?
    A. It cannot to be performed at home.
    B. It requires the administration of heparin during treatment.
    C. It is ineffective in the presence of multicystic dysplastic kidneys.
    D. It provides slower correction of metabolic abnormalities and hypervolemia.

14. A 1-kg, 2-day-old, 28-week gestational age infant develops a nonhemolyzed serum potassium level of 8.5 mEq/L. The rationale for administering sodium bicarbonate to this infant is to:
    A. shift potassium into the cells.
    B. decrease myocardial excitability.
    C. increase the renal excretion of potassium.
    D. create a metabolic acidosis to enhance potassium excretion.

15. While performing a physical examination on a newborn, the nurse detects an abdominal mass. The most common cause of such a mass in the newborn is:
    A. ascites.
    B. ovarian tumor.
    C. undescended testis.
    D. multicystic dysplastic kidney.

## Chapter 21

# Genetics and Congenital Anomalies

1. The parents of an infant with an autosomal dominant disorder ask the nurse about their chances of having another baby with the same disorder. The nurse should explain that:
   A. all future babies born to the parents will have the disorder.
   B. no future babies born to the parents will have this disorder.
   C. there is a 50% chance with each pregnancy of having another affected offspring.
   D. if the baby is a girl, she will be a carrier; if the baby is a boy, there is a 50% chance that he will have the disorder.

2. Loss of a chromosomal segment is called:
   A. deletion.
   B. mosaicism.
   C. translocation.
   D. nondisjunction.

3. The clinical features of VATER association include:
   A. abdominal mass, imperforate anus, and myelodysplasia.
   B. anal atresia, vertebral abnormalities, and cardiac defects.
   C. anal atresia, tracheoesophageal fistula, and dysplasia of the kidneys.
   D. abdominal mass, ventricular septal defect, and a single umbilical artery.

4. An infant is born with an amputated hand caused by amniotic bands. This defect is an example of which of the following?
   A. Sequence
   B. Disruption
   C. Deformation
   D. Malformation

5. An infant has been diagnosed with a genetic disorder. The mother of the infant does not exhibit the disorder but is a carrier. The mother's brother does have the disorder. What should the mother know about this disorder?
   A. It is considered an X-linked recessive disorder.
   B. It is considered an X-linked dominant disorder.
   C. It is considered an autosomal recessive disorder.
   D. It is considered an autosomal dominant disorder.

6. Which of the following congenital anomalies is *not* associated with an abnormal number of chromosomes?
   A. Patau syndrome
   B. Down syndrome
   C. Edwards syndrome
   D. Osteogenesis imperfecta

7. Chromosomal analysis of an infant has revealed a 47,XXY karyotype. This is defined as Klinefelter syndrome. This multifactorial disease is related to which of the following?
   A. Advanced parental age, monosomy, and paternal meiosis errors
   B. Advanced maternal age, monosomy, and maternal meiosis errors
   C. Advanced maternal age, partial trisomy, and paternal meiosis errors
   D. Advanced maternal age, parental nondisruption errors, and maternal meiosis errors

8. An infant is observed to have prominent epicanthal folds, a flat face, a protruding tongue, and a herniated umbilicus. What genetic disorder does this infant likely have?
   A. Trisomy 13
   B. Trisomy 18
   C. Trisomy 21
   D. Turner syndrome

9. Which of the following should be performed to confirm a diagnosis of DiGeorge syndrome?
   A. Rectal biopsy
   B. Electrocardiography
   C. Oxygen challenge test
   D. Fluorescence in situ hybridization (FISH) chromosomal analysis

10. A sequence is defined as a(n):
    A. nonrandom occurrence of multiple anomalies.
    B. set of anomalies that arises when a primary event or anomaly gives rise to a pattern of other events or anomalies.
    C. abnormality of morphogenesis caused by intrinsic problems within developing structures.
    D. abnormality of morphogenesis caused by disruptive forces acting on the developing structure.

# Chapter 22

# Immunologic Disorders and Infections

1. Which of the following cerebrospinal fluid (CSF) values is abnormal and could indicate meningitis?
   A. CSF protein level of 50 mg/dl
   B. CSF protein level of 70 mg/dl
   C. CSF glucose level of 25 mg/dl with a serum glucose level of 100 mg/dl
   D. CSF leukocyte count of 15/mm$^3$ with 40% polymorphonuclear cells

2. The American Academy of Pediatrics recommends that a healthy-appearing neonate born at 38 weeks' gestation to a mother who received 8 hours of intrapartum antimicrobial prophylaxis for suspected chorioamnionitis should:
   A. be observed for 48 hours.
   B. undergo a full diagnostic evaluation and receive empiric therapy for a minimum of 48 hours.
   C. undergo a limited evaluation initially with further diagnostic evaluation and empiric therapy if signs of neonatal sepsis develop.
   D. be eligible for discharge home after 24 hours if other discharge criteria are met and a caregiver is able to comply with instructions for home observation.

3. Which of the following statements regarding the use of C-reactive protein (CRP) as a marker for neonatal sepsis is most accurate?
   A. CRP levels have higher sensitivity and negative predictive values if the infant's gestational age is at least 37 weeks.
   B. CRP response is better in coagulase-negative Staphylococcus (CoNS) than gram-negative infections.
   C. Serial CRP measurements may improve sensitivity and positive predictive value.
   D. Sensitivity is highest when the CRP is obtained within 6 to 8 hours of the infective process.

4. Which of the following sets of hematologic values best predicts infection in a 1-hour-old term neonate?
   A. WBCs 8.25 × 10$^3$/mm$^3$; segs 52%; bands 12%
   B. WBCs 6.1 × 10$^3$/mm$^3$; segs 32%; bands 4%
   C. WBCs 15 × 10$^3$/mm$^3$; segs 17%; bands 3%
   D. WBCs 4.7 × 10$^3$/mm$^3$; segs 27%; bands 8%

5. Which of the following clinical factors is associated with a decreased total neutrophil count?
   A. Stressful labor
   B. Neonatal seizures
   C. Maternal hypertension
   D. Uncomplicated respiratory distress syndrome

6. An otherwise healthy-appearing term newborn has pustules localized to the axillae and groin. Laboratory analysis reveals gram-positive cocci and neutrophils. The lesions most likely represent:
   A. a benign newborn rash.
   B. Staphylococcus aureus infection.
   C. Candida diaper dermatitis.
   D. Staphylococcus epidermidis infection.

7. A 37-week gestational age infant is born with hydrocephalus, generalized intracranial calcifications, and chorioretinitis. What congenital infection is associated with these clinical findings?
   A. Herpes infection
   B. Rubella
   C. Toxoplasmosis
   D. Cytomegalovirus infection

8. Which of the following antimicrobials is contraindicated for use in newborns?
   A. Ticarcillin (Ticar)
   B. Amikacin (Amikin)
   C. Ceftazidime (Fortaz)
   D. Sulfamethoxazole/trimethoprim (Bactrim)

9. Which of the following measures is the most effective in preventing nosocomial infections in preterm infants in the NICU?
   A. Hand washing
   B. Use of pooled intravenous immune globulin
   C. Antibiotic prophylaxis
   D. Routine use of gowns by nursery personnel

10. A preterm infant with a birth weight of 1800 g was delivered to a mother who was not tested during pregnancy for hepatitis B surface antigen (HBsAg). A maternal blood sample was drawn at delivery for HBsAg determination. While awaiting the results, and within 12 hours of birth, the infant should receive hepatitis B vaccine. When should the infant receive hepatitis B immune globulin?

A. At 1 month of age

B. Within 7 days of age if the mother tests positive for HBsAg

C. According to the recommendations for term infants

D. Within 12 hours of age if maternal status cannot be determined

11. Even with appropriate neonatal prophylaxis, breast-feeding poses additional risks for infants whose mothers test positive for:

A. human immunodeficiency virus (HIV).

B. hepatitis B surface antigen (HBsAg).

C. both HBsAg and HIV.

D. neither HBsAg nor HIV.

12. Which immunoglobulin (Ig) crosses the placenta in significant amounts?

A. IgA

B. IgE

C. IgG

D. IgM

13. What is the rate of transmission of syphilis to the fetus for a mother in the primary or secondary stage of disease?

A. Less than 10%

B. 10% to 25%

C. 30% to 54%

D. 60% or higher

14. The initial blood culture report on an infant with suspected sepsis reveals coagulase-positive, gram-positive cocci. The most likely organism is:

A. *Escherichia coli.*

B. *Staphylococcus aureus.*

C. *Listeria monocytogenes.*

D. *Staphylococcus epidermidis.*

15. What is the organism most commonly responsible for nosocomial bloodstream infection in NICU patients?

A. *Enterococcus*

B. Group B streptococci

C. *Staphylococcus aureus*

D. Coagulase-negative staphylococci

16. An infant receiving zidovudine (Retrovir) for prevention of maternal-fetal human immunodeficiency virus transmission should be monitored for:

A. anemia.

B. neutrophilia.

C. hypotension.

D. hypokalemia.

17. A 7-day-old infant with a postmenstrual age of 24 weeks has a history of hyperglycemia and is receiving steroids for treatment of hypotension. The nurse caring for the patient notices erosive skin lesions with serous drainage and crusting on the infant's back. Suspicion should be raised for infection with which of the following organisms?

A. Candidiasis

B. Parvovirus B19

C. *Escherichia coli*

D. *Staphylococcus epidermidis*

---

Chapter 23

# Dermatologic Disorders

1. A 750-g infant is born at 26 weeks' gestation. Which nursing intervention is most appropriate in providing skin care to this preterm infant?

A. Bathe the infant daily with soap and water.

B. Provide environmental humidity to the incubator.

C. Use a chemical solvent to remove adhesives from the skin.

D. Allow povidone-iodine or chlorhexidine solutions to remain on the skin following invasive procedures.

2. The removal of tape or electrodes can cause damage to the skin of a 24-week gestational age infant because of what characteristic of preterm skin?

A. Immature sweat glands

B. Fewer layers of stratum corneum

C. Thinner layer of subcutaneous fat

D. Diminished cohesion between the dermis and epidermis

3. A full-term infant is diagnosed with epidermolysis bullosa. When planning care for this infant, what

potential complication should the nurse anticipate?
A. Jaundice
B. Secondary infection
C. Neurologic dysfunction
D. Extremely dry and scaly skin

4. A newborn has a small strawberry hemangioma located on the scalp. What information should the nurse provide to the parents about this condition?
A. There is no treatment for this permanent condition.
B. Oral antibiotic therapy will be necessary to prevent infection.
C. The hemangioma is likely to increase in size before it regresses.

D. Genetic testing should be performed to assess for hereditary syndromes.

5. Which neonatal skin disorder is infectious, requiring isolation and antibiotic therapy?
A. Cutis aplasia
B. Erythema toxicum
C. Pustular melanosis
D. Scalded skin syndrome

6. A male infant is born with congenital ichthyosis. In discussing this condition with the parents, the nurse can best describe its cause as:
A. zinc deficiency.
B. a genetic disorder.
C. an infectious process.
D. prenatal exposure to mercury.

## Chapter 24

# Auditory and Ophthalmologic Disorders

1. A neonate with which of the following characteristics is at highest risk of developing retinopathy of prematurity?
A. 27 weeks' gestation, weighing 950 g, requiring mechanical ventilation
B. 32 weeks' gestation, mild respiratory distress syndrome, receiving oxygen by nasal cannula
C. 36 weeks' gestation, maternal diabetes, requiring phototherapy
D. 40 weeks' gestation, pneumothorax, receiving 100% oxygen by hood

2. A preterm infant receives mydriatic eye drops before an eye examination to assess for retinopathy of prematurity. The nurse should evaluate this infant for which potential complication of this procedure?
A. Lethargy
B. Bradycardia
C. Hypotension
D. Subconjunctival hemorrhage

3. The neonatal nurse is planning for the discharge of a full-term infant. What action is most appropriate when the nurse discovers that the hearing screening has not yet been completed?
A. Perform the hearing screening before the infant's discharge.
B. Perform the hearing screening only if the infant received antibiotic therapy.

C. Inform the parents that hearing screening is necessary only for preterm infants.
D. If there is a family history of hearing loss, refer the infant for outpatient testing.

4. A full-term infant received ampicillin and gentamicin for suspected sepsis. Before discharge, the infant fails hearing screening in both ears. What information should the nurse provide to the parents at this time?
A. Further evaluation of auditory function will be necessary.
B. Immediate treatment for permanent hearing loss is required.
C. Failing the hearing screening is a temporary side effect of antibiotic therapy.
D. The hearing screening will be repeated until the infant passes the test in at least one ear.

5. What is an important nursing consideration when caring for a newborn whose mother had a *Chlamydia trachomatis* infection at the time of delivery?
A. Observe the infant for eyelid edema and purulent discharge.
B. Administer silver nitrate drops to prevent chlamydial conjunctivitis.
C. Delay eye prophylaxis for 24 hours to determine if conjunctivitis develops.
D. Administer erythromycin ointment, but further assessment is unnecessary.

# MULTISYSTEM CONSIDERATIONS

## Chapter 25

# Maternal-Fetal Complications

1. A 35-year-old G1P0 woman has class A2 gestational diabetes that has been well controlled with glyburide. She develops preeclampsia and delivers at 37 weeks' gestation. In preparing to care for this infant of a diabetic mother, the nurse should anticipate which of the following in the newborn?
   A. Apnea
   B. Anemia
   C. Jaundice
   D. Hyperglycemia

2. A pregnant woman at term has a history of seizures and has been treated throughout her pregnancy with phenobarbital with good results. Neonatal care providers should anticipate which of the following infant responses at birth?
   A. Listlessness
   B. Hyperreflexia
   C. Hypoventilation
   D. Abnormal clotting and hemorrhage

3. A woman who developed severe hypothyroidism in early pregnancy that was untreated until late in the second trimester delivers a full-term infant. Which of the following neonatal outcomes should the nurse anticipate?
   A. Tachycardia
   B. Neonatal goiter
   C. Hyperthyroidism
   D. Neurodevelopmental delay

**Questions 4 and 5 refer to the following scenario:**
A pregnant woman with heart disease has been found to have a significant decrease in cardiac output during the late second trimester. Prenatal history includes the use of warfarin sodium (Coumadin) during the first 5 months of pregnancy. The woman is now at 38 weeks' gestation.

4. The nurse should anticipate that this woman's infant is at greatest risk for:
   A. congestive heart failure.
   B. intracranial hemorrhage.
   C. respiratory distress syndrome.
   D. intrauterine growth restriction.

5. A history of warfarin sodium use early in pregnancy is particularly worrisome for the development of which of the following in the infant?
   A. Hypotension
   B. Microcytic anemia
   C. Ambiguous genitalia
   D. Congenital anomalies

6. A term infant is born to a mother with a history of severe asthma that has been treated by bronchodilator use. Maternal asthma has been well controlled both antepartum and intrapartum. The neonatal nurse should anticipate an infant with:
   A. low birth weight.
   B. respiratory distress.
   C. pulmonary hypoplasia.
   D. normal respiratory function.

7. Women with phenylketonuria who are of reproductive age and have discontinued their special diet to prevent hyperphenylalaninemia are at high risk of having offspring with:
   A. renal agenesis and blindness.
   B. macrosomia and hypocalcemia.
   C. microcephaly and/or mental retardation.
   D. intrauterine growth restriction and hearing impairment.

8. A 24-year-old woman is in labor at 36 weeks' gestation. She has smoked a pack of cigarettes per day throughout her pregnancy. She gives birth to a 2200-g male infant with Apgar scores of 6 and 9 at 1 and 5 minutes respectively. The neonatal nurse should anticipate which of the following neonatal problems?
   A. Seizures
   B. Loose stools
   C. Respiratory depression
   D. Withdrawal-like symptoms

9. A 1680-g infant born at 35 weeks' gestation is admitted to the NICU following placental abruption. The infant is irritable with tachycardia and poor feeding. Substance abuse is suspected, but the mother denies drug use. The most accurate

means of determining the infant's exposure to cocaine is through screening of:

A. maternal urine or blood.

B. neonatal hair or meconium.

C. neonatal urine or meconium.

D. maternal blood or breast milk.

10. The offspring of obese women are at increased risk of:

A. prematurity.

B. macrosomia.

C. microcephaly.

D. congenital heart defects.

11. Which of the following placental abnormalities carries the greatest risk of adverse fetal outcome?

A. Placenta accreta

B. Circumvallate placenta

C. Complete placenta previa

D. Succenturiate lobe of placenta

12. An infant is born at 36 weeks' gestation after induction of labor because of severe maternal preeclampsia. Magnesium sulfate was administered during labor. Which of the following neonatal signs would the nurse expect following birth?

A. Hypotonia

B. Hypotension

C. Hypertension

D. Hyperglycemia

13. A woman is a primigravida at 29 weeks' gestation with preterm labor. The neonatal nurse knows that

a single course of corticosteroid treatment for this woman will have what potential impact on the preterm infant?

A. Reduce the risk of low birth weight

B. Increase the risk of adrenal suppression

C. Increase the risk of intraventricular hemorrhage

D. Reduce the risk of respiratory distress syndrome

14. Which of the following fetal surveillance findings would cause the most concern for fetal well-being at 36 weeks' gestation?

A. Nonreactive result on the nonstress test

B. Biophysical profile score of 7

C. Negative result on the contraction stress test

D. Reversal of diastolic flow on umbilical artery velocity testing

15. A woman at 34 weeks' gestation receives intravenous fentanyl for pain relief and gives birth a few minutes later. Maternal history is negative for substance abuse. The infant is apneic and has a heart rate of 60 upon delivery. The heart rate improves with positive pressure ventilation. Which of the following interventions would be most appropriate in responding to continued respiratory depression noted in the neonate in the delivery room?

A. Administration of naloxone

B. Administration of intravenous dextrose

C. Administration of epinephrine

D. Placement of an umbilical artery catheter

## Chapter 26

# Pain Assessment and Management

1. Which of the following statements is true regarding the feasibility and clinical utility of pain measures?

A. *Feasibility* refers to the consistency, accuracy, and precision of the measure.

B. *Feasibility* refers to the extent to which the items in a measure accurately reflect the content of the topic.

C. *Clinical utility* refers to relevance: does the measure really measure what it claims to measure?

D. *Clinical utility* refers to the extent to which the score on a measure can be used to direct pain management.

2. Which factor contributes to an inconsistent, less robust pattern of pain response in infants?

A. Opioid use

B. Neurologic integrity

C. Developmental maturity

D. Intraventricular hemorrhage

3. The nurse reports a change in an infant's pain response after a surgical procedure. Previously the infant's pain scores were low, but now the scores are high in response to gentle handling. Which of the following explanations needs to be considered first?

A. The infant is experiencing withdrawal.

B. The infant's opioid dose needs to be increased.
C. The infant may be experiencing a wind-up phenomenon.
D. The infant's pain needs to be assessed using a measure specific for postoperative pain.

4. The parent of a 4-day-old male infant born at 26 weeks' gestation does not want his infant to receive pain medication for a chest tube insertion for fear that his son will become addicted. Based on the knowledge of opioids, the nurse would:
   A. suggest sucrose as an alternative intervention.
   B. respect the parent's decision and not provide pain medication.
   C. explore the parent's beliefs about pain and pain medication.
   D. tell the parent that addiction is a psychologic dependence on a drug and preterm infants cannot become addicted.

5. A 30-day-old infant born at 33 weeks' gestation is being cared for in the NICU. Planning for pain management after an extensive bowel resection should be based on the knowledge that:
   A. adequate preemptive analgesia eliminates the need for postoperative pain management.
   B. neuroanatomy, neurophysiology, and neurochemical systems are insufficiently developed in the bowel.
   C. activation of descending pathways that exert inhibitory effects on pain transmission is less developed in preterm infants.
   D. the response of neurotransmitters such as adenosine triphosphate, glutamate, neurokinin A, and substance P is exaggerated after bowel surgery.

6. A 6-week-old female infant with severe retinopathy of prematurity is scheduled for her third eye examination. Her mother indicates that the infant required reintubation after her last examination. Which of the following is the best action?
   A. Provide 24% sucrose 2 minutes before the examination.
   B. Ask the mother to watch her daughter's response to the examination while the nurse assists the ophthalmologist.
   C. Instruct the mother to provide her daughter with containment while softly speaking to her during the procedure.
   D. Ask the mother if she knows what makes her daughter comfortable during painful procedures and explain that facilitated tucking, containment, or offering of pacifiers may reduce pain.

7. Which of the following statements about sucrose is true?
   A. Sucrose can be used to calm irritable infants.
   B. Sucrose is safe and effective in single doses.
   C. Sucrose modulates pain through nonopioid pathways.
   D. Sucrose reduces pain in infants exposed to methadone before birth.

8. Which of the following statements is true regarding pain assessment in infants?
   A. Physiologic measures are more specific than behavioral measures.
   B. Pain is a subjective experience that cannot be communicated by infants.
   C. Pain responses and irritability-agitation are similar and cannot be distinguished from each other.
   D. The frequency with which the infant experiences painful procedures in the NICU will affect the infant's subsequent responses to pain.

9. When planning pain management for a 14-day-old term infant who undergoes daily ventricular taps, the nurse would consider pain assessment every 4 hours and:
   A. application of EMLA (eutectic mixture of local anesthetics) at the site.
   B. a continuous opioid infusion.
   C. comfort measures during the procedure.
   D. documentation of the infant's pain response.

10. A 3-day-old male infant born at 34 weeks' gestation is scheduled to receive a vaccine. His mother does not want him to receive sucrose, and she is not able to hold him during the procedure. Nonnutritive sucking on a pacifier is recommended based on the knowledge that:
    A. sucking reduces pain transmission through opioid pathways.
    B. sucking reduces pain transmission through nonopioid pathways.
    C. the pain-relieving properties of sucking increase with gestational age.
    D. the pain-relieving properties of sucking are effective after the pacifier is removed.

11. In an emergency situation in which immediate pain relief is desired, the nurse will administer:
    A. fentanyl.
    B. morphine.
    C. midazolam (Versed).
    D. meperidine (Demerol).

# Chapter 27

# Perinatal Substance Abuse

1. A newborn exhibits the following characteristics: small for gestational age, dysmorphic facial features, and central nervous system abnormalities. These characteristics were most likely caused by perinatal exposure to:
   A. heroin.
   B. alcohol.
   C. cocaine.
   D. amphetamines.

2. When caring for a full-term infant whose mother used cocaine during her pregnancy, the nurse should assess the infant for complications including:
   A. macrosomia.
   B. absence of the startle reflex.
   C. neonatal abstinence syndrome.
   D. central nervous system irritability.

3. When providing care for an infant who was prenatally exposed to heroin, the nurse demonstrates appropriate use of the Neonatal Abstinence Scoring System by:
   A. scoring the infant twice daily until symptoms subside.
   B. determining a treatment plan based on the initial score.
   C. initiating pharmacologic treatment when the score is less than 8.
   D. scoring the infant every 4 hours to monitor the progression of symptoms.

4. An infant is receiving oral morphine for treatment of neonatal abstinence syndrome. Which finding indicates to the nurse that the morphine is effective in controlling signs of withdrawal?

   A. Tremors subside with swaddling.
   B. The respiratory rate is less than 55 breaths/minute.
   C. The infant remains in a drowsy state.
   D. Neonatal Abstinence Scoring System scores are between 4 and 8.

5. Which medication would most likely be used in the treatment of neonatal abstinence syndrome?
   A. Fentanyl (Sublimaze)
   B. Clonidine (Catapres)
   C. Naloxone (Narcan)
   D. Midazolam (Versed)

6. What information should be included in discharge education for the parents of a full-term newborn who is experiencing the effects of perinatal cocaine exposure?
   A. Use of a prone infant sleeping position to decrease irritability
   B. Correct method of administering methadone to treat withdrawal symptoms
   C. Omission of bottle feedings if the infant exhibits poor suck and swallow
   D. Calming strategies, such as swaddling and decreasing environmental stimuli

7. What is the most accurate and effective strategy for assessing neonates for perinatal exposure to drugs?
   A. Neonatal meconium analysis
   B. Use of the Neonatal Abstinence Scoring System
   C. Maternal history and self-report
   D. Neonatal urine toxicologic screening

# PROFESSIONAL CARING AND ETHICAL PRACTICE

## Chapter 28

# Family Integration

1. Which of the following is a psychologic task a mother and family must accomplish to establish a healthy parent-child relationship after the crisis of the birth of a premature or sick infant?
   A. Refusing to participate in the infant's care
   B. Discussing the infant with family members
   C. Adapting to the intensive care environment
   D. Allowing friends and family to touch and hold the infant

2. Which term describes the grief frequently seen in parents of a chronically ill or disabled child?
   A. Denied grief
   B. Chronic grief
   C. Unresolved grief
   D. Anticipatory grief

3. A mother is spending time with her preterm infant in the NICU. Which of the following is a predictor of good maternal parenting outcome?
   A. The mother's time spent in the NICU is short.
   B. The mother has limited verbal interaction with staff.
   C. The mother makes positive eye contact with the infant.
   D. The mother does not seek out information related to the infant's condition.

4. During a parents' visit to the NICU, it is important for the nurse to encourage family-infant bonding by:
   A. modeling nurturing parenting behavior.
   B. speaking only to the adult members of the family.
   C. discouraging parents' participation in care because the baby is too sick.

   D. quickly explaining all of the medical conditions and equipment in great detail.

5. A full-term infant is born with multiple congenital anomalies. Despite adequate prenatal care, the anomalies were undiagnosed. The mother sits at the bedside and cries, but the father continues his usual work schedule. The mother is angry that the father is not more involved. The nurse caring for these parents should recognize that these parents are experiencing which of the following?
   A. Delayed grief
   B. Abnormal grief
   C. Incongruent grief
   D. Anticipatory grief

6. When working with the family of a full-term infant diagnosed with a fatal disorder, the nurse should:
   A. avoid discussing end-of-life care.
   B. collect mementos and offer them to the family.
   C. keep the family in the middle of the room so they can be monitored carefully.
   D. tell the family not to bring in the infant's siblings because it would be too upsetting to them.

7. A preterm infant is diagnosed with a significant intraventricular hemorrhage. The physicians have explained the damage to the brain and are discussing treatment options with the adolescent parents. The maternal grandmother insists on telling the mother the best treatment plan for the infant. The mother and father do not want the grandmother telling them what to do. The parents' reactions are not unusual, because as adolescents they:
   A. feel like the staff will not accept their decision.
   B. are able to think abstractly and anticipate future problems.

C. are capable of decision making without the help from adults.

D. may be trying to take on adult responsibilities and feel they are being treated like children.

8. An infant is brought to the special care nursery to be treated for sepsis. The infant's mother is single and a victim of domestic abuse. The nurses have noticed that the mother comes in infrequently and stays only a short time. She avoids feeding times and rarely wants to hold the baby. This mother's behavior is consistent with:
A. adaptation.
B. normal parenting.
C. inadequate bonding.
D. positive attachment behavior.

9. An infant of 26 weeks' gestation is born at an outlying hospital. The baby has been intubated because of respiratory distress. The transport team from the regional NICU is on the way to transfer the baby to their hospital 50 miles away. Which of the following interventions is most appropriate for the referring hospital staff to perform?
A. Keep the family in the waiting room.
B. Close the curtain to the nursery viewing window.
C. Avoid giving information about the transfer process.
D. Periodically assess the parents' understanding of their infant's condition.

10. After the birth and admission of a 28-week gestational age infant to the NICU, the infant's father screams, "This is all your fault!" at the physician and storms out of the room, while the mother sits crying. What stage of grief is the father experiencing?
A. Shock
B. Denial
C. Anger
D. Acceptance

## Chapter 29

# Discharge Planning and Transition to Home

1. Effective transitional planning ensures that the process of care:
A. follows structured protocols.
B. remains coordinated and continuous.
C. is established 1 week before discharge.
D. is relinquished to a competent home care company.

2. Preterm infants in medically stable condition who remain in the hospital at 2 months of age should:
A. not receive vaccines while they remain hospitalized.
B. receive all routinely recommended vaccines appropriate for their corrected age.
C. receive less than the full dose of routinely recommended vaccines based on the infant's weight.
D. receive all routinely recommended vaccines at the same chronologic age as full-term infants.

3. Which group of infants should undergo a period of observation in a car safety seat before hospital discharge to monitor for possible apnea, bradycardia, or oxygen desaturation?
A. Only those infants with known respiratory compromise

B. All infants born prematurely at less than 35 weeks' gestation
C. All infants born prematurely at less than 37 weeks' gestation
D. Infants with a corrected age of less than 40 weeks at discharge

4. An infant born at 27 weeks' gestation remains in the NICU at 2 months of age with a diagnosis of bronchopulmonary dysplasia. Which of the following vaccines should be administered?
A. Hepatitis B (HepB), diphtheria/tetanus/acellular pertussis (DTaP), inactivated poliovirus (IPV), *Haemophilus influenzae* type b (Hib), hepatitis A (HepA)
B. DTaP, Hib, IPV, pneumococcal conjugate (PCV), HepB
C. DTaP, Hib, oral poliovirus (OPV), PCV, HepB
D. DTaP, Hib, influenza, IPV, PCV

5. An infant born at 32 weeks' gestation is discharged at 6 weeks of age, receiving exclusively breast milk. It is recommended that, in addition to human milk, the infant receive:
A. folic acid, 50 mcg/day.
B. vitamin E, 25 IU/day.

C. vitamin D, 400 IU/day.

D. human milk fortifier in one supplemental bottle per day.

6. A male baby who was born at 26 weeks' gestation and is now 4 months old is brought to the emergency department by his frightened parents. The parents describe an episode of apnea, cyanosis, and limpness after the infant choked on a feeding. The baby is stimulated and given about 1 minute of rescue breathing. The infant now appears well. The episode can most appropriately be called:

A. a near-miss sudden infant death syndrome.

B. an aborted crib death.

C. an apparent life-threatening event.

D. obstructive apnea.

7. A highly cooperative parent of 8-week-old, 28-week gestation twins who has been visiting regularly refuses to attend discharge planning meetings and cardiopulmonary resuscitation classes in preparation for discharge. The nurse caring for the infants should recognize that the parent:

A. has not formed a bond with the babies.

B. should not be expected to participate in discharge planning.

C. is likely frightened of having the infants out of intensive care and at home.

D. has developed conflict with the health care team as discharge approaches.

8. An infant born at 31 weeks' gestation who is now at a corrected age of 40 weeks is being discharged home. Which of the following tests do not need to be performed before discharge?

A. Blood typing and screening

B. Hearing evaluation and/or screening

C. Metabolic screening and thyroid function tests

D. Cranial ultrasonography for intraventricular hemorrhage

9. When teaching parents infant cardiopulmonary resuscitation, it is important to emphasize that the most common cause of cardiac arrest in infants is which of the following?

A. Infection

B. Heart disease

C. Breathing problems

D. Abnormal heart rhythms

10. Hospitalized preterm infants should be kept predominately in the supine position beginning at least:

A. at a postmenstrual age of 32 weeks.

B. at a postmenstrual age of 34 weeks.

C. 1 week before anticipated discharge.

D. when the infant is older than 34 weeks postmenstrual age and all monitoring has been discontinued.

## Chapter 30

# Patient Safety

1. Which of the following statements about medication errors in the NICU is true?

A. Wrong dose is the most common error in the NICU.

B. Because of unit dose dispensing, errors occur less frequently in the NICU.

C. Errors are underreported in the NICU compared with other areas of the hospital.

D. Compared with other areas of the hospital, the NICU has an increased frequency of medication errors, and these errors result in more harm to the patient.

2. Double-checking a medication with another RN before administration is considered an:

A. effective method of reducing medication errors regardless of how it is performed.

B. ineffective method of reducing medication errors.

C. unnecessary step because the pharmacy serves as the double-check.

D. effective method of reducing medication errors when performed independently.

3. The NICU that has a "culture of safety" is focused on which of the following?

A. Promoting a no-blame approach to error reporting

B. Focusing on individual performance with each error event

C. Sharing error reports as a method of learning and improving

D. Measuring the effectiveness of safety efforts by a reduction in the number of errors reported

4. A nonpunitive approach to patient safety errors means that health care providers:
   A. are human and mistakes happen.
   B. are the focus of patient safety efforts.
   C. are accountable for safety procedures.
   D. will not receive disciplinary action for an error regardless of the circumstances.

5. Distractions during medication administration:
   A. can be easily reduced.
   B. are not a major contributing factor in errors.
   C. are a major contributing factor in errors.
   D. are caused mostly by patients and their families.

6. In the NICU, patients are particularly at risk of which of the following types of errors?
   A. Wrong-drug
   B. Wrong-dose
   C. Wrong-route
   D. Misidentification (wrong-patient)

7. The majority of patient safety events in the NICU are:
   A. harmless.
   B. preventable.
   C. voluntarily reported.
   D. the result of human error.

## Chapter 31

# Research

1. The results of a recent study demonstrated that the incidence of necrotizing enterocolitis (NEC) in preterm infants increased as the number of nosocomial infections increased. In this study, NEC is the:
   A. dependent variable.
   B. extraneous variable.
   C. antecedent variable.
   D. independent variable.

2. The extent to which the findings of a research study can be applied to populations beyond the study's sample is termed the study's:
   A. validity.
   B. reliability.
   C. testability.
   D. generalizability.

3. An investigation into the effect of co-bedding on weight gain in preterm infants used a process in which each baby had an equal chance of being assigned to either an experimental group or a control group. This process is referred to as:
   A. blinding.
   B. control.
   C. anonymity.
   D. randomization.

4. Evidence-based practice involves making decisions about patient care by integrating research, clinical expertise, and what other element to achieve improved outcomes?
   A. Corporate directives
   B. Clinician preferences
   C. Patient-family values and expectations
   D. Quality improvement and cost-cutting measures

5. A study determined that tympanic membrane temperature recordings provide consistent temperature readings in preterm neonates in stable condition. This study demonstrated that the instrument used to record tympanic membrane temperatures has which of the following attributes?
   A. Validity
   B. Accuracy
   C. Precision
   D. Reliability

6. Which of the following represent the highest level of evidence on which to base nursing practice?
   A. Descriptive studies
   B. Case-control studies
   C. Reports from expert committees
   D. Systematic reviews or meta-analyses

## Chapter 32

# Legal Issues

1. Which of the following elements must be proven by the plaintiff in a medical malpractice case?
   A. Negligence, intent, harm, breach
   B. Duty, harm, accountability, negligence
   C. Duty, breach of duty, harm, proximal cause
   D. Intent, proximal cause, harm, accountability

2. A neonatal nurse is asked to write an institutional policy for a new procedure. The nurse is concerned that this procedure may not be in a nurse's scope of practice. Where can the nurse go to obtain scope of practice information?
   A. Standards of care
   B. Practice guidelines
   C. State nurse practice act
   D. American Nurses Association

3. The nurse notes that a neonate's blood pressure is dropping dangerously low and calls the hospital operator to have the physician paged; the nurse then documents the current blood pressure and call to the physician. After 15 minutes the physician has not returned the call. The nurse pages the physician again and records: "1300—BP continues to fall. Dr. paged with no return call after 15 minutes. Paged again. Infant's condition unstable and worsening." This documentation:
   A. demonstrates critical thinking.
   B. shifts all responsibility to the physician.
   C. indicates that the nursing process is being followed.
   D. places the nurse and physician at risk for legal action.

4. The number one cause of all patient injuries is which of the following?
   A. Unfamiliarity with institutional protocol
   B. Lack of sufficient orientation and training
   C. Lack of comprehensive standards of care
   D. Failure to follow the five steps in the nursing process

5. Which of the following is best defined as "what the average, reasonable, and prudent nurse would do under similar circumstances"?
   A. Standard of care
   B. Nursing process
   C. Scope of practice
   D. Policy and procedure

6. The parent of a neonate gives informed consent for a procedure. The physician signs the consent and asks the nurse to sign as a witness. The nurse's signature indicates that the:
   A. signature is the parent's and was voluntary.
   B. nurse agrees with the need for the procedure.
   C. physician gave all required information to the parents.
   D. nurse confirms that the parents understand all risks, benefits, and alternatives.

7. Which of the following major principles is an integral part of the informed consent process?
   A. Justice
   B. Autonomy
   C. Beneficence
   D. Nonmaleficence

## Chapter 33

# Ethical Issues

1. Determining the most morally desirable course of action in health care is termed:
   A. ethics.
   B. bioethics.
   C. narrative ethics.
   D. principle-based ethics.

2. What are the four major principles of biomedical ethics?
   A. Fidelity, truth telling, confidentiality, privacy
   B. Veracity, confidentiality, privacy, fidelity
   C. Do no harm, do good, be truthful, be respectful
   D. Autonomy, beneficence, nonmaleficence, justice

3. The rule of double effect applies when a nurse gives:
   A. fentanyl (Sublimaze) for pain and respirations are slowed.
   B. antibiotics for an infection and anaphylaxis occurs.
   C. midazolam (Versed) for agitation and the baby becomes calm.
   D. a suppository for constipation and the baby has a stool.

4. A premature infant born at 24 weeks' gestation develops a grade IV intraventricular hemorrhage on day 10 of life. The neonatologist meets with the family and explains the very poor prognosis and recommends discontinuation of life support. Who can make the final decision to discontinue life support except in extreme conditions?
   A. The neonatologist
   B. The primary nurse
   C. The ethics committee
   D. The parents or legal guardian

5. *Nonmaleficence* is defined as:
   A. do no harm.
   B. do good.
   C. fairness.
   D. autonomy.

6. The nurse wants to consult the ethics committee regarding a critically ill infant with a diagnosis of trisomy 13. The family wants everything to be done to keep the baby alive despite the diagnosis. The nurse can expect the ethics committee to:
   A. mandate an action.
   B. give a written order.
   C. impact the plan of care.
   D. facilitate understanding of the issues and information about a case.

7. The best way to prevent ethical conflicts between families and the medical team is to:

A. chart accurately.
B. not tell the family how sick the baby is.
C. discuss issues only with the neonatologist and the primary nurse.
D. communicate openly with the family.

8. Obtaining an informed consent upholds the principle of:
   A. justice.
   B. autonomy.
   C. beneficence.
   D. nonmaleficence.

9. The neonatal team attends the delivery of a 24-week gestational age premature infant. The neonatologist has met with the family earlier to explain all the risks, benefits, and long-term outcomes related to care of an infant born at this gestational age. The family decides on a full resuscitation. At delivery, the baby has fused eyes and gelatinous skin, and the gestation time appears to be less than 24 weeks. The team must decide whether to initiate care or to approach the family after resuscitation regarding withdrawal of care. This situation represents:
   A. compassion.
   B. an ethical dilemma.
   C. a treatment dilemma.
   D. the principle of benevolence.

10. Magnetic resonance imaging results for a critically ill infant are given to the nurse. The nurse discusses the results with the physician and a family conference is arranged. During the conference, the physician does not share the results with the family because the mother is despondent. This violates what basic principle of health care ethics?
    A. Veracity
    B. Fidelity
    C. Autonomy
    D. Confidentiality

## Chapter 34

# AACN Synergy Model for Patient Care

## Introduction

The AACN Synergy Model for Patient Care is integrated into the AACN CCRN examination. The Synergy Model is a conceptual framework that emphasizes that the needs or characteristics of patients and families drive the competencies or characteristics of the nurse. Each patient brings a set of eight characteristics (needs) to the health care situation. These characteristics are stability, complexity, vulnerability, predictability, resiliency, participation in decision making, participation in care, and resource availability.

The Synergy Model also describes eight characteristics (competencies) that are essential for the nurse providing care to critically ill patients. These nurse characteristics are clinical judgment, advocacy and moral agency, caring practices, collaboration, response to diversity, clinical inquiry, facilitation of learning, and systems thinking. According to the Synergy Model, when patient needs and nurse competencies match, optimal patient outcomes are achieved. The Synergy Model is a blueprint for certified practice, and as such, AACN's CCRN examination is based on the Synergy Model. This chapter illustrates how test questions based on the Synergy Model cover application of the model, rather than the concepts themselves. The rationale for each question identifies the nurse characteristic demonstrated in the question.

1. A neonate with bilious vomiting is admitted from an outlying community hospital to the NICU at a tertiary care facility on the second day of life. Gastrointestinal studies reveal the presence of intestinal malrotation with volvulus, and surgical repair is undertaken. On postoperative day 1, the father insists that the neonate be transferred back to the community hospital because transportation to the tertiary care facility is a problem for the parents. The nurse should:
   A. request a consultation with the social worker.
   B. allow the parents to verbalize their frustrations.
   C. ask the pediatric surgeon to speak with the father.
   D. review the clinical aspects of malrotation and volvulus.

2. An electronic documentation system, including bedside computer work stations, is scheduled to be installed in a 30-bed level III NICU. An interdisciplinary team has been appointed by the pediatric administrator to coordinate the effort. The equipment vendor has planned for the installation of all of the work stations in one day. The NICU nurse serving on the team should take which of the following actions?
   A. Schedule a meeting with the NICU nurse manager.
   B. Request a staged installation of the computer terminals.
   C. Speak with the director of neonatology regarding the plan.
   D. Report the issue to the hospital administrator for further action.

3. A neonate is admitted to the NICU with a diagnosis of omphalocele. The mother did not receive prenatal care. The maternal history obtained immediately before delivery was reflective of recreational drug use. The mother expressed remorse on her first bedside visit to the infant in the NICU, claiming that she had "ruined" her baby. The nurse should:
   A. offer information regarding drug treatment programs.
   B. offer a counseling session with the NICU social worker.
   C. explain the anatomic basis for omphalocele development.
   D. refer the mother to the pediatric surgeon for further information.

4. A neonate experiences wound dehiscence after repair of a diaphragmatic hernia. The mother expresses anger toward the pediatric surgeon and nursing staff regarding the alteration in skin integrity, declaring that it results from deficient medical and nursing care. The nurse should:
   A. ask the pediatric surgeon to speak with the parents.
   B. contact the quality care coordinator for the hospital.
   C. schedule a team meeting to address the care concerns.
   D. refer the mother to a website addressing diaphragmatic hernias.

5. A nursing project is undertaken by the clinical practice task force of a tertiary care NICU that will examine the use of two different skin care products in extremely low birth weight neonates. For the project to be completed successfully, the nurse responsible for project coordination on the task force should:
   A. individually recruit parents to enroll their infants.
   B. notify the NICU nurse manager of noncompliant staff.
   C. schedule unit-based staff meetings to explain the project.
   D. display a poster with the names of the enrolled neonates.

6. A neonate with a large sacral teratoma is admitted to the NICU. The parents were informed of the diagnosis prenatally but are visibly upset during a bedside conversation with the neonatologist shortly after the infant's admission. After the neonatologist leaves the bedside, the mother begins to cry and the father expresses anger and frustration. The nurse should:
   A. request a visit from the hospital chaplain.
   B. ask the neonatologist to return to the bedside.
   C. allow the parents to verbalize their emotions.
   D. schedule a multidisciplinary team conference.

7. A nurse caring for a postterm neonate with persistent pulmonary hypertension of the newborn who is undergoing mechanical ventilation notices

decreasing oxygen saturation, tachycardia, and agitation with nursing care activities. The nurse on the previous shift had decreased the dosage of the fentanyl infusion per physician order. The nurse should:

A. notify the respiratory therapy staff of the desaturations.

B. increase the percentage of oxygen during cares activities.

C. speak with the physician regarding the sedation order.

D. perform nursing cares less frequently to allow for rest periods.

8. A neonate is admitted to the NICU with multiple congenital anomalies. Following subspecialty evaluation, it is determined that survival past the first 6 months of life is unlikely, and palliative and hospice care is recommended. The mother is 16 years of age and homeless, and the father is not involved. To facilitate an appropriate discharge plan for this neonate, the nurse should:

A. request a social work consultation.

B. contact a homeless shelter for placement.

C. contact child protective services for assistance.

D. schedule a team discharge planning conference.

9. A neonate with suspected congenital heart disease undergoes a hyperoxia test. The test reveals an arterial $Po_2$ of 52, pH of 7.31, and $Pco_2$ of 35. Based on these clinical findings, the nurse should:

A. repeat the arterial blood gas analysis.

B. administer a prostaglandin infusion.

C. prepare the neonate for echocardiography.

D. prepare for intubation and mechanical ventilation.

10. A premature neonate with respiratory distress is weaned from a conventional mechanical ventilator to nasal continuous positive airway pressure ventilation following surfactant administration on day 1 of life. On day 10, the neonate experiences a bout of sepsis and requires reintubation because of respiratory decompensation. The mother questions the nurse regarding the need for mechanical ventilation given the successful tolerance of nasal continuous positive airway pressure ventilation for the past 9 days of life. The nurse should:

A. refer the mother to the respiratory therapist.

B. explain the effect of surfactant administration.

C. ask the neonatologist to speak with the mother.

D. review the clinical aspects of respiratory distress.

# ANSWER KEY

## Section I: General Assessment and Management

### CHAPTER 1: ASSESSMENT OF FETAL WELL-BEING

1. **(B)** Fetal fibronectin (fFN) is uncommonly present in cervicovaginal secretions in the late second and early third trimesters. fFN is an extracellular glycoprotein that is thought to act as an adhesive between the fetal membrane and uterine wall and can be disrupted by inflammation. A preterm birth within 2 weeks is probable after a positive test result. Cervical ferritin is not a biomarker but an inflammatory marker whose presence provides support for the theory that infection is a mediator of preterm birth. Maternal plasma concentrations of corticotropin-releasing hormone are elevated in both term and preterm pregnancies. It appears to be a component of the common pathway of labor regardless of gestation. Placental α-microglobulin-1 is a protein found in amniotic fluid that is a biomarker for rupture of membranes.

**References:** Ramsey, P., Tsunenobu, T., Goldenberg, R., et al.: The preterm prediction study: Elevated cervical ferritin levels at 22 to 24 weeks of gestation are associated with spontaneous preterm delivery in asymptomatic women. *American Journal of Obstetrics and Gynecology,* 186(3):458-463, 2002.

Spong, C.Y.: Prediction and prevention of recurrent spontaneous preterm birth. *Obstetrics and Gynecology,* 110(2, part 1):405-415, 2007.

Weintraub, A., Sheiner, E., Mazor, M., et al.: Maternal serum ferritin concentration in patients with preterm labor and intact membranes. *Journal of Maternal Fetal Neonatal Medicine,* 18(3):163-166, 2005.

2. **(D)** Premature rupture of membranes is one of the most common complications of pregnancy resulting in a newborn's admission to the NICU. A bedside immunoassay test, AmniSure ROM, is simple, easy to perform, rapid (5-10 minutes), and minimally invasive. This test identifies a placental glycoprotein that is abundant in amniotic fluid but present in lower concentrations in maternal blood and cervicovaginal secretions. Prolactin is responsible for priming the breast tissue in preparation for lactation. α-Fetoprotein is assessed to identify neural tube defects (high) and Down syndrome (low). Fetal fibronectin is an extracellular glycoprotein that is thought to act as an adhesive between the fetal membranes and uterine wall and is a biomarker for predicting preterm birth.

**Reference:** Caughey, A., Robinson, J., Norwitz, E.: Contemporary diagnosis and management of preterm premature rupture of membranes. *Reviews in Obstetrics and Gynecology,* 1(1):11-22, 2008.

3. **(B)** Moderate fetal heart rate (FHR) variability is strongly associated with an arterial umbilical cord pH higher than 7.15. Normal FHR variability provides reassurance about fetal status and the absence of metabolic acidemia. FHR variability is the sign most predictive of fetal well-being. The most important single FHR characteristic is variability. FHR baseline is 110 to 160 beats/minute regardless of gestational age. Decelerations are a reflection of head compression, umbilical cord compression, or a transient interruption in oxygen transfer. Accelerations are highly predictive of the absence of fetal metabolic acidemia and form the basis of the nonstress test. They occur in association with fetal movement.

**References:** American College of Obstetricians and Gynecologists: *Intrapartum Fetal Heart Rate Monitoring: Nomenclature, Interpretation, and General Management Principles,* No. 106. Washington, D.C., American College of Obstetrics and Gynecologists, July 2009.

Freeman, R.K., Garite, T.J., Nageotte, M.P.: *Fetal Heart Rate Monitoring,* 3rd ed. Philadelphia, Lippincott Williams & Wilkins, 2003, pp. 63-89.

Tucker, S., Miller, D., Miller, L.: *Fetal Monitoring: A Multidisciplinary Approach,* 6th ed. St. Louis, Mosby, 2009, pp. 95-138.

4. **(A)** The biophysical profile (BPP) presumes that multiple indicators are better predictors of outcome than one indicator. The score for each indicator is either 0 if that component is absent or 2 points if it is present, and management depends on the total score. A score of 10 out of 10 indicates that fetal asphyxia is extremely unlikely. The BPP consists of a nonstress test using an electronic fetal monitor and real-time limited ultrasonography to observe the fetus for the other components. The components include fetal tone, fetal movement, fetal breathing, the nonstress test, and amniotic fluid index. Fetal position and fetal heart rate are not included in the BPP.

**References:** Freeman, R.K., Garite, T.J., Nageotte, M.P.: Antepartum fetal monitoring. In *Fetal Heart Rate Monitoring,* ed 3, Philadelphia, Lippincott Williams & Wilkins, 2003, pp. 181-202.

Richardson, B., Gagon, R.: Behavioral state activity and fetal health and development. In Creasy, R., Resnik, R. (Eds.): *Creasy and Resnik's Maternal-Fetal Medicine Principles and Practices,* 6th ed. Philadelphia, Saunders, 2009, pp. 171-181.

5. **(C)** Patients who are at low risk for developing gestational diabetes (<25 years, normal weight, member of an ethnic group with low prevalence of diabetes, no diabetes in a first-degree relative, no history of abnormal glucose tolerance, and no history of poor obstetric outcome) are tested between 24 and 28 weeks' gestation. Patients with risk factors (>35 years, body mass index >30, history of gestational diabetes, delivery of

a large-for-gestational-age infant, polycystic ovarian syndrome, strong family history of diabetes) should receive a plasma glucose screening at their first prenatal visit followed by one at 24 to 28 weeks.

**Reference:** Bowers, N., Curran, C., Freda, M.C., et al.: High risk pregnancy. In Simpson, K., Creehan, P. (Eds.): *Perinatal Nursing,* 3rd ed. Philadelphia, Lippincott Williams & Wilkins, 2008, pp. 189-207.

6. **(B)** Values of $P_{CO_2}$ are lower when women give birth in an upright position than when they give birth in the supine position. A supine position during labor should be avoided to prevent maternal hypotension and to enhance uteroplacental blood flow to keep the fetal pH within normal limits. Values of pH and $P_{O_2}$ are higher in women who give birth in the upright position. A normal pH, $P_{O_2}$, and $P_{CO_2}$ should reflect a normal base excess.

**References:** Simpson, K., James, D.: Efficacy of intrauterine resuscitation techniques in improving fetal oxygen status during labor. *Obstetrics and Gynecology,* 105:1362-1368, 2005.

Zwelling, E.: Overcoming the challenges: Maternal movement and positioning to facilitate labor progress. *MCN American Journal of Maternal Child Nursing,* 35(2):72-80, 2010.

7. **(B)** The major factor influencing pulmonary maturity in the infants of diabetic mothers is blood glucose control. In mothers with good control, fetal lung maturation is not delayed. Phosphatidylglycerol (PG) enhances the spread of phospholipids on alveoli and its presence indicates an advanced state of fetal lung development and function. The fetal lung maturity test reports in milligrams of surfactant per gram of albumin. The AmnioSTAT is the test that is used and uses 55 mg of surfactant/gram albumin as "mature." Lamellar bodies are lamellated phospholipids that represent a storage form of surfactant. The size of lamellar bodies is similar to that of platelets, so a lamellar body count can be obtained rapidly with the use of a platelet channel of a hematology analyzer. The fetal lung maturity cutoff is suggested to be 50,000 μL. The lecithin/sphingomyelin ratio is best used in combination with the PG test. It is the PG that indicates the advanced state of lung development.

**References:** Fischer, A., Dodia, C., Ruckert, P., et al.: The pathway to lamellar bodies for surface protein A. *American Journal of Physiology—Lung Cell Molecular Physiology,* 299(1):L51-58, 2010.

Mercer, B.: Assessment and induction of fetal pulmonary maturity. In Creasy, R., Resnik, R. (Eds.): *Creasy and Resnik's Maternal-Fetal Medicine Principles and Practices,* 6th ed. Philadelphia, Saunders, 2009, pp. 419-432.

Szallasi, A., Gronowski, A.M, Eby, C.S.: Lamellar body count in amniotic fluid: A comparative study of four different hematology analyzers. *Clinical Chemistry,* 49:994-997, 2003.

8. **(D)** A late deceleration of the fetal heart rate reflects a transient interruption of oxygen transfer from the environment to the fetus resulting in transient fetal hypoxemia. It can be corrected by changing the environment. *Fetal distress* is an imprecise term, and the National Institute of Child Health and Human Development Task Force has recommended that this term be abandoned. Acceleration reflects a sympathetic

nervous system response and results in an increase in the fetal heart rate. Rapid descent through the pelvis may cause a parasympathetic response that results in prolonged deceleration or fetal bradycardia, but not in late deceleration.

**Reference:** Tucker, S., Miller, D., Miller, L.: *Fetal Monitoring: A Multidisciplinary Approach,* 6th ed. Philadelphia, Mosby, 2009, pp. 95-138.

9. **(C)** Amnioinfusion has been used to attempt to resolve variable fetal heart rate decelerations by correcting umbilical cord compression as a result of oligohydramnios. During amnioinfusion, normal saline or lactated Ringer solution is infused into the uterus either by gravity flow or through an infusion pump. Amnioinfusion may assist with oligohydramnios (amniotic fluid index <5 cm) to provide additional fluid to cushion the umbilical cord and prevent variable decelerations from occurring. Careful monitoring and documentation of fluid infused is important to avoid iatrogenic polyhydramnios. Amnioinfusion has been shown to significantly improve fetal heart rate patterns characterized by variable decelerations but does not affect late decelerations or patterns with minimal to absent variability. Amnioinfusion does not affect decreased fetal heart variability.

**References:** Regi, A., Alexander, N. Jose, R., et al.: Amnioinfusion for the relief of recurrent severe and moderate variable decelerations in labor. *Journal of Reproductive Medicine,* 54(5):295-302, 2009.

Simpson, K.R.: Intrauterine resuscitation during labor: review of the current methods and supportive evidence. *Journal of Midwifery and Women's Health,* 52(3):229-237, 2007.

10. **(D)** Nifedipine (Procardia) works by inhibiting voltage-dependent channels of calcium entry into smooth muscle cells, acting to decrease intracellular calcium and decrease the release of stored calcium. It is rapidly absorbed after oral administration, which makes it convenient to use. It should not be used in combination with either magnesium sulfate or β-sympathomimetics (terbutaline). Magnesium sulfate is an anticonvulsant and acts to relax the smooth muscle of the uterus by substituting itself in place of calcium. Ketorolac (Toradol) is an antiinflammatory and an antiprostaglandin generally used for pain management. Its use can cause oligohydramnios and premature closure of the ductus arterious. Terbutaline is a β-sympathomimetic that supplements or mimics the effects of norepinephrine and epinephrine.

**Reference:** Iams, J.D., Romero, R., Creasy, R.K.: Preterm labor and birth. In Creasy, R., Resnik, R. (Eds.): *Creasy and Resnik's Maternal-Fetal Medicine: Principles and Practice,* 6th ed. Philadelphia, Saunders, 2009, pp. 545-582.

## CHAPTER 2: ADAPTATION TO EXTRAUTERINE LIFE

1. **(C)** Systemic vascular resistance in the aorta normally increases postnatally with the removal of the placenta. Pulmonary vascular resistance normally decreases postnatally with the onset of ventilation and the dilation of the pulmonary vasculature, which increases pulmonary blood flow to the lungs. An increase in pulmonary vascular resistance after birth

would further decrease blood flow to the lungs. Increased pulmonary vascular resistance can develop from cardiac defects (e.g., ventricular septal defect, single ventricle) or in infants with persistent pulmonary hypertension.

**References:** Kenny, P.A., Hoover, D., Williams, L.C., et al.: Cardiovascular diseases and surgical interventions. In Gardner, S.L., Carter, B.S., Enzman-Hines, M., et al. (Eds.): *Merenstein and Gardner's Handbook of Neonatal Intensive Care*, 7th ed. St. Louis, Mosby, 2011, pp. 678-716.

Verklan, M.T.: Adaptation to extrauterine life. In Verklan, M., Walden, M. (Eds.): *Core Curriculum for Neonatal Intensive Care Nursing*, 4th ed. St. Louis, Saunders, 2010, pp. 72-90.

2. **(C)** During fetal life, the ductus arteriosus is responsible for shunting blood away from the lungs to the aorta. This shunt functionally closes during the transition period following delivery. The foramen ovale is an opening between the left and right atria. Following delivery, as pressures increase on the left side of the heart and decrease on the right side of the heart, this connection functionally closes. Changes in an infant's condition can open this connection and allow blood to shunt in either direction. The ductus venosus is responsible for shunting blood from the umbilical vein to the inferior vena cava so that blood bypasses the liver. A Blalock-Taussig shunt is a surgical procedure performed to connect the subclavian artery to the pulmonary artery.

**References:** Kenny, P.A., Hoover, D., Williams, L.C., et al.: Cardiovascular diseases and surgical interventions. In Gardner, S.L., Carter, B.S., Enzman-Hines, M., et al. (Eds.): *Merenstein and Gardner's Handbook of Neonatal Intensive Care*, 7th ed. St. Louis, Mosby, 2011, pp. 678-716.

Verklan, M.T.: Adaptation to extrauterine life. In Verklan, M., Walden, M. (Eds.): *Core Curriculum for Neonatal Intensive Care Nursing*, 4th ed. St. Louis, Saunders, 2010, pp. 72-90.

3. **(B)** A scaphoid abdomen is the classic appearance of an infant with a diaphragmatic hernia. The majority of diaphragmatic hernias generally occur on the left side, resulting in breath sounds greater on the right side. The degree of respiratory distress varies depending on the size of the herniation. Respiratory distress can increase when the infant is bag-and-mask ventilated, because some air enters the stomach and passes to the intestine. Bowel sounds can sometimes be audible in the chest on the affected side. Bag-and-mask ventilation should be stopped and the infant intubated if assisted ventilation is required. Respiratory distress generally accompanies a pneumothorax. Breath sounds are diminished or absent on the affected side and the abdomen appears normal. The presence of a scaphoid abdomen is a hallmark pointing to a different diagnosis. Although respiratory distress can occur in an infant with a tracheoesophageal fistula, the presence of excessive oral secretions is usually the primary presenting symptom. Abdominal distention, rather than a scaphoid abdomen, would be expected in an infant with a gastrointestinal obstruction. When the abdomen is palpated, the infant can experience pain and may show some guarding.

**References:** Bradshaw, W.T.: Gastrointestinal disorders. In Verklan, M., Walden, M. (Eds.): *Core Curriculum for Neonatal*

*Intensive Care Nursing*, 4th ed. St. Louis, Saunders, 2010, pp. 589-637.

Lovvorn, H.N. III, Glenn, J.B., Pacetti, A.S., et al.: Neonatal surgery. In Gardner, S.L., Carter, B.S., Enzman-Hines, M., et al. (Eds.): *Merenstein and Gardner's Handbook of Neonatal Intensive Care*, 7th ed. St. Louis, Mosby, 2011, pp. 812-847.

Verklan, M.T.: Adaptation to extrauterine life. In Verklan, M., Walden, M. (Eds.): *Core Curriculum for Neonatal Intensive Care Nursing*, 4th ed. St. Louis, Saunders, 2010, pp. 72-90.

4. **(B)** Vacuum-assisted delivery places the infant at a higher risk for developing a subgaleal hemorrhage. A subgaleal hemorrhage can result in massive blood loss, leading to shock and death. Any changes in vital signs, level of consciousness, or swelling that is extending to the eyes and neck requires the caregiver to transfer the infant into an intensive care environment so that the delivery of blood products and hemodynamic stabilization are not delayed. Preparation may also be needed to transfer this infant to a higher level of care. A cephalohematoma can be unilateral or bilateral but does not cross the suture line; it will usually resolve within weeks after birth. A cephalohematoma generally does not require the infant to be cared for in an NICU unless there is significant blood loss or a fractured skull is suspected and the baby needs further evaluation. Otherwise, these infants can stay with their mothers in the labor and delivery department. However, they must be assessed for hyperbilirubinemia, for which they are at a higher risk. Caput succedaneum is caused by contact of the presenting part (scalp) with the cervix. The swelling is fluid in the subcutaneous tissues of the scalp. The swelling usually resolves within 1 to 2 days after birth. These infants can stay with their mothers in the labor and delivery department.

**References:** Karlsen, K.: *The S.T.A.B.L.E. Program*, 5th ed. Park City, Utah, American Academy of Pediatrics, 2006, pp. 147-148.

Verklan, M.T., Lopez, S.M.: Neurological disorders. In Gardner, S.L., Carter, B.S., Enzman-Hines, M., et al. (Eds.): *Merenstein and Gardner's Handbook of Neonatal Intensive Care*, 7th ed. St. Louis, Mosby, 2011, pp. 748-786.

5. **(D)** The Centers for Disease Control and Prevention (CDC) currently recommends that infants born to mothers whose hepatitis B surface antigen (HBsAg) status is unknown receive hepatitis B vaccine within 12 hours of birth. The mother should have blood drawn to determine her HBsAg status. If the mother is HBsAg positive, the infant should receive hepatitis B immune globulin (HBIG) as soon as possible and no later than 1 week of age. The administration of monovalent hepatitis B vaccine (single-antigen formulation that does not contain the preservative thimerosal) to all infants before discharge is the CDC recommendation. However, the mother's HBsAg status must be obtained to determine when hepatitis B immunization should be performed and whether or not HBIG should also be given. The mother's hepatitis status is usually assessed in the prenatal period. Hepatitis B is a serious illness if the infant contracts it from the mother.

**Reference:** Centers for Disease Control and Prevention: Recommended childhood and adolescent immunization schedule—United States, 2010. *MMWR Morbidity and Mortality Weekly Report*, 58:1-4, 2010.

6. **(C)** These assessment findings are normal during the transition period (first 4-6 hours) following birth. The petechiae on the face are the result of the precipitous delivery. Because the lungs are attempting to clear the fluid, infants can often have moist-sounding breath sounds, intermittently elevated respiratory rates, and occasional grunting. Transfer to the special care nursery/neonatal intensive care unit should be considered if the infant has a sudden deterioration in respiratory status, difficulty maintaining temperature, or changes in neurologic status. The pediatric provider should be contacted if the respiratory status changes with sustained grunting, increased work of breathing, and/or central color change. The peripheral cyanosis is normal during the transition period after birth due to vasomotor instability. The risk of aspiration occurring is very rare in this circumstance. Feeding should be delayed if the elevated respiratory rate is sustained.

**References:** Sielski, L.A., McKee-Garrett, T.M.: Nursery care of the well newborn. In Cloherty, J., Eichenwald, E., Stark, A. (Eds.): *Manual of Neonatal Care,* 2nd ed. Boston, Little, Brown, 2007, pp. 72-77.

Verklan, M.T.: Adaptation to extrauterine life. In Verklan, M., Walden, M. (Eds.): *Core Curriculum for Neonatal Intensive Care Nursing,* 4th ed. St. Louis, Saunders, 2010, pp. 72-90.

7. **(B)** Coarctation of the aorta has the classic finding of decreased perfusion and pulses in the lower extremities. These infants can develop temperature instability and poor feeding. Congenital heart disease should be suspected when infants present with an increase in respiratory rate in the absence of any other respiratory signs of distress and cyanosis. The physician should be notified immediately and the infant transferred to the nursery for further evaluation and stabilization. Infants with sepsis usually present with signs and symptoms of infection within 12 hours of birth. Clinical findings can include hypoglycemia, poor feeding, lethargy, temperature instability, respiratory distress, weak pulses in all extremities, and cyanosis. Normal transition occurs in the first 4 to 6 hours after birth, so this baby has completed transition. The infant's poor perfusion in the lower extremities and tachypnea suggest a pathologic process for which the infant should be assessed. Severe meconium aspiration that leads to persistent pulmonary hypertension usually presents itself in the delivery room. Respiratory distress presents with tachypnea and an increase work of breathing that can include grunting, flaring, and retractions.

**References:** Sadowski, S.L.: Cardiovascular disorders. In Verklan, M., Walden, M. (Eds.): *Core Curriculum for Neonatal Intensive Care Nursing,* 4th ed. St. Louis, Saunders, 2010, pp. 534-588.

Verklan, M.T.: Adaptation to extrauterine life. In Verklan, M., Walden, M. (Eds.): *Core Curriculum for Neonatal Intensive Care Nursing,* 4th ed. St. Louis, Saunders, 2010, pp. 72-90.

8. **(D)** Norepinephrine is a stress hormone that is activated in response to cold stress. The release of norepinephrine sends a signal to the nerve endings in the brown fat causing it to be metabolized. Brown fat is located in the axillary area, mediastinum, kidneys, adrenals, and nape of the neck. This metabolic process is referred to as *nonshivering thermogenesis.* The energy that is produced from this metabolic process heats the blood as it circulates past the areas where the brown fat is stored. Insulin regulates glucose. Infants who are cold stressed are also at risk for developing hypoglycemia and should be monitored closely. Vasopressin is created by the hypothalamus and prompts the pituitary gland to release a hormone that helps maintain blood pressure and water and electrolyte balance. It does not play a role in thermoregulation. Epinephrine is produced within the adrenal glands and works with norepinephrine to produce the "fight or flight" response by increasing the supply of oxygen to the brain and muscles. It does not play a role in thermoregulation.

**References:** Brand, M.C., Boyd, H.A.: Thermoregulation. In Verklan, M., Walden, M. (Eds.): *Core Curriculum for Neonatal Intensive Care Nursing,* 4th ed. St. Louis, Saunders, 2010, pp. 110-119.

Brown, V.D., Landers, S.: Heat balance. In Gardner, S.L., Carter, B.S., Enzman-Hines, M., et al. (Eds.): *Merenstein and Gardner's Handbook of Neonatal Intensive Care,* 7th ed. St. Louis, Mosby, 2011, pp. 113-133.

Karlsen, K.: *The S.T.A.B.L.E. Program,* 5th ed. Park City, Utah, American Academy of Pediatrics, 2006, pp. 46-47.

Soll, R.: Heat loss prevention in neonates. *Journal of Perinatology,* 28:S57-S59, 2008.

9. **(D)** Surfactant is produced by type II alveolar pneumocytes and coats the inner lining of the alveoli. Surfactant decreases surface tension and allows alveoli to remain open at the end of expiration, which prevents alveolar collapse. Surfactant increases lung compliance. The increase in catecholamines at birth is responsible for decreasing the secretions and improving absorption through the lymphatic system.

**References:** Gardner, S.L., Enzman-Hines, M., Dickey, L.A.: Respiratory diseases. In Gardner, S.L., Carter, B.S., Enzman-Hines, M., et al. (Eds.): *Merenstein and Gardner's Handbook of Neonatal Intensive Care,* 7th ed. St. Louis, Mosby, 2011, pp. 581-677.

Verklan, M.T.: Adaptation to extrauterine life. In Verklan, M., Walden, M. (Eds.): *Core Curriculum for Neonatal Intensive Care Nursing,* 4th ed. St. Louis, Saunders, 2010, pp. 72-90.

10. **(D)** Provided the baby remains asymptomatic, breast-feeding should be attempted immediately. Glucose level should be assessed approximately 30 minutes to 1 hour after the feed. A glucose level of 33 mg/dl is low, and treatment with an early feeding should not be delayed. Glucose water is no longer recommended as a treatment for hypoglycemia because it can cause rebound hypoglycemia. If the infant becomes symptomatic and is unable to feed, an infusion of dextrose 10% in water at 80 ml/kg/day is appropriate. This infusion would provide glucose at 5.5 mg/kg/minute.

**References:** Armentrout, D.: Glucose management. In Verklan, M., Walden, M. (Eds.): *Core Curriculum for Neonatal Intensive Care Nursing,* 4th ed. St. Louis, Saunders, 2010, pp. 172-181.

McGowan, J.E., Rozance, P.J., Price-Douglas, W., et al.: Glucose homeostasis. In Gardner, S.L., Carter, B.S., Enzman-Hines, M., et al. (Eds.): *Merenstein and Gardner's Handbook of Neonatal Intensive Care,* 7th ed. St. Louis, Mosby, 2011, pp. 353-377.

Karlsen, K.: *The S.T.A.B.L.E. Program,* 5th ed. Park City, Utah, American Academy of Pediatrics, 2006, pp. 12-20.

Verklan, M.T.: Adaptation to extrauterine life. In Verklan, M., Walden, M. (Eds.): *Core Curriculum for Neonatal Intensive Care Nursing*, 4th ed. St. Louis, Saunders, 2010, pp. 72-90.

11. **(D)** The right hand is always preductal, because the right subclavian artery is the first branch off the aorta that originates from the left ventricle carrying oxygenated blood. The ductus arteriosus usually inserts into the aorta distal to the right subclavian artery. Preductal and postductal saturations are used to assess for the presence of right-to-left shunting associated with certain congenital cardiac defects or pulmonary hypertension. In the presence of a right-to-left shunt across the ductus arteriosus, blood distal to the ductus is a mixture of oxygenated and deoxygenated blood. Both the left and right feet are always postductal, because they are perfused by the descending aorta. Although the ductus arteriosus usually inserts into the aorta distal to the right subclavian artery, it may be inserted across from or near the left subclavian artery. The left hand may or may not be preductal, because this depends on where the ductus arteriosus inserts into the aorta in relation to the left subclavian branch off the aortic arch.

**Reference:** Karlsen, K.: *The S.T.A.B.L.E. Program*, 5th ed. Park City, Utah, American Academy of Pediatrics, 2006, pp. 79-80.

## CHAPTER 3: NEONATAL RESUSCITATION

1. **(D)** Along with infant condition, interventions and gestational age significantly impact what the Apgar score will be. Interventions such as positive pressure ventilation will change the Apgar score. Differences in gestational age will affect the infant's tone, reflexes, and respirations. The Apgar scoring tool is a numerical objective scoring tool with specific operational definitions. Although the Apgar score is not assessed until 1 minute of age, it could be a guide to further resuscitation if it were not influenced by interventions, gestational age, and infant condition. Ethnicity is not one of the indicators tallied in the Apgar score.

**Reference:** Pappas, B.E., Walker, B.: Neonatal delivery room resuscitation. In Verklan, M., Walden, M. (Eds.): *Core Curriculum for Neonatal Intensive Care Nursing*, 4th ed. St. Louis, Saunders, 2010, pp. 95-97.

2. **(C)** Because the infant is vigorous, intubation is not necessary. The initial steps of resuscitation are required. The infant's airway should be suctioned with a bulb syringe or large-bore catheter and the infant closely observed. Suctioning of the trachea is not indicated. Because the amniotic fluid is meconium stained, positive pressure ventilation is indicated only if the condition of the infant requires it.

**References:** Kattwinkel, J., Bloom, R.S., American Heart Association, American Academy of Pediatrics: (2006). *Textbook of Neonatal Resuscitation*, 5th ed. Dallas, American Heart Association, 2006, pp. 2-7.

Pappas, B.E., Walker, B.: Neonatal delivery room resuscitation. In Verklan, M., Walden, M. (Eds.): *Core Curriculum for Neonatal Intensive Care Nursing*, 4th ed. St. Louis, Saunders, 2010, p. 98.

3. **(D)** The most common presenting signs of a congenital diaphragmatic hernia are barrel chest, scaphoid abdomen, diminished breath sounds, and bowel sounds in the chest cavity. Signs of a left pneumothorax include diminished or absent breath sounds on the left side. Bowel sounds heard in the chest are not characteristic of a pneumothorax. Presenting symptoms of a tracheoesophageal fistula are respiratory distress and excessive salivation. Although meconium aspiration syndrome can present with respiratory distress and a barrel chest, bowel sounds would not be able to be heard in the chest cavity.

**Reference:** Pappas, B.E., Walker, B.: Neonatal delivery room resuscitation. In Verklan, M., Walden, M. (Eds.): *Core Curriculum for Neonatal Intensive Care Nursing*, 4th ed. St. Louis, Saunders, 2010, p. 104.

4. **(C)** The most effective way to address severe respiratory distress related to a diaphragmatic hernia is to intubate the patient and provide direct ventilation to the lungs through the endotracheal tube. Providing oxygen via high-flow nasal cannula, bag-and-mask ventilation, or continuous positive airway pressure to a patient with diaphragmatic hernia will result in gastric dilation and increased difficulty in lung expansion.

**Reference:** Pappas, B.E., Walker, B.: Neonatal delivery room resuscitation. In Verklan, M., Walden, M. (Eds.): *Core Curriculum for Neonatal Intensive Care Nursing*, 4th ed. St. Louis, Saunders, 2010, p. 104.

5. **(D)** Epinephrine is a cardiac stimulant that increases the heart rate and the strength of contractions, causes peripheral vasoconstriction, and increases blood flow through the coronary arteries and the brain.

**Reference:** Pappas, B.E., Walker, B.: Neonatal delivery room resuscitation. In Verklan, M., Walden, M. (Eds.): *Core Curriculum for Neonatal Intensive Care Nursing*, 4th ed. St. Louis, Saunders, 2010, p. 102.

6. **(C)** Pallor despite good oxygenation, a low-normal blood pressure, and diminished tone are all signs of shock. According to the Neonatal Resuscitation Program, the first treatment of shock is to give a 10-ml/kg bolus of a volume expander—generally normal saline. If the infant shows signs of acute blood loss, administration of O-negative blood may be appropriate. Because normal saline is readily available, it is the preferred volume expander for a newly born infant in shock. While starting a maintenance intravenous infusion of 80 ml/kg/day would be standard treatment for an infant admitted to the NICU, treatment of shock would be a higher priority. Because the blood glucose level is 50 mg/dl, the infant is not hypoglycemic. A push of dextrose 10% in water is not necessary.

**Reference:** Pappas, B.E., Walker, B.: Neonatal delivery room resuscitation. In Verklan, M., Walden, M. (Eds.): *Core Curriculum for Neonatal Intensive Care Nursing*, 4th ed. St. Louis, Saunders, 2010, p. 102.

7. **(C)** High-resolution ultrasonography will reveal the presence of pleural effusion and ascites. These findings can significantly impact the respiratory status of the newborn. Amniocentesis allows the chromosomes to be analyzed for fetal defects but will not

significantly impact care at the delivery. The Kleihauer-Betke test is sometimes useful to rule out fetomaternal hemorrhage. It would give an idea of a potential cause for the hydrops but is not useful at delivery. The glycosylated hemoglobin test provides an indication of the mother's glucose control during the pregnancy.

**Reference:** Bradshaw, W.: Gastrointestinal disorders. In Verklan, M., Walden, M. (Eds.): *Core Curriculum for Neonatal Intensive Care Nursing,* 4th ed. St. Louis, Saunders, 2010, p. 634.

8. **(B)** Because of the generalized edema and respiratory distress experienced by most hydropic babies, provision of respiratory support would be the most immediate need. Pericardiocentesis may be necessary if the infant has a pericardial effusion, but this would come after respiratory support. Placement of an umbilical arterial line can occur in the NICU. A bilateral tube thoracotomy may be necessary for pleural effusion, but this would come after respiratory support.

**Reference:** Bradshaw, W.: Gastrointestinal disorders. In Verklan, M., Walden, M. (Eds.): *Core Curriculum for Neonatal Intensive Care Nursing,* 4th ed. St. Louis, Saunders, 2010, p. 635.

9. **(A)** Choanal atresia commonly presents with cyanosis upon delivery that resolves with crying due to the blockage of one or both nares. Although infants with Pierre Robin syndrome present with cyanosis, they also have stridor and apnea. The jaw is characteristically small and pushed back, which results in obstruction of the airway by the tongue. Infants with congenital cardiac disease would become more cyanotic with crying. Respiratory distress syndrome (RDS) is most frequently seen in premature infants. In addition to cyanosis, infants with RDS normally have other signs of respiratory distress such as retractions and flaring.

**Reference:** Pappas, B.E., Walker, B.: Neonatal delivery room resuscitation. In Verklan, M., Walden, M. (Eds.): *Core Curriculum for Neonatal Intensive Care Nursing,* 4th ed. St. Louis, Saunders, 2010, p. 103.

10. **(B)** Because there is no chest rise, breath sounds are heard over the stomach, and the infant has never responded to the positive pressure ventilation via the endotracheal tube, one must assume that the endotracheal is in the wrong position—most likely in the esophagus. If the tube were on the carina, there might be no appreciable sign of this. The infant would likely become pink, chest rise would be visible, and breath sounds would be audible. In many situations, the only way this would be noticed would be through indications on the confirmatory radiograph and the finding of a higher tip-to-lip measurement than expected. If the tube were in the correct position, the infant would have a positive response to the positive pressure ventilation. The color would improve and chest rise would be visible. Generally air would not be heard over the stomach. In addition, if a $CO_2$ detector were used, it would show color change. If the tube were in the right mainstem bronchus, the infant's color would show no improvement. Breath sounds would be diminished or absent over the left side of the chest and not audible over the stomach.

**Reference:** Kattwinkel, J., Bloom, R.S., American Heart Association, American Academy of Pediatrics: *Textbook of Neonatal Resuscitation,* 5th ed. Dallas, American Heart Association, 2006, pp. 5-24.

## CHAPTER 4: PHYSICAL ASSESSMENT

1. **(A)** Checking the infant's hips is most likely to elicit crying and should be left until the last step of the examination. Reflexes are tested as the examiner moves through the head-to-toe examination. Pulses are difficult to palpate if the infant is crying and therefore should be left until last. The spinal examination is less likely to elicit crying and therefore can be performed before checking the hips.

**Reference:** Honeyfield, M.A.: Principles of physical assessment. In Tappero, E.P., Honeyfield, M.A. (Eds.): *Physical Assessment of the Newborn: A Comprehensive Approach to the Art of Physical Examination,* 4th ed. Santa Rosa, Calif., NICU Ink, 2009, pp. 1-8.

2. **(D)** Magnesium sulfate crosses the placenta and may cause hypermagnesemia. Signs of elevated serum magnesium include respiratory depression, hypotonia, poor suck, weakness, and lethargy. Magnesium does not interfere with red cell production and does not cause red blood cell hemolysis. Magnesium depresses rather than exaggerates deep tendon reflexes. Diminished deep tendon reflexes would be an expected finding in a newborn whose mother received magnesium sulfate. Hypernatremia in newborns usually results from inadequate fluid intake leading to decreased plasma fluid volume. Sodium and fluid volume are not affected by hypermagnesemia. Magnesium does not alter blood glucose levels.

**Reference:** Broussard, A.B., Hurst, H.M.: Antepartum-intrapartum complications. In Verklan, M.T., Walden, M. (Eds.): *Core Curriculum for Neonatal Intensive Care Nursing,* 4th ed. St. Louis, Saunders, 2010, pp. 20-40.

3. **(D)** Subgaleal hemorrhage occurs when blood vessels below the aponeurotic membrane tear, which allows a large amount of blood to collect in the connective tissue at the back of the head and in the neck. Subgaleal hemorrhages occur most commonly after vacuum- or forceps-assisted deliveries. Symptoms include a fluctuant mass at the back of the head that increases in size after delivery. There are two types of skull fractures in newborns: linear and depressed. Linear skull fractures are usually asymptomatic, whereas depressed skull fractures present as an indentation that does not cross the suture line. A cephalohematoma results from bleeding under the periosteal lining of the skull. It increases in size after birth but is bounded by suture lines and feels firm to the touch. Subdural hematoma is an intracranial bleed that presents with neurologic signs such as seizures, decreased level of consciousness, and asymmetry of motor function.

**Reference:** Lynam, L., Verklan, M.T.: Neurologic disorders. In Verklan, M.T., Walden, M. (Eds.): *Core Curriculum for Neonatal Intensive Care Nursing,* 4th ed. St. Louis, Saunders, 2010, pp. 749-781.

4. **(B)** The infant's size in comparison to gestational age indicates that the infant is small for gestational age

(SGA). The incidence of hypoglycemia in SGA infants is approximately 15%. This occurs because SGA infants lack the glycogen stores necessary for maintaining blood glucose levels after birth. Some SGA babies may be polycythemic because of chronic intrauterine hypoxia. Anemia is not a risk factor. Prematurity and lung disease requiring mechanical ventilation and supplemental oxygen are risk factors for chronic lung disease. Because growth restriction enhances fetal lung maturity, the risk of chronic lung disease is reduced. Intrauterine growth restriction has been shown to enhance fetal lung maturity. The risk of respiratory distress syndrome is lower in an SGA infant than in an appropriately sized infant of the same gestational age.

**Reference:** Trotter, C.W.: Gestational age assessment. In Tappero, E.P., Honeyfield, M.A. (Eds.): *Physical Assessment of the Newborn: A Comprehensive Approach to the Art of Physical Examination*, 4th ed. Santa Rosa, Calif., NICU Ink, 2009, pp. 21-39.

5. **(C)** Intrauterine growth restriction (IUGR) has traditionally been described as symmetric (non–head sparing) and asymmetric (head sparing), with asymmetric the most common. In symmetric IUGR, the head and length are at the same or similar percentile as the weight on the growth curve. At 34 weeks, an infant exceeding the 90th percentile, the definition of *large for gestational age*, would weigh more than 2800 g. The 10th percentile for 34 weeks' gestation is 1600 g; therefore, an infant of 1500 g would not be appropriately grown. With asymmetric growth restriction, brain growth is preserved, which results in a head circumference in the normal range and a weight that falls below the third percentile for gestational age.

**Reference:** Trotter, C.W.: Gestational age assessment. In Tappero, E.P., Honeyfield, M.A. (Eds.): *Physical Assessment of the Newborn: A Comprehensive Approach to the Art of Physical Examination*, 4th ed. Santa Rosa, Calif., NICU Ink, 2009, pp. 21-39.

6. **(A)** Meconium aspiration is more common in postterm infants. Low Apgar scores reflect intrauterine hypoxia, which is associated with meconium aspiration. Radiographic findings in meconium aspiration include hyperinflation and patchy infiltrates. Infants with respiratory distress syndrome present at birth or within hours with clinical signs of respiratory distress that include tachypnea, grunting, retractions, and cyanosis accompanied by increasing oxygen requirements. The chest radiograph is characterized by atelectasis, air bronchograms, and diffuse granular infiltrates that often progresses to severe bilateral opacity. Infants with congenital heart disease do not usually initially demonstrate respiratory distress. Transient tachypnea is more common in late preterm infants and term infants born by cesarean section. Infants with transient tachypnea of the newborn often have chest radiographic findings that include overexpansion, haziness, increased vascular markings, and fluid in the fissure.

**Reference:** Askin, D.F.: Respiratory distress. In Verklan, M.T., Walden, M. (Eds.): *Core Curriculum for Neonatal Intensive Care Nursing*, 4th ed. St. Louis, Saunders, 2010, pp. 453-483.

7. **(B)** Down syndrome, or trisomy 21, is the most common chromosomal aberration recognized at birth.

Among the features associated with Down syndrome are Brushfield spots, small ears, simian creases, excess skin at the nape of the neck, upslanting palpebral fissures, hypotonia, large protruding tongue, and cardiac anomalies. Features of trisomy 18 include a prominent occiput, low-set malformed ears, small eyes and jaw, clenched hands with overlapping fingers, and rocker-bottom feet. Infants with Turner syndrome, which occurs in phenotypic females, are usually small for gestational age with a broad chest, widely spaced nipples, edema of the extremities, and a short neck. Klinefelter syndrome occurs in males and results in long limbs, elbow dysplasia, and clinodactyly involving the fifth finger. Hypospadias, hypogonadism, and cryptorchidism are usually present.

**Reference:** Sterk, L.: Congenital anomalies. In Verklan, M.T., Walden, M. (Eds.): *Core Curriculum for Neonatal Intensive Care Nursing*, 4th ed. St. Louis, Saunders, 2010, pp. 782-812.

8. **(B)** Infants with congenital diaphragmatic hernia typically present with dramatic cyanosis and severe respiratory distress secondary to pulmonary hypoplasia. Because the abdominal viscera are dislocated through a defect into the chest, the abdominal contour can appear scaphoid. Breath sounds are diminished or absent, and because the mediastinal structures have been displaced, the heart sounds are heard in the right chest. Congenital diaphragmatic hernia occurs more frequently on the left side, causing a displacement of structures to the right side of the chest. A large or tension pneumothorax can cause a shift in heart sounds away from the affected side as well as unilaterally decreased breath sounds. The shape of the abdomen is unaffected. Depending on the amount of oxygenated blood moving into the aorta, cyanotic heart disease may result in significant cyanosis. Breath sounds are unaffected, as is the shape of the abdomen. Severe respiratory distress syndrome is uncommon in term infants and is not associated with alterations in the shape of the abdomen.

**References:** Askin, D.F.: Respiratory distress. In Verklan, M.T., Walden, M. (Eds.): *Core Curriculum for Neonatal Intensive Care Nursing*, 4th ed. St. Louis, Saunders, 2010, pp. 453-483.

Bradshaw, W.T.: Gastrointestinal disorders. In Verklan, M.T., Walden, M. (Eds.): *Core Curriculum for Neonatal Intensive Care Nursing*, 4th ed. St. Louis, Saunders, 2010, pp. 589-637.

9. **(C)** The infant's signs and symptoms are consistent with hydrops. Immune hydrops results from the destruction of fetal red blood cells by maternal antibodies (usually Rhesus or Rh) that cross the placenta. Parvovirus infection results in nonimmune hydrops because it also causes hemolysis of fetal red cells leading to the development of capillary leak and edema. Maternal alcohol ingestion during pregnancy results in growth and central nervous system abnormalities but has not been reported to cause hydrops. *HELLP syndrome* refers to a maternal condition causing low platelets and elevated liver enzyme levels. It does not result in fetal hydrops. In the newborn, infection with group B streptococcus can cause respiratory distress, shock, or meningitis. Pleural effusions may be seen in group B streptococcus disease, but ascites and generalized edema are not reported.

**Reference:** Bradshaw, W.T.: Gastrointestinal disorders. In Verklan, M.T., Walden, M. (Eds.): *Core Curriculum for Neonatal Intensive Care Nursing,* 4th ed. St. Louis, Saunders, 2010, pp. 589-637.

10. **(D)** Transposition of the great vessels occurs when septation and migration of the truncus arteriosus is interrupted during development. As a result, the aorta arises from the right ventricle and the pulmonary artery arises from the left ventricle. Marked cyanosis is a presenting feature of transposition, because the aorta carries deoxygenated blood from the right ventricle to the systemic circulation. Atrial septal defects (ASDs) account for 5% to 10% of all congenital heart defects and are usually asymptomatic at birth. A soft systolic ejection murmur may be audible, but cyanosis does not occur with an ASD. Patent ductus arteriosus is an acyanotic heart defect resulting from a failure of the ductus arteriosus to close after birth. Simple ventricular septal defect (VSD) is the single most common congenital heart malformation, accounting for about 20% to 25% of all cases of congenital cardiac anomalies. Small VSDs are usually asymptomatic at birth, whereas with moderate to larger defects, left-to-right shunting eventually leads to congestive heart failure. Cyanosis is not present in the newborn period.

**Reference:** Wright Lott, J.W.: Cardiovascular system. In Kenner, C.A., Wright Lott, J.W. (Eds.): *Comprehensive Neonatal Care: An Interdisciplinary Approach.* St. Louis, Saunders, 2007, pp. 32-64.

11. **(A)** Weak pulses signal conditions of vascular collapse, such as sepsis, hypovolemic shock, or congestive heart failure. Decreased pulses in the lower extremities with normal pulses in the upper extremities result from obstruction to aortic flow. The differential diagnosis starts with coarctation of the aorta and includes aortic or femoral thrombosis or spasm. Although a small patent ductus arteriosus may be symptomatic, larger defects allow shunting of blood from the aorta into the pulmonary system, which causes symptoms of pulmonary edema and congestive heart failure. Following birth, right ventricular pressures are higher than those on the left side of the heart. In the presence of a ventricular septal defect, blood is initially shunted from right to left. As the pulmonary pressures drop after birth, the flow of blood is reversed, which leads to symptoms of congestive heart failure. Decreased femoral pulses are not part of the initial presentation. Persistent pulmonary hypertension occurs when the pressure in the pulmonary vasculature fails to drop after birth. This allows the foramen ovale and ductus arteriosus to remain patent, which results in the shunting of blood away from the lungs. Hypoxia and respiratory distress result. Although systemic perfusion is affected, femoral pulses do not differ significantly from brachial pulses.

**Reference:** Wright Lott, J.W.: Cardiovascular system. In Kenner, C.A., Wright Lott, J.W. (Eds.): *Comprehensive Neonatal Care: An Interdisciplinary Approach.* St. Louis, Saunders, 2007, pp. 32-64.

12. **(B)** *Candida albicans* infection, a common fungal skin disorder, is usually found in the groin area. A moist rash with satellite pustules and areas of skin breakdown are common presenting signs. Herpes simplex infections in the newborn present in one of three patterns: skin and eye findings, central nervous system disease, and systemic infection. A herpes skin rash presents as a cluster of vesicles or pustules on an erythematous base. Ulcerated and crusting lesions are also common. Scalded skin syndrome, caused by a staphylococcal infection, appears as a generalized area of erythema followed by peeling of the epidermis. Erythema toxicum is a benign rash found in up to 70% of newborns. It presents as small white or yellow papules on a reddened base. The rash often fades and reappears on a different part of the body.

**Reference:** Witt, C.L.: Skin assessment. In Tappero, E.P., Honeyfield, M.A. (Eds.): *Physical Assessment of the Newborn: A Comprehensive Approach to the Art of Physical Examination,* 4th ed. Santa Rosa, Calif., NICU Ink, 2009, pp. 41-55.

13. **(B)** Dermal sinuses, markers for spina bifida, can occur anywhere along the spine but are most common in the lumbar region of the spine. The sacral region of the spine is a common location for dimples but a less common location for dermal sinuses. Dermal sinuses are not commonly found over the cervical or thoracic spine.

**Reference:** Heaberlin, P.D.: Neurologic assessment. In Tappero, E.P., Honeyfield, M.A. (Eds.): *Physical Assessment of the Newborn: A Comprehensive Approach to the Art of Physical Examination,* 4th ed. Santa Rosa, Calif., NICU Ink, 2009, p. 177.

14. **(B)** A cephalohematoma is a collection of blood under the periosteum. Most commonly found over the parietal or occipital bones, a cephalohematoma is bounded by suture lines. It is usually present at birth but increases in size over the first few hours following delivery. Resolution is usually complete but may take weeks to months. An increased risk of jaundice is the only clinical consideration. Skull fractures are rare in newborns. When present, they may be linear or depressed. Linear fractures are often asymptomatic, whereas with depressed fractures, an indentation over the affected bone may be palpated. Caput succedaneum is commonly seen after vaginal delivery, causes scalp edema, crosses cranial suture lines, and gives the head an elongated shape. It usually resolves during the first few days of life. A subdural hematoma is a collection of blood in the subdural space within the cranium. Presentation is one of altered tone, altered alertness, or seizures.

**Reference:** Johnson, P.: Head, ears, mouth and neck. In Tappero, E.P., Honeyfield, M.A. (Eds.): *Physical Assessment of the Newborn: A Comprehensive Approach to the Art of Physical Examination,* 4th ed. Santa Rosa, Calif., NICU Ink, 2009, pp. 57-74.

15. **(D)** The harlequin color change or harlequin sign is thought to result from an imbalance in the autonomic nervous system that disrupts blood flow to the cutaneous vasculature. It occurs on the dependent side of the body and is rarely seen after 10 days of life. It is a benign finding that lasts from a few seconds to 30 minutes and usually reverses when the infant's position is changed. Cold stress or hypothermia results in pallor in the extremities or a mottled appearance of the skin. Hypovolemia results in generalized pallor that is

not isolated to one side of the body. Overstimulation may cause the infant to have generalized pallor.

**Reference:** Blackburn, S.T.: *Maternal, Fetal, and Neonatal Physiology: A Clinical Perspective.* St. Louis, Saunders, 2007, p. 531.

16. **(C)** The landmarks for the tricuspid valve are the fourth intercostal space and the left sternal angle. The pulmonic valve is best heard at the second intercostal space, left sternal angle. The aortic valve is best heard at the second intercostal space, right sternal angle. The mitral area is found at the fifth intercostal space, mid-clavicular line.

**Reference:** Vargo, L.: Cardiovascular assessment. In Tappero, E.P., Honeyfield, M.A. (Eds.): *Physical Assessment of the Newborn: A Comprehensive Approach to the Art of Physical Examination,* 4th ed. Santa Rosa, Calif., NICU Ink, 2009, pp. 87-103.

17. **(A)** Risk factors for late-onset sepsis in premature infants include the presence of a central line or other invasive devices, and the use of total parenteral nutrition. Clinical signs of infection include temperature instability, lethargy, poor tone, respiratory distress, and glucose instability. A pneumothorax or air leakage into the pleural cavity from a ruptured alveolus results in increased respiratory distress, cyanosis, decreased oxygen saturation, tachycardia, and diminished breath sounds on the affected side. If large, it may also shift the apex of the heart away from the affected side. Systemic signs such as temperature instability are not found with a pneumothorax. Failure of the ductus arteriosus to close is common in low birth weight infants. As the initial period of respiratory distress resolves and pulmonary artery pressures decrease, blood is allowed to flow from the aorta across the ductus to the pulmonary arteries and into the lungs. This increased blood flow results in tachypnea, respiratory distress, and signs of congestive heart failure. Poor tone, hyperglycemia, and temperature instability are not common findings in infants with a patient ductus arteriosus. Clinical manifestations of acute severe intraventricular hemorrhage can include seizures, metabolic acidosis, bulging fontanelle, temperature instability, lethargy, coma, and hypotension. Often there is an unexpectedly low hematocrit or a hematocrit that does not rise as expected after transfusion, and an abnormally "tight" popliteal angle.

**Reference:** Lott, J.W.: Immunology and infectious disease. In Verklan, M.T., Walden, M. (Eds.): *Core Curriculum for Neonatal Intensive Care Nursing,* 4th ed. St. Louis, Saunders, 2010, pp. 694-723.

18. **(B)** Fracture of the clavicles is the most common fracture associated with delivery. An infant with shoulder dystocia is at increased risk of fracturing the clavicle. Bell palsy results from damage to the facial nerve caused by pressing against the maternal pelvis. Phrenic nerve paralysis may be unilateral or bilateral. Unilateral damage, usually on the right side, is more common. Symptoms include respiratory distress. Fracture of the cervical vertebrae would affect movement in all limbs and may also impact breathing.

**Reference:** Askin, D.F.: Chest assessment. Tappero, E.P., Honeyfield, M.A. (Eds.): *Physical Assessment of the Newborn: A Comprehensive Approach to the Art of Physical Examination,* 4th ed. Santa Rosa, Calif., NICU Ink, 2009, p. 84.

19. **(A)** First published in 1979 and modified in 1991, the Ballard assessment uses six physiologic and six neuromuscular criteria to estimate gestational age. The Finnegan score and the Neonatal Abstinence Scoring System are two tools used to quantify the behaviors associated with neonatal narcotic withdrawal. Several tools have been developed to assess the behavioral characteristics of the preterm infant, including the Newborn Behavioral Assessment Scale and the Assessment of Preterm Infant Behavior. In 1967, Battaglia and Lubchenko used length, weight, and head circumference percentiles to construct intrauterine growth charts. These charts defined criteria for identifying large-for-gestational-age, appropriate-for-gestational-age, and small-for-gestational-age infants.

**Reference:** Trotter, C.W.: Gestational age assessment. In Tappero, E.P., Honeyfield, M.A. (Eds.): *Physical Assessment of the Newborn: A Comprehensive Approach to the Art of Physical Examination,* 4th ed. Santa Rosa, Calif., NICU Ink, 2009, pp. 21-39.

20. **(C)** Café au lait spots, more common in black infants, are flat macules that are tan or light brown. They are usually less than 3 cm in diameter. When six or more lesions of larger than 0.5 cm are present, there is an increased risk of neurofibromatosis. Salmon patches, a type of hemangioma, are usually found at the back of the neck, over the eyelids, or on the glabella. Mongolian spots are gray-blue in appearance and are usually found over the buttocks and lower back. These lesions are more common in black, Asian, and Native American infants. Congenital melanocytic nevi are brown to black pigmented lesions that may be macular or plaquelike in appearance.

**Reference:** Blackburn, S.T.: *Maternal, Fetal, and Neonatal Physiology: A Clinical Perspective.* St. Louis, Saunders, 2007, p. 532.

21. **(B)** As a result of central nervous system immaturity, seizures in neonates are more subtle than those seen in children and adults. Neonatal seizures are more likely to arise from areas of the brain that are more mature (temporal lobe, limbic area). These areas initiate behaviors such as chewing, sucking, and ocular movements, behaviors common in subtle seizures. Jerky movements of the limbs are frequently seen in normal newborns, but when they occur in a repetitive and rhythmic pattern, are more likely to represent a clonic seizure. Jitteriness or tremulous movements that cease with flexion are common in infants and can be confused with seizure activity. Normal newborns, especially premature infants, startle easily and respond with disorganized or jerky movements.

**Reference:** Blackburn, S.T.: *Maternal, Fetal, and Neonatal Physiology: A Clinical Perspective.* St. Louis, Saunders, 2007, p. 587.

22. **(B)** Hypoxic injury (hypoxic-ischemic encephalopathy, or HIE) is the most common cause of neonatal seizures. Risk factors for HIE include birth after due date, low Apgar scores, and abnormal fetal heart rate patterns. The majority of seizures secondary to hypoxic injury begin within 6 to 12 hours after delivery. Although a serum sodium level of 133 mEq/L is low, this level is unlikely to precipitate a seizure. Risk factors for subdural hemorrhage include large fetal

head, vaginal breech delivery, malpresentation, and forceps or vacuum extraction. Subdural hematomas are usually asymptomatic in the first 24 hours. Intraventricular hemorrhages (IVH) are uncommon in post-mature infants. Seizures are a late sign of an IVH.

**Reference:** Lynam, L., Verklan, T.: Neurologic disorders. In Verklan, M.T., Walden, M. (Eds.): *Core Curriculum for Neonatal Intensive Care Nursing,* 4th ed. St. Louis, Saunders, 2010, pp. 748-781.

23. **(D)** The optimal test for postural tone is the pull-to-sit maneuver. In a normal response, the newborn contracts the shoulder and arm muscles and flexes the neck. Turning the head from side to side is useful in assessing range of motion in the neck but does not address postural tone. Stimulating a newborn's palm should elicit the grasp reflex. An intact grasp reflex is one indication of a healthy brachial plexus. Touching the newborn's feet to a firm surface should result in the infant's taking a step. The stepping reflex is most active after 72 hours of age.

**Reference:** Heaberlin, P.D.: Neurologic assessment. In Tappero, E.P., Honeyfield, M.A. (Eds.): *Physical Assessment of the Newborn: A Comprehensive Approach to the Art of Physical Examination,* 4th ed. Santa Rosa, Calif., NICU Ink, 2009, pp. 153-183.

24. **(A)** Signs of a tension pneumothorax include decreased breath sounds on the affected side, a shift in the heart sounds, increasing respiratory distress, and hypoxia. Severe respiratory distress is consistent with pulmonary hypoplasia but is more likely to be present at birth. A pneumothorax may occur as a result of pulmonary hypoplasia. When inserted too deeply, the endotracheal tube is most likely to pass into the right mainstem bronchus, which results in louder breath sounds on the right and diminished sounds on the left. Congenital cystic adenomatoid malformation (CCAM) may be asymptomatic at birth or cause some degree of respiratory distress. Acute deterioration in respiratory status is not an expected finding in CCAM.

**Reference:** Askin, D.F.: Respiratory distress. In Verklan, M.T., Walden, M. (Eds.): *Core Curriculum for Neonatal Intensive Care Nursing.* St. Louis, Saunders, 2010, pp. 453-483.

25. **(D)** The incidence of tracheoesophageal fistulas is estimated to be 1 in 1000 to 2500 live births. Of the five types of esophageal malformations, esophageal atresia with a tracheal fistula connecting to the lower esophagus is most common. A history of polyhydramnios, drooling, excessive oral secretions, and choking with feeding is common. Pyloric stenosis presents with projectile vomiting after feeding. An olive-sized mass may be palpated in the epigastric region. Symptoms usually begin after 3 weeks of age. Regurgitation after feeds is common in newborn infants. Pathologic reflux resulting in respiratory distress or esophagitis is more likely in premature infants. Polyhydramnios and excessive oral secretions are not findings in reflux. Duodenal atresia occurs in 1 per 7000 live births, and a history of polyhydramnios is present. Presentation at birth is more likely to include abdominal distention and bilious vomiting.

**Reference:** Bradshaw, W.T.: Gastrointestinal disorders. In Verklan, M.T., Walden, M. (Eds.): *Core Curriculum for Neonatal*

*Intensive Care Nursing,* 4th ed. St. Louis, Saunders, 2010, pp. 589-637.

26. **(D)** During pregnancy, antilupus antibodies cross the placenta resulting in neonatal lupus erythematous (NLE), which is characterized by congenital heart block, a cutaneous lupus rash, and pancytopenia. These antibodies persist in the neonatal circulation for several weeks after delivery, followed by resolution of the NLE. Maternal diabetes predisposes the fetus and newborn to cardiomyopathy. Sustained bradycardia is not a feature of cardiomyopathy. Preeclampsia is sometimes treated with magnesium sulfate, which can cause respiratory depression in the newborn. Chorioamnionitis usually presents with an increased heart rate and decreased heart rate variability.

**Reference:** Blackburn, S.T.: *Maternal, Fetal, and Neonatal Physiology: A Clinical Perspective.* St. Louis, Saunders, 2007, p. 489.

27. **(D)** Talipes equinovarus is a developmental deformity of the hindfoot. Commonly known as *clubfoot,* talipes equinovarus is bilateral in 50% of cases, with males being affected twice as often as females. The sole of the foot is turned medially and inverted, with varus deformity of the hindfoot and equinus of the ankle. The deformity can be positional or structural, and radiographs are helpful in identifying a bony defect. Genu recurvatum, or congenital hyperextension of the knee, may result from frank breech positioning. Webbing of the fingers or toes is referred to as *syndactyly.* External rotation, or knock-knee, usually presents in older children.

**Reference:** Tappero, E.: Musculoskeletal assessment. In Tappero, E.P., Honeyfield, M.A. (Eds.): *Physical Assessment of the Newborn: A Comprehensive Approach to the Art of Physical Examination,* 4th ed. Santa Rosa, Calif., NICU Ink, 2009, pp. 133-157.

28. **(A)** The presence of peritoneal fluid in the scrotum results in the formation of a hydrocele. The scrotum is nontender but swollen and appears translucent when transilluminated. The testes can be felt in the scrotal sac. Inguinal hernias, more common in premature infants, result when one or more loops of intestine herniate through the processus vaginalis. In the presence of a hernia, crepitus may be felt in the scrotal sac, and it is impossible to feel the entire perimeter of the testes. The scrotal sac does not transilluminate. Cryptorchidism results from failure of one or both testes to descend into the scrotum and presents as a hypoplastic or empty scrotal sac. Testicular torsion or twisting of the testes presents as a hard, swollen scrotum that is red or blue in appearance.

**Reference:** Cavaliere, T.A.: Genitourinary assessment. In Tappero, E.P., Honeyfield, M.A. (Eds.): *Physical Assessment of the Newborn: A Comprehensive Approach to the Art of Physical Examination,* 4th ed. Santa Rosa, Calif., NICU Ink, 2009, pp. 115-132.

29. **(A)** Erb palsy results when the brachial plexus is injured at C5 or C6. Upper-arm paralysis results in the arm being adducted and internally rotated with pronation of the forearm and flexion of the wrist. The Moro reflex is absent on the affected side. Bell palsy results from compression of the facial nerve and presents with facial drooping. Neonatal stroke most commonly

presents with seizures and may affect alertness and global tone. Absence of the radius occurs more often in males than in females and may be found in infants with VACTERAL association (*v*ertebral, *a*nal, *c*ardiovascular, *t*racheal, *e*sophageal, *r*enal, and *l*imb abnormalities). The hand and wrist are deviated 90 degrees or more, and the forearm is shortened and may be bowed.

**Reference:** Tappero, E.: Musculoskeletal assessment. In Tappero, E.P., Honeyfield, M.A. (Eds.): *Physical Assessment of the Newborn: A Comprehensive Approach to the Art of Physical Examination,* 4th ed. Santa Rosa, Calif., NICU Ink, 2009, pp. 133-157.

30. **(C)** Occurring at a rate of 1 in 800 live births, developmental dysplasia of the hip (DDH) is more common in infants born in frank breech position. DDH occurs more often in females (80% of cases). Oligohydramnios, which limits fetal movement, increases the risk of DDH; polyhydramnios does not limit fetal movement. Genetically the risk of DDH is higher in white than in black newborns.

**References:** Sterk, L.: Congenital anomalies. In Verklan, M.T., Walden, M. (Eds.): *Core Curriculum for Neonatal Intensive Care Nursing,* 4th ed. St. Louis, Saunders, 2010, pp. 782-812.

McCarthy, J.J.: Developmental dysplasia of the Hip. Emedicine. 2009. Available from http://emedicine.medscape.com/article/1248135-overview.

31. **(D)** The anterior fontanelle is normally 0.6 to 3.6 cm across in white infants and 1.4 to 4.7 cm in black newborns. A large fontanelle is a finding in congenital hypothyroidism. Craniosynostosis results from premature fusion of one or more of the sutures in the skull. Depending on which bones are affected, the skull assumes an abnormal shape. Features of Turner syndrome include webbing of the neck and lymphedema of the extremities. A large fontanelle is not a reported association. Maternal diabetes may result in fetal macrosomia and a large head. The head size is usually proportionate to the body size.

**Reference:** Johnson, C.B.: Head, eyes, ears, nose, mouth, and neck assessment. In Tappero, E.P., Honeyfield, M.A. (Eds.): *Physical Assessment of the Newborn: A Comprehensive Approach to the Art of Physical Examination,* 4th ed. Santa Rosa, Calif., NICU Ink, 2009, pp. 57-74.

32. **(A)** Malrotation, or volvulus, must be urgently ruled out in any infant presenting with bilious emesis. A volvulus results when the bowel is rotated and wrapped around the mesentery, which obstructs the flow of blood to the bowel. Pyloric stenosis presents with an olive-shaped mass in the epigastric region of the abdomen. Projectile nonbilious vomiting and visible peristaltic waves are also present. Surgical correction is required but not emergent. Duodenal atresia or obstruction of the duodenum presents with abdominal distention and bilious emesis. It is not a surgical emergency. The absence of ganglion cells, usually in the large bowel (Hirschsprung disease), results in diminished peristalsis, abdominal distention, and failure to pass meconium.

**Reference:** Goodwin, P.: Gastrointestinal assessment. In Tappero, E.P., Honeyfield, M.A. (Eds.): *Physical Assessment of the Newborn: A Comprehensive Approach to the Art of Physical Examination,* 4th ed. Santa Rosa, Calif., NICU Ink, 2009, pp. 105-114.

33. **(B)** Turner syndrome occurs in 1 in 2500 live-born female infants. The absence of the second X chromosome (45, X) results in widely spaced nipples, a short webbed neck, and edema of the hands and feet. Trisomy 13 occurs in 1 in 5000 births. Findings include cleft lip, polydactyly, microphthalmia, and microcephaly. DiGeorge syndrome, a 22q11 chromosomal deletion, includes physical findings of small abnormally shaped ears, dysmorphic facial features, and congenital heart defects. Features of trisomy 21 (Down syndrome) include hypotonia, excessive skin at the back of the neck, upturned palpebral fissures, simian crease, and a wide space between the first and second toes.

**Reference:** Bennett, M., Meier, S.: Assessment of the dysmorphic Infant. In Tappero, E.P., Honeyfield, M.A. (Eds.): *Physical Assessment of the Newborn: A Comprehensive Approach to the Art of Physical Examination,* 4th ed. Santa Rosa, Calif., NICU Ink, 2009, pp. 201-217.

34. **(A)** Heroin exposure in pregnancy results in typical symptoms of narcotic withdrawal, usually beginning about 48 hours after delivery. Symptoms of neonatal abstinence syndrome include increased tone and reflexes, tremors, tachypnea, yawning, sneezing, nasal stuffiness, poor feeding, and vomiting. In newborns, the onset of alcohol withdrawal is usually seen between birth and 12 hours of age and includes hypertonia, tremors, and a poor feeding pattern. Excessive crying and exaggerated sucking is reported. Restlessness, irritability, and tremors have been described in cocaine-exposed newborns. These effects are thought to be direct effects of the drug rather than signs of withdrawal. After an initial period of hyperalertness, infants often become drowsy or lethargic. Reported effects of selective serotonin reuptake inhibitors on newborns include seizures, respiratory distress, hypoglycemia, and problems with temperature regulation.

**Reference:** Pitts, K.: Perinatal substance abuse. In Verklan, M.T., Walden, M. (Eds.): *Core Curriculum for Neonatal Intensive Care Nursing,* 4th ed. St. Louis, Saunders, 2010, pp. 41-71.

35. **(D)** Low-set ears are found in conjunction with a number of genetic syndromes. If a line drawn toward the ear from the inner canthus through to the outer canthus of the eye falls above the insertion of the ear, the ear is low set. The size and shape of the nose may vary according to the infant's size and race. It is not used to determine correct ear position. The orientation of the eyebrow is not relevant in determining ear position. A line from the outer eye to the mastoid process normally bisects the lower portion of the ear.

**Reference:** Johnson, C.B.: Head, eyes, ears, nose, mouth, and neck assessment. In Tappero, E.P., Honeyfield, M.A. (Eds.): *Physical Assessment of the Newborn: A Comprehensive Approach to the Art of Physical Examination,* 4th ed. Santa Rosa, Calif., NICU Ink, 2009, pp. 57-74.

36. **(A)** A diffuse petechial rash is suggestive of thrombocytopenia. A low platelet count would be an expected finding. If internal bleeding accompanies petechiae, a low hematocrit may result, but it would not cause the petechial rash. When significant blood loss accompanies thrombocytopenia, anemia may result but is not a contributing factor. Low white blood

cell counts are found in newborns with infection, but infection is not a common cause of petechiae.

**Reference:** Furdon, S.A., Benjamin, K.: Physical assessment. In Verklan, M.T., Walden, M. (Eds.): *Core Curriculum for Neonatal Intensive Care Nursing,* 4th ed. St. Louis, Saunders, 2010, pp. 120-155.

37. **(C)** The rash seen in skin infections caused by the herpes simplex virus is often vesicular and may occur first over the area of the body presenting at birth. Disruption of skin integrity provides a portal of entry for the virus. *Candida* skin infection usually occurs in the diaper area and is characterized by white or yellow pustules on an erythematous base. *Klebsiella*, a waterborne pathogen, usually causes pneumonia and is not implicated in newborn skin infections. *Staphylococcus aureus* causes omphalitis abscesses, impetigo, and scalded skin infections in the newborn. Presenting signs include erythema, warmth, tenderness, or bullous lesions. When present, blisters usually begin in the groin area.

**Reference:** Witt, C.L.: Neonatal dermatology. In Verklan, M.T., Walden, M. (Eds.): *Core Curriculum for Neonatal Intensive Care Nursing,* 4th ed. St. Louis, Saunders, 2010, pp. 813-831.

38. **(D)** Port-wine stains in infants with Sturge-Weber syndrome are confined to the area of the face innervated by the trigeminal nerve, including the eyes and nose. Vascular lesions on the neck are most commonly nevus simplex, or "stork bites." These lesions usually fade with time and have no associated pathology. Port-wine stains can occur on any part of the body, but only those on the face are markers for Sturge-Weber syndrome. Vascular birthmarks on the buttocks are usually mongolian spots, bluish purple lesions resembling bruises.

**Reference:** Witt, C.L.: Neonatal dermatology. In Verklan, M.T., Walden, M. (Eds.): *Core Curriculum for Neonatal Intensive Care Nursing,* 4th ed. St. Louis, Saunders, 2010, pp. 813-831.

39. **(A)** Infants with trisomy 18 have a third copy of chromosome 18. The clinical features include syndactyly, rocker-bottom feet, a narrow pelvis, clenched fists with overlapping fingers, and a short sternum. Infants with trisomy 21, or Down syndrome, have a variety of physical findings, including a fat pad at the back of the neck, epicanthal folds, almond-shaped eyes, and a simian crease. DiGeorge syndrome, or velocardiofacial syndrome, results from a 22q11 deletion. These infants usually have microcephaly, cleft palate, a long face with a prominent nose, and hyperextensible fingers. Six types of osteogenesis imperfecta (OI) have been identified, with effects ranging from macrocephaly and altered dentition to severe growth deficiency with kyphoscoliosis and limb deformities. Clenched hands and rocker-bottom feet are not reported in OI.

**Reference:** Sterk, L.: Congenital anomalies. In Verklan, M.T., Walden, M. (Eds.): *Core Curriculum for Neonatal Intensive Care Nursing,* 4th ed. St. Louis, Saunders, 2010, pp. 782-812.

40. **(C)** Although only 5% to 10% of infants with congenital cytomegalovirus (CMV) infection are symptomatic at birth, chorioretinitis is the single most common symptom. Infants with congenital CMV infection are usually small for gestational age rather than macrosomic. Microphthalmia is a characteristic finding in congenital rubella but is not reported in CMV infection. Pleural effusions are a common manifestation of congenital parvovirus infection, which causes anemia that results in the development of non-immune hydrops.

**Reference:** Askin, D.F., Diehl-Jones, W.: Ophthalmologic and auditory disorders. In Verklan, M.T., Walden, M. (Eds.): *Core Curriculum for Neonatal Intensive Care Nursing,* 4th ed. St. Louis, Saunders, 2010, pp. 832-849.

41. **(B)** Among infants with omphalocele, 45% to 55% have accompanying anomalies. Fifty percent of these anomalies involve the heart and 40% involve the neural tube. Only 10% to 15% of infants with gastroschisis have associated anomalies. These usually involve the gastrointestinal system. The incidence of pyloric stenosis is 3 in 1000 live births, but associated anomalies are rare. Hirschsprung disease may be associated with colonic atresia or imperforate anus, but these conditions are not common.

**Reference:** Bradshaw, W.T.: Gastrointestinal disorders. In Verklan, M.T., Walden, M. (Eds.): *Core Curriculum for Neonatal Intensive Care Nursing,* 4th ed. St. Louis, Saunders, 2010, pp. 589-637.

42. **(B)** Erythema toxicum, a benign transient neonatal skin condition, consists of patches of erythematous skin with a yellow or white central pustule. It appears between 24 and 72 hours after birth and can affect any area of the body except the palms or soles. Milia appear as small yellow-white cysts usually found on the cheeks, forehead, and nose. They occur in clusters. Candidiasis is usually found in the groin area and presents as an area of generalized erythema with pebbly white satellite lesions. Transient neonatal pustular melanosis is usually present at birth. It occurs most commonly on the face, hands, and soles of the feet. It is most frequently seen in black infants.

**References:** Blackburn, S.T.: *Maternal, Fetal, and Neonatal Physiology. A Clinical Perspective.* St. Louis, Saunders, 2007, p. 531

Lund, C.H., Kuller, J.M.: Integumentary system. In Kenner, C., Wright Lott, J. (Eds.): *Comprehensive Neonatal Care: An Interdisciplinary Approach,* 4th ed. St. Louis, Saunders, 2007, p. 71.

## CHAPTER 5: GESTATIONAL AGE ASSESSMENT

1. **(D)** Low birth weight is classified as birth weight less than 2500 g. Extremely low birth weight is classified as birth weight less than 1000 g. Very low birth weight is classified as birth weight less than 1500 g.

**Reference:** Furdon, S.A., Benjamin, K.: Physical assessment. In Verklan, M.T., Walden, M. (Eds.): *Core Curriculum for Neonatal Intensive Care Nursing,* 4th ed. St. Louis, Saunders, 2010, p. 127.

2. **(C)** Measuring the infant crown to heel is the correct way to determine length. Measuring hip to hip does not determine the length of the infant. Measuring head to toe does not ensure an accurate length, because the toes can flex or extend, which causes the length measurement to potentially vary. Measuring the infant shoulder to shoulder determines the infant's width, not the infant's length.

**Reference:** Furdon, S.A., Benjamin, K.: Physical assessment. In Verklan, M.T., Walden, M. (Eds.): *Core Curriculum for Neonatal Intensive Care Nursing*, 4th ed. St. Louis, Saunders, 2010, p. 127.

3. **(C)** An infant whose weight is greater than the 90th percentile is a large-for-gestational-age infant. An infant whose weight is at the 50th percentile is an appropriate-for-gestational-age infant. An infant whose weight is less than the 10th percentile is a small-for-gestational-age infant. An infant whose weight is between the 10th and 90th percentiles is an appropriate-for-gestational-age infant.

**Reference:** Furdon, S.A., Benjamin, K.: Physical assessment. In Verklan, M.T., Walden, M. (Eds.): *Core Curriculum for Neonatal Intensive Care Nursing*, 4th ed. St. Louis, Saunders, 2010, p. 130.

4. **(B)** An infant whose weight is less than the 10th percentile is a small-for-gestational-age infant. An infant whose weight is at the 50th percentile is an appropriate-for-gestational-age infant. An infant whose weight greater than the 90th percentile is a large-for-gestational-age infant. An infant whose weight is within the 10th and 90th percentile is an appropriate-for-gestational-age infant.

**Reference:** Furdon, S.A., Benjamin, K.: Physical assessment. In Verklan, M.T., Walden, M. (Eds.): *Core Curriculum for Neonatal Intensive Care Nursing*, 4th ed. St. Louis, Saunders, 2010, p. 130.

5. **(D)** An infant whose weight is between the 10th and 90th percentiles is an appropriate-for-gestational-age infant. Although an infant whose weight is at the 50th percentile is an appropriate-for-gestational-age (AGA) infant, a wider range of weight is considered AGA. An infant whose weight is less than the 10th percentile is a small-for-gestational-age infant. An infant whose weight is greater than the 90th percentile is a large-for-gestational-age infant.

**Reference:** Furdon, S.A., Benjamin, K.: Physical assessment. In Verklan, M.T., Walden, M. (Eds.): *Core Curriculum for Neonatal Intensive Care Nursing*, 4th ed. St. Louis, Saunders, 2010, p. 130.

6. **(A)** Head circumference is an indicator of brain growth, and a circumference greater than the 90th percentile or below the 10th percentile can signal intracranial pathology. Head circumference does not indicate brain function, anatomy, or physiology of the brain. Brain function can be determined via neurologic tests and assessments. The anatomy of the brain can be determined via imaging tests. The physiology of the brain can be determined through the combination of neurologic and imaging tests.

**Reference:** Furdon, S.A., Benjamin, K.: Physical assessment. In Verklan, M.T., Walden, M. (Eds.): *Core Curriculum for Neonatal Intensive Care Nursing*, 4th ed. St. Louis, Saunders, 2010, pp. 123, 130.

7. **(C)** Late-preterm infants are those whose gestational age falls between 34 and 36 6/7 weeks. Term infants are infants whose gestational age falls between 37 and 40 weeks. Posterm infants are those whose gestational age is longer than 40 weeks. "Extremely preterm" is not a recognized gestational category.

**Reference:** Furdon, S.A., Benjamin, K.: Physical assessment. In Verklan, M.T., Walden, M. (Eds.): *Core Curriculum for Neonatal Intensive Care Nursing*, 4th ed. St. Louis, Saunders, 2010, p. 127.

8. **(D)** Lanugo covers the entire body beginning at 20 weeks' gestation. Lanugo does not start disappearing until 28 weeks' gestation. Lanugo is expected to be seen on premature infants.

**Reference:** Furdon, S.A., Benjamin, K.: Physical assessment. In Verklan, M.T., Walden, M. (Eds.): *Core Curriculum for Neonatal Intensive Care Nursing*, 4th ed. St. Louis, Saunders, 2010, p. 135.

9. **(B)** A head disproportionately large for the trunk is the typical appearance of an infant with intrauterine growth restriction (IUGR). An infant with IUGR is born with little or no vernix on the skin. The umbilical cord of an infant with IUGR is thin with decreased Wharton jelly. The anterior fontanelles of an infant with IUGR are typically large with cranial sutures wide or overlapping.

**Reference:** Furdon, S.A., Benjamin, K.: Physical assessment. In Verklan, M.T., Walden, M. (Eds.): *Core Curriculum for Neonatal Intensive Care Nursing*, 4th ed. St. Louis, Saunders, 2010, pp. 130-131.

10. **(A)** As gestation progresses beyond 38 weeks, the subcutaneous tissue decreases, which causes the skin to wrinkle. At term gestation, the breast tissue nodule measures up to 10 mm. There is cartilage present in the pinna, which allows it to spring back from being folded. In the preterm infant, the skin is usually transparent, breast tissue is imperceptible or barely imperceptible, and the pinna has little cartilage, which causes the pinna to stay folded on itself. In the late-preterm infant, the subcutaneous tissue has not decreased to the point of causing the skin to wrinkle, the breast tissue nodule measures only 1 to 2 mm, and the pinna may or may not stay folded on itself, depending on the gestational age. "Very postterm" is not a recognized gestational category.

**Reference:** Furdon, S.A., Benjamin, K.: Physical assessment. In Verklan, M.T., Walden, M. (Eds.): *Core Curriculum for Neonatal Intensive Care Nursing*, 4th ed. St. Louis, Saunders, 2010, p. 126.

11. **(C)** An infant whose weight is between the 10th and 90th percentiles is appropriate for gestational age. An infant whose weight less than the 10th percentile is small for gestational age. An infant whose weight is greater than the 90th percentile is large for gestational age.

**Reference:** Furdon, S.A., Benjamin, K.: Physical assessment. In Verklan, M.T., Walden, M. (Eds.): *Core Curriculum for Neonatal Intensive Care Nursing*, 4th ed. St. Louis, Saunders, 2010, p. 130.

12. **(D)** Meconium aspiration is associated with term and postterm infants. The postterm infant's skin is leathery, cracked, and wrinkled. In the postterm infant male, the scrotum becomes more pendulous and is completely covered with rugae. The testes have completely descended. The preterm infant's skin is gelatinous, red, and translucent with visible veins. In the premature infant male, the scrotum is not completely covered with rugae and the testes have not yet

descended into the scrotum. The late-preterm infant's skin is smooth and pink with few visible veins and has superficial peeling. In the late-preterm infant male, the scrotum is not completely covered with rugae and the testes have descended high into the scrotum. The term infant's skin is cracking and pale in areas with no visible veins, but not leathery or wrinkled. In the term infant male, the scrotum is completely covered with rugae and the testes are completely descended, but not pendulous.

**Reference:** Gardner, S.L., Hernandez, J.A.: Initial nursery care. In Gardner, S.L., Carter, B.S., Enzman-Hines, M. et al.: *Merenstein and Gardner's Handbook of Neonatal Intensive Care,* 7th ed. St. Louis, Mosby, 2011, pp. 88-92.

13. **(D)** For the term infant, the square window angle would be 0 degrees, the popliteal angle would be 90 degrees, and in scarf sign testing, the elbow could not be pulled over the infant's body. The preterm infant's posture would be flexed, skin would be cracking with no visible veins, and creases would be noted on the plantar surface. The square window angle would be greater than 90 degrees, the popliteal angle would be 180 degrees, and in scarf sign testing, the elbow could be pulled past the midline of the infant's body. The preterm infant's posture would be hypotonic, skin would be gelatinous with visible veins, and no creases would be noted on the plantar surface. For the late-preterm infant, the square window angle would be about 45 degrees, the popliteal angle would be 110 to 140 degrees, and in scarf sign testing, the elbow could be pulled to the midline of the infant's body. The infant's posture would be slightly flexed, skin would be cracking with rare visible veins, and anterior transverse creases would be noted on the plantar surface.

**Reference:** Furdon, S.A., Benjamin, K.: Physical assessment. In Verklan, M.T., Walden, M. (Eds.): *Core Curriculum for Neonatal Intensive Care Nursing,* 4th ed. St. Louis, Saunders, 2010, p. 124-126.

14. **(B)** Positioning the infant supine, taking the infant's hand and pulling it across the infant's chest and around the neck as far posterior as possible toward the opposite shoulder, and observing the elbow position relative to the midline of the infant's body is the correct way to test for the scarf sign. Positioning the infant supine, flexing the infant's arms for 5 seconds, then fully extending the infant's arms by pulling the hands downward and releasing is the technique for performing the arm recoil test. Flexing the infant's hand on the forearm between the examiner's thumb and index finger, using enough pressure to get full flexion, and visually measuring the angle between the hypothenar eminence and the ventral aspect of the forearm is the correct way to perform the square window test. Positioning the infant supine with the pelvis flat on a surface, holding the infant's thigh in knee-chest position with the left index finger and thumb, placing the right index finger behind the infant's ankle and extending the leg gently, and measuring the angle between the lower leg and thigh is the correct way of determining popliteal angle.

**Reference:** Furdon, S.A., Benjamin, K.: Physical assessment. In Verklan, M.T., Walden, M. (Eds.): *Core Curriculum for Neonatal Intensive Care Nursing,* 4th ed. St. Louis, Saunders, 2010, pp. 124-125.

15. **(A)** Positioning the infant supine, flexing the infant's arms for 5 seconds, then fully extending the infant's arms by pulling the hands downward and releasing is the technique for testing arm recoil. Positioning the infant supine, taking the infant's hand and pulling it across the infant's chest and around the neck as far posterior as possible toward the opposite shoulder, and observing the elbow position relative to the midline of the infant's body is the correct way to test for the scarf sign. Flexing the infant's hand on the forearm between the examiner's thumb and index finger, using enough pressure to get full flexion, and visually measuring the angle between the hypothenar eminence and the ventral aspect of the forearm is the correct way to perform the square window test. Positioning the infant supine with the pelvis flat on a surface, holding the infant's thigh in knee-chest position with the left index finger and thumb, placing the right index finger behind the infant's ankle and extending the leg gently, and measuring the angle between the lower leg and thigh is the correct way of determining popliteal angle.

**Reference:** Furdon, S.A., Benjamin, K.: Physical assessment. In Verklan, M.T., Walden, M. (Eds.): *Core Curriculum for Neonatal Intensive Care Nursing,* 4th ed. St. Louis, Saunders, 2010, pp. 124-125.

16. **(C)** Flexing the infant's hand on the forearm between the examiner's thumb and index finger, using enough pressure to get full flexion, and visually measuring the angle between the hypothenar eminence and the ventral aspect of the forearm is the correct way to perform the square window test. Positioning the infant supine, flexing the infant's arms for 5 seconds, then fully extending the infant's arms by pulling the hands downward and releasing is the technique for testing arm recoil. Positioning the infant supine, taking the infant's hand and pulling it across the infant's chest and around the neck as far posterior as possible toward the opposite shoulder, and observing the elbow position relative to the midline of the infant's body is the correct way to test for the scarf sign. Positioning the infant supine with the pelvis flat on a surface, holding the infant's thigh in knee-chest position with the left index finger and thumb, placing the right index finger behind the infant's ankle and extending the leg gently, and measuring the angle between the lower leg and thigh is the correct way of determining popliteal angle.

**Reference:** Furdon, S.A., Benjamin, K.: Physical assessment. In Verklan, M.T., Walden, M. (Eds.): *Core Curriculum for Neonatal Intensive Care Nursing,* 4th ed. St. Louis, Saunders, 2010, pp. 124-125.

17. **(C)** Clinical care such as blood glucose testing, timing of diagnostic studies, and feeding pathways are based on the gestational age and size-date plotting. Early (second-trimester) ultrasonograms are often

used for dating. The dates obtained are often compared with last menstrual period dating and the findings of the gestational age examination to determine the gestational age. Late ultrasonograms may be less accurate, but are used when menstrual cycle dating is not available. Neurodevelopmental outcome is very hard to predict, and although gestational age can influence it, gestational age assessment examinations are not useful for this purpose.

**Reference:** Trotter, C.: Gestational age assessment. In Tappero, E., Honeyfield, M.E. (Eds.): *Physical Assessment of the Newborn,* 4th ed. Santa Rosa, Calif., NICU Ink, 2009, pp. 21-40.

18. **(A)** Babies who fall between the 10th and the 90th percentiles are appropriate-for-gestational-age infants, which means that they have grown in utero as expected and are therefore at less risk for problems such as hypoglycemia, infection, and poor neurodevelopmental outcomes. Babies who fall above the 90th percentile are large for gestational age (LGA) infants. LGA babies are at risk for birth trauma and hypoglycemia. Babies who fall below the 10th percentile have not grown as expected and may need further evaluation to assess the possible cause(s) of abnormal growth. These babies can have problems with blood glucose level (i.e., hypoglycemia).

**Reference:** Furdon, S.A., Benjamin, K.: Physical assessment. In Verklan, M., Walden, M. (Eds.): *Core Curriculum for Neonatal Intensive Care Nursing,* 4th ed. St. Louis, Saunders, 2010, pp. 120-155.

19. **(C)** As a baby matures, the pinnae of the ears will mature and the cartilage will eventually firm up, the genitalia will mature, the skin will thicken, and subcutaneous fat will become deposited. Very preterm babies will develop cartilage in their ears after birth and will not necessarily have deformed ears. The internal structure of a preterm infant's ears will form normally. Hearing loss in preterm infants may be related to exposure to ototoxic antibiotics (e.g., aminoglycoside). Growth and development continue after birth, so preterm babies will develop cartilage in their ears. Hearing is impacted by familial issues, ototoxic medications, and congenital infections.

**Reference:** Trotter, C.: Gestational age assessment. In Tappero, E., Honeyfield, M.E. (Eds.): *Physical Assessment of the Newborn,* 4th ed. Santa Rosa, Calif., NICU Ink, 2009, pp. 21-40.

20. **(D)** Preterm infants have smooth plantar surfaces, which develop creases as they mature, and large amounts of lanugo over the shoulders and back, which will eventually slough off into the amniotic fluid as they get close to term. Vernix covers preterm fetuses, but sloughs off into the amniotic fluid as the fetus develops, so that by term it is left only in folds like the groin and in the axilla. The skin of preterm infants is thin with little subcutaneous fat, which allows veins to be visible on the abdomen. Palpable breast buds and stippling of the areolae would be apparent in the full-term infant.

**Reference:** Trotter, C.: Gestational age assessment. In Tappero, E., Honeyfield, M.E. (Eds.): *Physical Assessment of the Newborn,* 4th ed. Santa Rosa, Calif., NICU Ink, 2009, pp. 21-40.

21. **(D)** As the placenta ages, it does not effectively provide nutrition to the fetus, which leads to weight loss and loss of subcutaneous tissue, not of bony structures. Weight loss from loss of subcutaneous fat may be evident and cause weight to be less than the 10th percentile. Circumference of the head (a bony structure) is not affected by the aging of the placenta. The head and length remain appropriate for gestational age, because bone growth at this stage is not affected by placental insufficiency.

**Reference:** Furdon, S.A., Benjamin, K.: Physical assessment. In Verklan, M., Walden, M. (Eds.): *Core Curriculum for Neonatal Intensive Care Nursing,* 4th ed. St. Louis, Saunders, 2010, pp. 120-155.

22. **(D)** Neurologic examination findings can be altered by neurologic disorders or asphyxic injury, which can affect tone and responsiveness, and therefore may not be reliable. Posture and flexion increases with advancing gestational age, as tone and muscle mass increase; however, counterintuitively, the wrist and ankle joints increase in flexibility, which decreases the number of degrees of the angle when tested with gentle pressure. The values of neurologic indicators are accurate in preterm infants; the tools account for gestational age.

**Reference:** Furdon, S.A., Benjamin, K.: Physical assessment. In Verklan, M., Walden, M. (Eds.): *Core Curriculum for Neonatal Intensive Care Nursing,* 4th ed. St. Louis, Saunders, 2010, pp. 120-155.

23. **(C)** Small-for-gestational-age (SGA) infants may have hypoglycemia due to inadequate glycogen stores. SGA infants are at risk for polycythemia, not anemia. They are at risk for hypothermia, not hyperthermia. Brachial plexus palsy is a form of birth injury that can be seen with shoulder dystocia and large-for-gestational-age infants.

**Reference:** Gardner, S.L., Hernandez, J.A.: Initial nursery care. In Gardner, S.L., Carter, B.S., Enzman-Hines M., et al. (Eds.): *Merenstein and Gardner's Handbook of Neonatal Intensive Care,* 7th ed. St. Louis, Mosby, 2011, p. 92.

24. **(B)** An infant born at 40 weeks' gestation weighing 2000 g is well below the 10th percentile for weight and would be classified as small for gestational age (SGA). SGA infants are at risk for polycythemia, hypoglycemia, and congenital infection, and may have experienced fetal distress. Large-for-gestational-age infants are at risk for birth trauma. An SGA infant who has experienced intrauterine growth restriction has low glycogen and fat stores in addition to increased substrate utilization. Premature infants are at risk for respiratory distress syndrome.

**Reference:** Furdon, S.A., Benjamin, K.: Physical assessment. In Verklan, M., Walden, M. (Eds.): *Core Curriculum for Neonatal Intensive Care Nursing,* 4th ed. St. Louis, Saunders, 2010, pp. 120-155.

25. **(D)** Full-term infants who are large for gestational age are at risk for birth trauma, polycythemia, and hypoglycemia, and have an increased risk of being born by cesarean section. Preterm infants and infants with intrauterine growth restriction are at risk for

hypothermia. Sodium and potassium homeostasis are not affected by size classification.

**Reference:** Furdon, S.A., Benjamin, K.: Physical assessment. In Verklan, M., Walden, M. (Eds.): *Core Curriculum for Neonatal Intensive Care Nursing,* 4th ed. St. Louis, Saunders, 2010, pp. 120-155.

26. **(D)** Female genitalia are assessed based on the prominence of the clitoris and the development of the labia majora and minora. Female genitalia develop with advancing age, and by term, the labia majora and minora completely cover the clitoris. Subcutaneous fat increases as gestational age increases, unless the fetus goes beyond 40 weeks' gestation and experiences placental insufficiency and growth restriction, at which time fat stores diminish. Skin thickness increases as gestational age increases; the skin becomes parchment-like and sloughs if gestation continues beyond 40 weeks. Lanugo peaks at 28 to 30 weeks and then decreases as gestational age increases. Breasts are assessed for amount of breast tissue and nipple size. Both nipple and breast tissue development progress with advancing age.

**Reference:** Trotter, C.: Gestational age assessment. In Tappero, E., Honeyfield, M.E. (Eds.): *Physical Assessment of the Newborn,* 4th ed. Santa Rosa, Calif., NICU Ink, 2009, pp. 21-40.

27. **(D)** Extremely premature infants do not have plantar creases. In the absence of these creases, foot length (heel to toe) is the characteristic scored for the plantar surface physical maturity sign. The extremely premature infant can be expected to have a heel-to-toe length of 40 to 50 mm. At the earliest gestations, the eye-ear maturity sign is based on fusion of the eyelids. The extremely premature infant can be expected to have fused eyelids. Lanugo development peaks at 28 to 30 weeks' gestation, and then lanugo disappears. The extremely premature infant can be expected to have no or sparse lanugo. As the fetus matures, the skin becomes dry and paperlike. The skin of an extremely premature infant is sticky, friable, gelatinous, and transparent.

**Reference:** Trotter, C.: Gestational age assessment. In Tappero, E., Honeyfield, M.E. (Eds.): *Physical Assessment of the Newborn,* 4th ed. Santa Rosa, Calif., NICU Ink, 2009, pp. 21-40.

28. **(B)** In postterm infants, the skin is cracked and wrinkled, plantar creases cover the entire foot sole, and the skin is mostly bald of lanugo. The ears are stiff with thick cartilage. The labia majora cover the labia minora as well as the clitoris. Breast areolae are full with 5- to 10-mm buds.

**Reference:** Trotter, C.: Gestational age assessment. In Tappero, E., Honeyfield, M.E. (Eds.): *Physical Assessment of the Newborn,* 4th ed. Santa Rosa, Calif., NICU Ink, 2009, pp. 21-40.

29. **(D)** There are three accepted methods of determining gestational age: (1) calculation of dates based on the mother's last menstrual period, (2) evaluation of obstetric parameters (e.g., detection of fetal heart tones by Doppler stethoscope, determination of fundal height), and (3) physical examination of the newborn. The latter includes assessment of neuromuscular and physical criteria (e.g., using the Dubowitz or Ballard

tools) and examination of the anterior capsule of the vascular lens of the eye. Although birth weight is used to assess intrauterine growth, birth weight is not used to determine gestational age. Ultrasonography is useful to evaluate obstetric parameters. Ultrasonography is most accurate for determining gestational age when performed before 20 weeks' gestation.

**Reference:** Trotter, C.: Gestational age assessment. In Tappero, E., Honeyfield, M.E. (Eds.): *Physical Assessment of the Newborn,* 4th ed. Santa Rosa, Calif., NICU Ink, 2009, pp. 21-40.

30. **(C)** There are limitations based on subjective scoring methods. Findings of the gestational age examination can be affected by neurologic disorders; intrauterine events such as asphyxia, breech position, and positional deformities; and maternal medications (e.g., magnesium sulfate). The estimate based on gestational age examination is accurate within plus or minus 2 weeks of gestation. The interrater reliability is not perfect, so the examination may be performed by two individuals to improve accuracy.

**Reference:** Furdon, S.A., Benjamin, K.: Physical assessment. In Verklan, M., Walden, M. (Eds.): *Core Curriculum for Neonatal Intensive Care Nursing,* 4th ed. St. Louis, Saunders, 2010, pp. 120-155.

31. **(B)** The best accuracy is obtained when the examination is performed on infants in an awake and alert state and within 48 hours of life. Performing the examination past 5 days of life leads to inaccuracy. The combined score of the physical and neurologic components has a higher correlation than either component used separately.

**Reference:** Furdon, S.A., Benjamin, K.: Physical assessment. In Verklan, M., Walden, M. (Eds.): *Core Curriculum for Neonatal Intensive Care Nursing,* 4th ed. St. Louis, Saunders, 2010, pp. 120-155.

32. **(A)** A 4.5-kg infant born at 38 weeks' gestation is well above the 90th percentile for weight and would be classified as full term and large for gestational age (LGA). Full-term LGA infants are at risk for birth trauma, polycythemia, and hypoglycemia, and have an increased risk of being born by cesarean section. Erb palsy results from injury to cervical nerves I and IV, which causes paralysis of the arm. Small-for-gestational-age infants, not LGA infants, are at risk for hypothermia and congenital anomalies. Preterm infants are at risk for respiratory distress syndrome.

**References:** Furdon, S.A., Benjamin, K.: Physical assessment. In Verklan, M., Walden, M. (Eds.): *Core Curriculum for Neonatal Intensive Care Nursing,* 4th ed. St. Louis, Saunders, 2010, pp. 120-155.

Lynam, L., Verklan, M.T.: Neurological disorders. In Verklan, M., Walden, M. (Eds.): *Core Curriculum for Neonatal Intensive Care Nursing,* 4th ed. St. Louis, Saunders, 2010, p. 765.

## CHAPTER 6: THERMOREGULATION

1. **(B)** Conduction is heat loss from direct contact. Convection is heat transfer via air currents. Evaporation is the loss of heat via the conversion of liquid into vapor. Radiation is the transfer of radiant energy (heat) without direct contact through absorption and emission of infrared rays.

Reference: Brand, M.C., Boyd, H.A.: Thermoregulation. In Verklan, M.T., Walden, M. (Eds.): *Core Curriculum for Neonatal Intensive Care Nursing*, 4th ed. St. Louis, Saunders, 2010, p. 113.

2. **(A)** Convection is heat transfer via air currents. Conduction is heat loss from direct contact. Evaporation is the loss of heat via the conversion of liquid into vapor. Radiation is the transfer of radiant energy (heat) without direct contact through absorption and emission of infrared rays.

Reference: Brand, M.C., Boyd, H.A.: Thermoregulation. In Verklan, M.T., Walden, M. (Eds.): *Core Curriculum for Neonatal Intensive Care Nursing*, 4th ed. St. Louis, Saunders, 2010, p. 114.

3. **(C)** Evaporation is the loss of heat via the conversion of liquid into vapor. Convection is heat transfer via air currents. Conduction is heat loss from direct contact. Radiation is the transfer of radiant energy (heat) without direct contact through absorption and emission of infrared rays.

Reference: Brand, M.C., Boyd, H.A.: Thermoregulation. In Verklan, M.T., Walden, M. (Eds.): *Core Curriculum for Neonatal Intensive Care Nursing*, 4th ed. St. Louis, Saunders, 2010, p. 114.

4. **(D)** Radiation is the transfer of radiant energy (heat) without direct contact through absorption and emission of infrared rays. Convection is heat transfer via air currents. Conduction is heat loss from direct contact. Evaporation is the loss of heat via the conversion of liquid into vapor.

Reference: Brand, M.C., Boyd, H.A.: Thermoregulation. In Verklan, M.T., Walden, M. (Eds.): *Core Curriculum for Neonatal Intensive Care Nursing*, 4th ed. St. Louis, Saunders, 2010, p. 114.

5. **(A)** A balance of heat loss, heat gain, and heat production is the definition of thermoregulation. Thermal instability is when the temperature of the body is out of the expected normal range. The inability to maintain core temperature above that of the environment is termed *poikilothermia*. A physiologic response to changes in ambient temperature in an attempt to maintain normal core is termed *homeothermia*.

Reference: Brand, M.C., Boyd, H.A.: Thermoregulation. In Verklan, M.T., Walden, M. (Eds.): *Core Curriculum for Neonatal Intensive Care Nursing*, 4th ed. St. Louis, Saunders, 2010, p. 111.

6. **(B)** Thermal instability is defined as the state in which the temperature of the body is out of the expected normal range. A balance of heat loss, heat gain, and heat production is the definition of thermoregulation. The inability to maintain core temperature above that of the environment is the definition of *poikilothermia*. A physiologic response to changes in ambient temperature in an attempt to maintain normal core is the definition of *homeothermic*.

Reference: Brand, M.C., Boyd, H.A.: Thermoregulation. In Verklan, M.T., Walden, M. (Eds.): *Core Curriculum for Neonatal Intensive Care Nursing*, 4th ed. St. Louis, Saunders, 2010, p. 110.

7. **(D)** Infants do not have the full capability to dissipate heat, which makes them prone to hyperthermia. A large body surface area, limited glycogen stores, and limited brown fat stores increase the infant's risk of hypothermia.

8. **(B)** A neutral thermal environment promotes minimal consumption of oxygen and glucose. A neutral thermal environment enables, not limits, the neonate's ability to maintain normothermia. It minimizes, not increases, the neonate's metabolic rate. It enables the neonate to minimize, not maximize, glucose consumption.

Reference: Brand, M.C., Boyd, H.A.: Thermoregulation. In Verklan, M.T., Walden, M. (Eds.): *Core Curriculum for Neonatal Intensive Care Nursing*, 4th ed. St. Louis, Saunders, 2010, p. 114.

9. **(D)** Increased body surface area, in combination with decreased brown fat stores, decreased subcutaneous fat, and decreased glycogen stores, makes the infant prone to experiencing hypothermia. Increased muscle tone, glycogen stores, and brown fat stores decrease the infant's risk of hypothermia.

Reference: Brand, M.C., Boyd, H.A.: Thermoregulation. In Verklan, M.T., Walden, M. (Eds.): *Core Curriculum for Neonatal Intensive Care Nursing*, 4th ed. St. Louis, Saunders, 2010, p. 111.

10. **(A)** Infection increases the infant's body temperature. Because the infant has limited ability to dissipate heat, the infant is at risk of hyperthermia. Prematurity increases the infant's risk of hypothermia. Infants have limited ability to dissipate heat. Hypermetabolism of drugs increases the infant's risk of hyperthermia.

Reference: Brand, M.C., Boyd, H.A.: Thermoregulation. In Verklan, M.T., Walden, M. (Eds.): *Core Curriculum for Neonatal Intensive Care Nursing*, 4th ed. St. Louis, Saunders, 2010, p. 111.

11. **(B)** Placing the infant on a warming mattress reduces the potential for heat loss to occur from direct contact. Thoroughly drying the infant reduces evaporative heat loss. Putting a knit cap on the infant reduces convective heat loss.

Reference: Brand, M.C., Boyd, H.A.: Thermoregulation. In Verklan, M.T., Walden, M. (Eds.): *Core Curriculum for Neonatal Intensive Care Nursing*, 4th ed. St. Louis, Saunders, 2010, p. 115.

12. **(C)** Putting a knit cap on the infant decreases the potential for heat loss to occur due to air currents. Thoroughly drying the infant reduces evaporative heat loss. Placing the infant on a warming mattress reduces conductive heat loss.

Reference: Brand, M.C., Boyd, H.A.: Thermoregulation. In Verklan, M.T., Walden, M. (Eds.): *Core Curriculum for Neonatal Intensive Care Nursing*, 4th ed. St. Louis, Saunders, 2010, p. 116.

13. **(B)** The polyethylene bag helps keep the infant warm by reducing evaporative heat loss and conductive heat loss. The infant should be placed in the polyethylene bag prior to drying. The infant's head remains out of the bag when the bag is applied. Therefore, the use of the polyethylene bag should not interfere with intubation. The bag maintains heat during the intubation procedure. The use of the polyethylene bag is not determined by the infant's respiratory status.

Reference: Brand, M.C., Boyd, H.A.: Thermoregulation. In Verklan, M.T., Walden, M. (Eds.): *Core Curriculum for Neonatal Intensive Care Nursing*, 4th ed. St. Louis, Saunders, 2010, p. 116.

14. **(C)** The infant is receiving warmth from direct contact with the mother's skin. This decreases conductive heat loss. It does not decrease radiant heat loss, convective heat loss, or evaporative heat loss.

**Reference:** 1Brand, M.C., Boyd, H.A.: Thermoregulation. In Verklan, M.T., Walden, M. (Eds.): *Core Curriculum for Neonatal Intensive Care Nursing,* 4th ed. St. Louis, Saunders, 2010, p. 115.

15. **(C)** The body responds to cold stress by peripherally vasoconstricting to decrease the amount of heat loss. The body responds to cold stress by depleting glycogen stores rather than increasing the storage of glycogen; by increasing the consumption of brown adipose tissue; and by increasing oxygen consumption.

**Reference:** Brand, M.C., Boyd, H.A.: Thermoregulation. In Verklan, M.T., Walden, M. (Eds.): *Core Curriculum for Neonatal Intensive Care Nursing,* 4th ed. St. Louis, Saunders, 2010, p. 113.

16. **(A)** A dislodged skin temperature probe will sense the ambient temperature and attempt to bring the temperature it is sensing to the skin temperature that has been set on the incubator, which could lead to the neonate experiencing hyperthermia. A skin temperature probe covered by an insulated probe cover enables continuous monitoring of the infant's skin temperature, which decreases the potential for the neonate to experience hyperthermia. The placement of the skin temperature probe away from brown adipose tissue areas enables accurate continuous monitoring of skin temperature, which decreases the potential for the neonate to experience hyperthermia. The continuous monitoring of the skin temperature of a neonate using a servocontrolled incubator decreases the potential for the neonate to experience hyperthermia.

**Reference:** Brand, M.C., Boyd, H.A.: Thermoregulation. In Verklan, M.T., Walden, M. (Eds.): *Core Curriculum for Neonatal Intensive Care Nursing,* 4th ed. St. Louis, Saunders, 2010, p. 111.

17. **(C)** Tachypnea, tachycardia, irritability, dehydration, a flushed look, and hypernatremia are signs of hyperthermia. Signs of hypothermia do not include tachypnea, tachycardia, irritability, dehydration, a flushed look, and hypernatremia. Signs of poikilothermia would be similar to the signs of hypothermia. Signs of normothermia do not include tachypnea, tachycardia, irritability, dehydration, a flushed look, and hypernatremia.

**Reference:** Brand, M.C., Boyd, H.A.: Thermoregulation. In Verklan, M.T., Walden, M. (Eds.): *Core Curriculum for Neonatal Intensive Care Nursing,* 4th ed. St. Louis, Saunders, 2010, p. 112.

18. **(D)** Once the infant is in a warm environment in the nursery, the polyethylene wrap must be removed. This reduces the potential for the infant to experience hyperthermia. The infant should not be dried before being placed in the polyethylene wrap. The infant's head should not be covered with the polyethylene wrap. The polyethylene bag should be used once the infant is born, prior to drying, in order to reduce evaporative heat loss and help with the infant's thermoregulation.

**Reference:** Brand, M.C., Boyd, H.A.: Thermoregulation. In Verklan, M.T., Walden, M. (Eds.): *Core Curriculum for Neonatal Intensive Care Nursing,* 4th ed. St. Louis, Saunders, 2010, p. 116.

19. **(A)** Use of an unwarmed blanket promoted conductive heat loss, transfer of the infant without a cap promoted convective heat loss, and placement of the warmer by the drafty windows promoted radiant heat loss. The infant was dried thoroughly, which reduced the risk of evaporative heat loss.

**Reference:** Brand, M.C., Boyd, H.A.: Thermoregulation. In Verklan, M.T., Walden, M. (Eds.): *Core Curriculum for Neonatal Intensive Care Nursing,* 4th ed. St. Louis, Saunders, 2010, pp. 114-116.

20. **(C)** Removing the positioning devices can help relieve the hyperthermia by increasing skin exposure and allowing heat loss to occur. It is important to intervene quickly when finding an infant to be hyperthermic, because a delay can lead to complications caused by hyperthermia. Turning off the incubator promotes, rather than relieves, the infant's hyperthermia. The incubator needs to be on for air within the incubator to be circulated. Turning off the phototherapy interrupts hyperbilirubinemia treatment.

**Reference:** Brand, M.C., Boyd, H.A.: Thermoregulation. In Verklan, M.T., Walden, M. (Eds.): *Core Curriculum for Neonatal Intensive Care Nursing,* 4th ed. St. Louis, Saunders, 2010, p. 118.

21. **(C)** Once the infant is under the radiant warmer, it is essential to change the mode from manual to servocontrolled to decrease the risk that the infant will become overheated. Alarms should not be turned off, particularly when equipment is in use. The warmer needs to be on; turning it off causes the radiant warmer to lose the heat obtained during prewarming. The radiant warmer should be set to servocontrolled mode when it is being used to warm an infant.

**Reference:** Brand, M.C., Boyd, H.A.: Thermoregulation. In Verklan, M.T., Walden, M. (Eds.): *Core Curriculum for Neonatal Intensive Care Nursing,* 4th ed. St. Louis, Saunders, 2010, p. 111.

## CHAPTER 7: FLUID AND ELECTROLYTES

1. **(D)** Sodium is the main extracellular ion and, with its salts, constitutes more than 90% of the total amount of solutes in the extracellular space. Chloride is the main inorganic anion in the extracellular fluid. Magnesium is distributed primarily in the intracellular space and skeleton. Potassium is found primarily in the intracellular space.

**Reference:** Collin, J.F., Liqun, B., Xu, H., et al.: Molecular aspects and regulation of gastrointestinal function during postnatal development. In Barrett, K.B., Ghishan, F.K., Merchant, J.L., et al. (Eds.): *Physiology of the Gastrointestinal Tract,* 4th ed. Burlington, Mass., Elsevier Academic Press, 2006, pp. 376-394.

2. **(D)** An infant's fluid and electrolyte status partially reflects the mother's fluid and electrolyte status. Excessive administration of oxytocin or hypotonic intravenous fluid to the mother may cause hyponatremia in the neonate by expanding extracellular fluid. Antenatal steroids do not cause hyponatremia. Placental dysfunction does not directly affect neonatal sodium levels. Uncontrolled maternal diabetes may cause hypocalcemia in the neonate, but does not cause hyponatremia.

**Reference:** Ambalavanan, N.: Fluid, Electrolyte, and Nutrition Management of the Newborn. May 25, 2010. Available at: http://emedicine.medscape.com/article/976386-overview. Accessed 05/31/10.

3. **(A)** Increasing gestational age reduces insensible water loss (IWL) because the infant's skin becomes thicker as gestation increases, and therefore there is decreased IWL. Environmental factors influence IWL; heat may be transferred through four basic mechanisms: convection, conduction, radiation, and evaporation. Maintaining thermoneutrality is difficult and requires close monitoring. IWL increases with high minute ventilation, although there may be negligible IWL via the lungs if the baby is on a ventilator or continuous positive airway pressure, because warm humidified gas is used in the ventilation system. Use of a radiant warmer increases IWL. Low relative ambient humidity will increase IWL from the infant's immature skin.

**References:** Jones, J.E., Hayes, R.D., Starbuck, A.L., et al.: Fluid and electrolyte management. In Gardner, S.L., Carter, B.S., Enzman-Hines, M., et al. (Eds.): *Merenstein and Gardner's Handbook of Neonatal Intensive Care*, 7th ed. St. Louis, Mosby, Elsevier, 2011, pp. 333-352.

Sherman, T.I., Greenspan, J.S., St. Clair, N., et al.: Optimizing the neonatal thermal environment. *Neonatal Network*, 25:251-260, 2006.

4. **(A)** Because of poor keratinization of the skin, high water content of the extremely low birth weight infant, diminished amount of subcutaneous fat, and large surface area, the infant has high evaporative losses in an environment with a low humidity of 45%. The humidity is set too low to minimize insensible water loss. Without enough humidity, infants will experience high insensible water losses. Recommended humidity is 70% to 80%. Preterm infants should lose between 10% and 15% of total body mass within the initial 72 hours of life; the infant has lost 140 g (more than 15%), and therefore needs an increase in fluids in addition to an increase in the humidity in the incubator. Changing the incubator without increasing humidity would not influence insensible fluid loss. Increasing fluid intake does influence insensible fluid loss. Because of the excessive weight loss, the baby needs increased fluids in addition to increased humidity. The weight loss is excessive and requires immediate action.

**References:** Chiou, Y.B., Blume-Peytavi, U.: Stratum corneum maturation: A review of neonatal skin function. *Skin Pharmacology and Physiology*, 17(2):57-66, 2004.

Jones, J.E., Hayes, R.D., Starbuck, A.L., et al.: Fluid and electrolyte management. In Gardner, S.L., Carter, B.S., Enzman-Hines, M., et al. (Eds.): *Merenstein and Gardner's Handbook of Neonatal Intensive Care*, 7th ed. St. Louis, Mosby, Elsevier, 2011, pp. 333-352.

5. **(B)** Renal blood flow increases from 5% of cardiac output at 12 hours after delivery to 10% at 5 to 7 days of age; this results in an increased glomerular flow rate and improved renal function, which affects clearance of medications. Renal blood flow does not decrease unless there is an insult from hypoxia, infection, or other causes. Preterm infants cannot concentrate urine well, although they can dilute urine almost as well as term infants.

**Reference:** Kelly, L.K., Seri, I.: Renal developmental physiology: Relevance to clinical care. *NeoReviews*, 9:e150-e161, 2008.

6. **(D)** Gradual correction of chronic hyponatremia within 48 to 72 hours will prevent injury to brain cells. Discontinuation of diuretic therapy will diminish sodium loss, but allowing the sodium to increase without supplementation will take days or weeks, exposing the infant to the hazards of hyponatremia. Correcting hyponatremia rapidly over 24 to 48 hours may result in brain cell injury. Slower correction diminishes the chances for adverse effects.

**References:** Halbardier, B.H.: Fluid and electrolyte management. In Verklan, M., Walden, M. (Eds.): *Core Curriculum for Neonatal Intensive Care Nursing*, 4th ed. St. Louis, Saunders, 2010, p. 163.

Jones, J.E., Hayes, R.D., Starbuck, A.L., et al.: Fluid and electrolyte management. In Gardner, S.L., Carter, B.S., Enzman-Hines, M., et al. (Eds.): *Merenstein and Gardner's Handbook of Neonatal Intensive Care*, 7th ed. St. Louis, Mosby, Elsevier, 2011, pp. 333-352.

7. **(A)** Chronic hyponatremia may be asymptomatic, but apnea, irritability, twitching, or seizures occur if the Na concentration drops acutely or falls to less than 115 mEq/L. Severe dehydration is usually indicated by elevated sodium level. Hyponatremia is not associated with cardiopulmonary arrest until after seizures occur. Syndrome of inappropriate antidiuretic hormone is characterized by decreased urine output, decreased serum sodium level, urine osmolality greater than plasma osmolality, and normal renal and adrenal function.

**References:** Jones, J.E., Hayes, R.D., Starbuck, A.L., et al.: Fluid and electrolyte management. In Gardner, S.L., Carter, B.S., Enzman-Hines, M., et al. (Eds.): *Merenstein and Gardner's Handbook of Neonatal Intensive Care*, 7th ed. St. Louis, Mosby, Elsevier, 2011, pp. 333-352.

Moritz, M.L., Ayus, J.C.: Hyponatremia in neonates: Not a benign condition. *Pediatrics*, 124(5):e1014-e1016, 2009.

8. **(D)** The infant is being placed to the breast, but the intake is too low as evidenced by two wet diapers per day. The infant has signs of hypernatremia. Term infants have mature skin and very little insensible water loss. The infant has no medical reason for increased sodium loss and diminished urine output. Overhydration would result in many wet diapers (more than 10 per day).

**Reference:** Konetzny, G., Bucher, H.U., Arlettaz, R.: Prevention of hypernatraemic dehydration in breastfed newborn infants by daily weighing. *European Journal of Pediatrics*, 168(7):815-818, 2009.

9. **(A)** Hypokalemia potentiates digitalis toxicity, which is most likely causing heart block. Hyperkalemia may cause short QT interval, widening QRS complex and sine wave QRS/T, and ventricular tachycardia, not heart block. Hyponatremia is usually asymptomatic, but may present with apnea, twitching, and seizures. Hypernatremia may present with seizures and decreased urine output, but not heart block.

**Reference:** Young, T.E., Mangum, O.B.: *Neofax: Manual of Drugs Used in Neonatal Care*, 22nd ed. Raleigh, N.C., Thomson Reuters, 2009.

10. **(C)** Because 90% of potassium is intracellular, tissue destruction and bruising may cause the damaged cells to send potassium into the extracellular fluid compartment. Hypoperfusion and hemorrhage may decrease glomerular filtration rate (GFR), thereby increasing extracellular potassium. Metabolic acidosis may cause the intracellular potassium to shift out of the cells to the extracellular compartment and metabolic alkalosis may send potassium into the cells. Hypoperfusion and hemorrhage may cause decreased GFR, and therefore extracellular potassium may increase. Because 90% of potassium is intracellular, the normal shift is from the intracellular to the extracellular compartment.

**Reference:** Jones, J.E., Hayes, R.D., Starbuck, A.L., et al.: Fluid and electrolyte management. In Gardner, S.L., Carter, B.S., Enzman-Hines, M., et al. (Eds.): *Merenstein and Gardner's Handbook of Neonatal Intensive Care,* 7th ed. St. Louis, Mosby, Elsevier, 2011, pp. 333-352.

11. **(D)** Severe bruising may contribute to a rapid increase in potassium. Because 90% of potassium is intracellular, bruising may facilitate the movement of potassium from the intracellular to the extracellular compartment. Although there are myriad causes of hyperbilirubinemia, in premature infants tissue destruction and bruising may contribute to rapidly increasing hyperbilirubinemia, because one of the products released during red cell destruction is bilirubin. Within several hours after delivery there is significant loss of extracellular fluid, which may contribute to rapidly increasing bilirubin. By initiation of phototherapy at birth, the effect of tissue destruction, and thus hyperbilirubinemia, may be tempered; checking potassium and bilirubin levels at 12 hours allows time for physiologic changes to take place and thereby provides reliable measurements. An electrocardiogram would show later signs of hyperkalemia (widened QRS complex, short QT interval, and sine wave QRS/T), and electrocardiography is not an intervention that would decrease hyperbilirubinemia. Neonatal potassium levels at delivery are reflective of the mother's potassium levels. Bilirubin levels at delivery can give a false sense of low bilirubin, and the extensive bruising may cause a rather rapid rise in bilirubin by 12 hours of age. Clinical manifestations of hyperkalemia do not occur until late stages, and clinical assessment of hyperbilirubinemia is uncertain at best.

**References:** Jones, J.E., Hayes, R.D., Starbuck, A.L., et al.: Fluid and electrolyte management. In Gardner, S.L., Carter, B.S., Enzman-Hines, M., et al. (Eds.): *Merenstein and Gardner's Handbook of Neonatal Intensive Care,* 7th ed. St. Louis, Mosby, Elsevier, 2011, pp. 333-352.

Wong, R.J., Desandre, G.H., Sibley, E., et al.: Neonatal jaundice and liver disease. In Martin, R.J., Fanaroff, A.A., Walsh, M.C. (Eds.): *Fanaroff and Martin's Neonatal-Perinatal Medicine,* 8th ed. Philadelphia, Mosby, 2006, pp. 1419-1465.

12. **(C)** Glucose and insulin infusions will help shift potassium to the intracellular space, thus decreasing the extracellular effect of potassium on the heart; calcium gluconate lowers the cell membrane threshold, which allows easier shifting of potassium to the intracellular compartment.

**Reference:** Jones, J.E., Hayes, R.D., Starbuck, A.L., et al.: Fluid and electrolyte management. In Gardner, S.L., Carter, B.S., Enzman-Hines, M., et al. (Eds.): *Merenstein and Gardner's Handbook of Neonatal Intensive Care,* 7th ed. St. Louis, Mosby, Elsevier, 2011, pp. 333-352.

13. **(C)** Hypocalcemia manifests with jitteriness (increased neuromuscular irritability and activity) and seizures, both generalized and focal. Infants with hypocalcemia may also have poor feeding, vomiting, and abdominal distension. Hypokalemia may present as flattened T waves, prominent U waves, and ST depression on the electrocardiogram and manifest clinically with hypotonia and abdominal distention (ileus). Hyperkalemia manifests with ventricular tachycardia, peaked T waves, and widened QRS complex. Hypercalcemia may present as hypotonia, irritability, poor feeding, hematuria, and nephrocalcinosis.

**References:** Kalhan, S.C., Parimi, P.S.: Metabolic and endocrine disorders. In Martin, R.J., Fanaroff, A.A., Walsh, M.C. (Eds.): *Fanaroff and Martin's Neonatal-Perinatal Medicine,* 8th ed. Philadelphia, Mosby, 2006, pp. 1467-1596.

Shulman, R., O'Gorman, C., Sochett, E.: Case 1: Neonate with seizures and hypocalcemia. *Paediatrics and Child Health,* 13(3):197-200, 2008.

14. **(D)** Liver, intestinal, and skin necrosis have been reported with infusion of calcium via umbilical catheter (arterial or venous). Calcium gluconate should be given slowly via a syringe pump over 20 to 30 minutes. Calcium chloride is generally used during cardiopulmonary resuscitation. When calcium gluconate is administered, the patient should be monitored.

**Reference:** Young, T.E., Mangum, O.B.: *Neofax: Manual of Drugs Used in Neonatal Care,* 22nd ed. Raleigh, N.C., Thomson Reuters. 2009.

15. **(D)** DiGeorge syndrome is 22q11.2 deletion syndrome with congenital heart disease, hypocalcemia, and an absent thymus gland leading to immune problems. Trisomy 13, trisomy 18, and trisomy 21 are not associated with hypocalcemia.

**Reference:** Goldmuntz, E.: DiGeorge Syndrome: New insights. *Clinics in Perinatology,* 32(4):963-978, 2005.

16. **(D)** The minimal amount of glucose to administer to maintain homeostasis is 4 to 6 mg/kg/minute. The infant needs 90 to 100 ml/kg/day of fluid. At 70 ml/kg/day of dextrose 7.5%, the infant is receiving 2.5 ml/hour (70 ml/kg/day [24 hours]) and 3.6 mg/kg/minute of glucose (0.075 g/ml × 2.5 ml/hour ÷ 60 minutes/hour × 1000 mcg/mg ÷ 0.865 kg). A fluid infusion of dextrose 7.5% at 3.5 ml/hour is 97 ml/kg/day and a glucose load of 5 mg/kg/minute based on a weight of 0.865 kg).

**Reference:** McGowan, J.E., Rozance, P.J., Price-Douglas, W., et al.: In Gardner, S.L., Carter, B.S., Enzman-Hines, M., et al. (Eds.): *Merenstein and Gardner's Handbook of Neonatal Intensive Care,* 7th ed. St. Louis, Mosby, 2011, pp. 353-377.

17. **(C)** Water is the most abundant component of the body and is distributed in two main compartments:

intracellular and extracellular. Early in gestation, total body water (TBW) makes up 95% of the total body weight, with the majority (up to 65%) in extracellular compartments. TBW decreases to 80% at 8 months of gestation.

**References:** Jones, J.E., Hayes, R.D., Starbuck, A.L., et al.: Fluid and electrolyte management. In Gardner, S.L., Carter, B.S., Enzman-Hines, M., et al. (Eds.): *Merenstein and Gardner's Handbook of Neonatal Intensive Care*, 7th ed. St. Louis, Mosby, Elsevier, 2011, pp. 333-352.

Lorenz, J.M.: Fluid and electrolyte therapy in the very low birth weight neonate. *NeoReviews*, 9(3):e102-e108, 2008.

18. **(B)** In the diuretic phase, urine output is increased abruptly. Insensible water loss remains high, and body weight decreases 1% to 3% per day. It is normal to have an output of 6.9 ml/kg/hour during the diuretic phase. Urine output during the postdiuretic phase is expected to be 3 ml/kg/hour. Infants, especially premature infants, have a relative oliguria (less than 1 ml/kg/hour) during the prediuretic phase (birth to 48 hours). The prediuretic phase is birth to 48 hours, the diuretic phase is 1 to 5 days after birth, and the postdiuretic phase (homeostatic phase) is after 2 to 5 days.

**Reference:** Lorenz, J.M.: Fluid and electrolyte therapy in the very low birth weight neonate. *NeoReviews*, 9(3):e102-e108, 2008.

19. **(D)** The feedings are 50 ml/kg/day of 24-kcal formula, which equals 63.25 total ml/day × 0.8 kcal/ml = 50.6 kcal/day ÷ 1.265 kg = 40 kcal/kg/day. Total parenteral nutrition (TPN) 100 ml/kg/day of dextrose 15% equals 126.5 ml/day × 0.6 kcal/ml = 76 kcal/day ÷ 1.265 kg = 60 kcal/kg/day. 40 kcal/kg/day (formula) + 60 kcal/kg/day (TPN) = 100 kcal/kg/day. Caloric requirements for term or near-term infants are 105 to 120 kcal/kg/day enterally and 85 to 100 kcal/kg/day parentally. Requirements are greater for very low birth weight infants.

**Reference:** Kilbride, H.W., Leick-Rude, M.K., Olsen, S.LO., et al.: Total parental nutrition. In Gardner, S.L., Carter, B.S., Enzman-Hines, M., et al. (Eds.): *Merenstein and Gardner's Handbook of Neonatal Intensive Care*, 7th ed. St. Louis, Mosby, 2011, pp. 378-397.

20. **(B)** Generally, if an infant fails to respond to therapy for hypocalcemia, hypomagnesemia may be the problem, especially in infants of diabetic mothers. Calcium chloride is not routinely used to treat hypocalcemia outside of cardiopulmonary arrest. Neither normal saline nor potassium are indicated in the treatment of hypocalcemia.

**Reference:** Jones, J.E., Hayes, R.D., Starbuck, A.L., et al.: Fluid and electrolyte management. In Gardner, S.L., Carter, B.S., Enzman-Hines, M., et al. (Eds.): *Merenstein and Gardner's Handbook of Neonatal Intensive Care*, 7th ed. St. Louis, Mosby, Elsevier, 2011, pp. 333-352.

21. **(C)** Laboratory tests suggestive of metabolic bone disease are normal calcium, low phosphorus, high alkaline phosphatase, and high 1,25-dihydroxyvitamin D levels. The serum calcium level is usually normal, phosphorus level is low, and 1,25-dihydroxyvitamin D level is elevated in metabolic bone disease.

**Reference:** Vachharajani, A.J., Mathur, A.M., Rao, P.: Metabolic bone disease of prematurity. *NeoReviews*, 10:e402-e411, 2009.

## CHAPTER 8: NUTRITION MANAGEMENT

1. **(B)** Pumping as soon as possible after delivery (within the first 8 hours) results in higher prolactin levels. Higher prolactin levels are associated with higher amounts of milk production. Waiting until the mother has recovered or until she is ready does not promote successful lactation. The goal is to have the mother expressing her breasts within 8 hours after delivery.

**Reference:** Smith M., Durkin M., Hinton V.J., et al.: Initiating of breastfeeding among mothers of very low birth weight infants. *Pediatrics*, 111:1337-1342, 2003.

2. **(B)** Preterm infants fed human milk have a lower rate of a variety of infections, including necrotizing enterocolitis and urinary tract infections, and experience less feeding intolerance than those receiving formula. Although breast milk is the preferred enteral feeding, it requires fortification to adequately supply the preterm infant's need for protein, calcium, phosphorus, and calories. In addition, the nutritional value of breast milk changes during lactation. Although preterm breast milk is higher in protein than term breast milk, the protein content of preterm breast milk is low, and it will not provide enough protein for growth of the preterm infant.

**Reference:** Chauhan M., Henderson G., McGuire W.: Enteral feeding for very low birth weight infants: Reducing the risk of necrotising Enterocolitis. *Archives of Disease in Childhood—Fetal and Neonatal Edition*, 93:F162-F166, 2008.

3. **(C)** Providing skin-to-skin contact via holding has been shown to improve breast milk supply and promote successful breast-feeding. Early introduction of the breast for nonnutritive sucking (sucking at an emptied breast) is associated with longer breast-feeding after discharge. Infants allowed to suckle at the empty breast, nuzzle at the breast, and be held skin to skin breast-feed longer after discharge from the NICU. In addition, breast-feeding is easier and less stressful for the preterm infant than bottle feeding. Offering the bottle as a first nipple feeding reduces the opportunity for breast-feeding. Mothers should be encouraged to be continuously present as much as possible to facilitate frequent access to breast-feeding. Use of breast shields is recommended to improve milk transfer.

**References:** Dimenna, L.: Considerations for implementation of a neonatal kangaroo care protocol. *Neonatal Network*, 25:405-412, 2006

Meier, P.: Supporting lactation in mothers with very low birth weight infants. *Pediatric Annals*, 32:317-325, 2003.

4. **(C)** Healthy newborns require 100 to 120 kcal/kg/day for adequate growth and development.

**Reference:** American Academy of Pediatrics Committee on Nutrition: *Pediatric Nutrition Handbook*, 6th ed. Elk Grove Village, Ill., The Academy, 2009.

5. **(D)** Reducing substance in the stool is indicative of excessive sugar content, often associated with

carbohydrate malabsorption. However, the presence of reducing substance in the stool must be correlated with other signs of malabsorption, such as loose or diarrheal stools and poor weight gain. The presence of reducing substance in the stool is not indicative of hepatobiliary disease or slow gastrointestinal motility. Although associated with early signs of necrotizing enterocolitis, the presence of reducing substance in the stool is not diagnostic and must be evaluated in conjunction with other physical assessment findings.

**Reference:** American Academy of Pediatrics Committee on Nutrition: *Pediatric Nutrition Handbook,* 6th ed. Elk Grove Village, Ill., The Academy, 2009.

6. **(C)** Immature gastrointestinal motility is a significant factor in the successful provision of enteral nutrition to preterm infants. Although gastric capacity is small in preterm infants and gastroesophageal reflux is common, reduced gastrointestinal motility most often results in withholding of enteral feeds due to residuals. Residuals are commonplace in the preterm infant and alone do not serve as a signal of feeding intolerance. Unless malabsorption syndrome or other intestinal disease is present, absorption from the gastrointestinal tract of preterm newborns is not altered.

**References:** Ditzenberger, G.R.: Nutritional management. In Verklan, M. and Walden, M. (Eds) *Core Curriculum for Neonatal Intensive Care Nursing*, 4th ed. St. Louis, Saunders Elsevier, 2010, pp. 183.

Dollber, S., Kuint, J., Mazkereth, R., Mimouni, F.: Feeding tolerance in preterm infants: Randomized trial of bolus and continuous feeding. *Journal of the American College of Nutrition*, 19(6): 797-800, 2000.

Williams, A.: Early enteral feeding of the preterm infant *Arch Dis Child Fetal Neonatal Ed.*, 83(3):F219-20, 2000.

7. **(B)** Bone health requires the necessary components, such as an adequate supply of substrates like calcium and phosphorous. Prolonged nothing-by-mouth (NPO) status, poor nutritional status, and severe prematurity all increase the risk of osteopenia of prematurity from a diminished available substrate. The risk of osteopenia is not increased by near-term delivery or exposure to total parenteral nutrition for one week. Use of commercial formula is not a risk factor for osteopenia of prematurity. The use of fortified breast milk is protective.

**Reference:** Rauch, F., Schoenau, E.: Skeletal development in premature infants: A review of bone physiology beyond nutritional aspects. *Archives of Disease in Childhood—Fetal and Neonatal Edition*, 86(2):F82-F85, 2002.

8. **(C)** Total parenteral nutrition (TPN) is associated with cholestasis, and the most significant risk factor is duration of exposure. Other risk factors include young gestational age, low birth weight, and multiple sepsis episodes. Although the degree of lung disease may be an indicator of degree of illness, severe illness alone has not been identified as a predictor of TPN–associated cholestasis. Enteral feeding of any type is protective against cholestasis. Protein requirements for adequate growth in the preterm infant are 3 to 4 g/kg/day.

**Reference:** Hsieh M., Pai W., Tseng H., et al.: Parenteral nutrition-associated cholestasis in premature babies: Risk factors and predictors. *Pediatrics and Neonatology*, 50(5):202-207, 2009.

9. **(C)** Early minimal feeding of the premature newborn is associated with earlier attainment of full enteral feeds and earlier discharge without an increased risk of necrotizing enterocolitis. Early minimal feeding has not been found to be associated with intestinal perforation, apnea and bradycardia, or an increased risk of necrotizing enterocolitis.

**Reference:** Tyson, J., Kennedy, K.: Trophic feeding for parenterally fed infants. *Cochrane Database of Systematic Reviews*, Issue 3:CD000504, 2005.

10. **(D)** Carnitine is an essential nutrient for fat metabolism and the production of energy and is present in sufficient quantities in formula and human milk. Owing to poor stores, possible lack of necessary enzymes to synthesize carnitine, and nothing-by-mouth status, the preterm infant is carnitine deficient. This deficiency may lead to increased apnea and bradycardia, failure to thrive, and decreased muscle tone. Infants not being fed enterally are carnitine deficient and may benefit from supplementation via total parenteral nutrition. Carnitine supplementation is not associated with a reduced incidence of respiratory distress, feeding intolerance, or necrotizing enterocolitis.

**Reference:** Shah M., Shah S.: Nutrient deficiencies in the premature infant. *Pediatric Clinics of North America*, 56:1069-1083, 2009.

11. **(B)** Intravenous lipid administration is associated with many morbidities, including alteration in leukocyte function, decreased pulmonary diffusion of gases, and decrease in peripheral oxygenation. It is associated with displacement of bound bilirubin by free fatty acids, not increased binding of bilirubin, and with hyperphospholipidemia, not hypophospholipidemia.

**Reference:** Shulman, R., Phillips, S.: Parenteral nutrition in infants and children. *Journal of Pediatric Gastroenterology and Nutrition*, 36(5):587-607, 2003.

12. **(D)** Preterm infant formulas differ from term infant formulas in many ways. The preterm infant formula provides increased calcium and phosphorus, increased carnitine, increased medium-chain triglycerides as a fat source, a reduced amount of lactose, and increased protein content. These modifications are to enhance the digestibility and absorption of nutrients by infants with immature gut function. Preterm infant formulas are not soy based and have increased protein content. Although the fat source is different, the amount of fat in preterm formulas is the same as that found in term infant formulas.

**Reference:** American Academy of Pediatrics Committee on Nutrition: *Pediatric Nutrition Handbook,* 5th ed. Elk Grove Village, Ill., The Academy, 2009.

13. **(C)** Soy-based formulas are indicated for infants with immunoglobulin E–mediated reaction to cow's milk protein and for those with lactase deficiency or galactosemia. Soy-based formulas are not indicated for infants with bloody stools without further

investigation of the cause or for those with feeding intolerance. They are not recommended for infants with frequent emesis. Infants with frequent emesis need to be further evaluated for other problems, including gastroesophageal reflux, and changing formulas may delay this evaluation. Soy-based formulas are not recommended for infants weighing less than 1800 g because of an increased risk of osteopenia.

**Reference:** American Academy of Pediatrics Committee on Nutrition: *Pediatric Nutrition Handbook,* 5th ed. Elk Grove Village, Ill., The Academy, 2009.

**14. (D)** Multiple studies have demonstrated an improvement in expressed milk volume when mothers pump both breasts simultaneously, possibly due to an increase in prolactin levels. Although pumping simultaneously does reduce the time the mother spends pumping, the primary emphasis should be on breast milk production.

**Reference:** Renfrew M., Craig D., Dyson L., et al.: Breastfeeding promotion for infants in neonatal units: A systemic review and economic analysis. *Health Technology Assessment,* 13(40):1-160, 2009.

**15. (C)** Recently it has been found that very low birth weight infants fed exclusively fortified human milk do not receive the necessary protein for adequate growth. Very low birth weight infants fed preterm formula have better postnatal weight gain than infants fed fortified human milk, despite adequate intake. Fat intake is generally adequate in the preterm infant who is receiving normal intake. Although restricted intake can lead to poor growth, increasing intake may not improve growth without the addition of adequate protein. In general, preterm infants do not have an increased incidence of poor intestinal absorption of nutrients. Infants with short bowel syndrome or ileostomies experience poor intestinal absorption of nutrients.

**Reference:** Sertac A., Guido E., Ziegler, E.: Optimization of human milk fortification for preterm infants: New concepts and recommendations. *Journal of Perinatal Medicine,* 38(3):233-238, 2010.

**16. (D)** Use of the pacing technique, which involves leaving the nipple in the mouth and tipping the bottle to stop the flow of fluid, allows the infant with a disorganized feeding behavior time to breathe and swallow. When identified early, disorganized feeding behaviors can be treated with pacing to reduce the incidence of feeding-associated bradycardia, coughing, and feeding fatigue, and to improve feeding competence. Use of the pacing technique can be attempted first before abandoning the feeding attempt. Disorganized sucking does not improve over the feeding event and, if allowed to progress, results in bradycardia. Pulling the bottle out of the mouth disrupts the sucking pattern.

**Reference:** Law-Morstatt L., Judd D., Snyder P., et al.: Pacing as a treatment technique for transitional sucking patterns. *Journal of Perinatology,* 23:483-488, 2003.

**17. (B)** Initiating total parenteral nutrition (TPN) soon after birth in preterm infants has been shown to improve weight gain, reduce sepsis events, and increase albumin synthesis without apparent toxicity. Although blood urea nitrogen levels rise with early initiation of TPN, this higher level is considered clinically insignificant and does not result in acidosis.

**Reference:** Clarke R., Chace D., Spitzer A.: Effects of two different doses of amino acid supplementations on growth and blood amino acid levels on premature neonates admitted to the neonatal intensive care unit: A randomized controlled trial. *Pediatrics,* 120:1286-1296, 2007.

**18. (D)** Commercially available human milk fortifier provides increased protein, calcium, phosphorous, and calories. Currently available human milk fortifier does not provide a significant source of iron. There is no evidence that adding fortifier increases the incidence of feeding intolerance or necrotizing enterocolitis.

**References:** Ditzenberger, G.R. Nutritional management. In Verklan, M. and Walden, M. (Eds): *Core Curriculum for Neonatal Intensive Care Nursing,* 4th ed. St. Louis, Saunders Elsevier, 2010, pp. 198.

Kuschel, C., Harding, J.: Multicomponent fortified human milk for promoting growth in preterm infants. *Cochrane Database of Systematic Reviews,* Issue 1:CD000343, 2004.

**19. (B)** Bolus feedings have been shown to reduce the time required to establish full enteral feedings. Bolus feedings are physiologic and are associated with cyclical surges of gut hormones that increase gastric emptying time and intestinal transit time. Bolus feedings are not associated with an increased risk of feeding intolerance or necrotizing enterocolitis.

**Reference:** Premji, S., Chessell, L.: Continuous nasogastric milk feeding versus intermittent bolus milk feeding for premature infants less than 1500 grams. *Cochrane Database of Systematic Reviews,* Issue 4:CD001819, 2007.

**20. (B)** Gastric residuals should be considered in the context of the clinical condition of the infant, because residuals may be early signs of feeding intolerance or may be normal. As a single presentation sign, gastric residuals are not predictive of an abnormal gastrointestinal (GI) process. The presence of other clinical findings, such as increasing abdominal girth along with a gastric residual, is more likely to signal an abnormal GI process. A one-time gastric residual in an otherwise healthy preterm infant or when feedings are just beginning is often benign. Residuals may be a sign of feeding intolerance, but could also be related to poor GI motility. Withholding feedings may be indicated depending on the results of the physical assessment. Although the manifestations of necrotizing enterocolitis often include the development of residuals, additional signs occur as well, including increasing abdominal girth or bowel loops. Residuals should be evaluated carefully and in the context of the clinical presentation.

**Reference:** Patole, S.K., De Klerk, N.: Impact of standardised feeding regimens on incidence of neonatal necrotising enterocolitis: A systematic review and meta-analysis of observational studies. *Archives of Disease in Childhood—Fetal and Neonatal Edition,* 90:F147-F151, 2005.

**21. (D)** Nonnutritive sucking is associated with improved feeding behavior and decreased length of hospital stay. Other benefits include increased gastric emptying, reduced feeding intolerance, and improved feeding performance. Nonnutritive sucking includes not only the use of the pacifier but also suckling at the emptied breast. Nonnutritive sucking using a pacifier is not associated with reduced performance at the breast. There is no identified association between nonnutritive sucking and incidence of fatigue or bradycardia.

**Reference:** Pinelli J., Symington A.: Non-nutritive sucking for promoting physiologic stability and nutrition in preterm infants. *Cochrane Database of Systematic Reviews,* Issue 4:CD001071, 2005.

## CHAPTER 9: DEVELOPMENTAL SUPPORT

1. **(A)** Paced feeding supports feeding success by coordinating sucking, promoting swallowing, regulating breathing breaks, and increasing stability. The synactive model of infant behavior is a major theoretic framework for establishing physiologic stability as the foundation for the organization of motor, state, and attentive-interactive behaviors. In infant-led feeding, the baby determines when to be fed. *Interactive feeding* is a nonexistent term.

**Reference:** Carrier, C.T.: Developmental support. In Verklan, M., Walden, M. (Eds.): *Core Curriculum for Neonatal Intensive Care Nursing,* 4th ed. St. Louis, Saunders, 2010, pp. 209-227.

2. **(A)** Oral aversion can develop in response to repetitive invasive procedures, feeding on a schedule instead of on demand, and having multiple caregivers. Feeding strike occurs when a baby refuses to breastfeed and is not in the process of being weaned. *Feeding opposition* is a nonexistent term. Signs of feeding intolerance are abdominal distention, emesis, residuals, and blood in the stool.

**Reference:** Gardner S.L., Goldson, E.: The neonate and the environment: Impact on development. In Gardner, S.L, Carter, B.S., Enzman-Hines M., et al. (Eds.): *Merenstein and Gardner's Handbook of Neonatal Intensive Care,* 7th ed. St. Louis, Mosby, 2011, pp. 315, 420.

3. **(C)** Recommended noise levels are below 45 dB. Hearing damage occurs in adults at 85 dB. Noise increases avoidance behaviors, disturbs sleep, increases cerebral blood flow and intraventricular hemorrhage, increases cardiorespiratory instability, and increases sensorineural hearing loss. The human voice is the greatest contributor to excessive noise in the NICU. Incubators produce internal noise, and the sound of the doors closing is louder on the inside of an incubator.

**Reference:** Gardner S.L., Goldson, E.: The neonate and the environment: Impact on development. In Gardner, S.L, Carter, B.S., Enzman-Hines M., et al. (Eds.): *Merenstein and Gardner's Handbook of Neonatal Intensive Care,* 7th ed. St. Louis, Mosby, 2011, pp. 308-309.

4. **(A)** Kangaroo care has been reported to enhance parental bonding and increase confidence. Other beneficial effects are improved breast-feeding, improved sleep patterns, and lower infection rates. One dose is best described as one sleep-wake cycle, which is 65 minutes in preterm infants. Barriers remain to full implementation of kangaroo care due to issues of perceptions of infant and parent readiness, as well as staff time.

**Reference:** Ludington-Hoe, S., Morgan, K., Abouelfettoh, A.: A clinical guideline for implementation of kangaroo care with premature infants of 30 or more weeks' postmenstrual age. *Advances in Neonatal Care,* 8(3):S3-S23, 2008.

5. **(D)** Skin infection on the chest of the kangaroo care provider could potentially be transmitted to the infant, so kangaroo care should be avoided until the skin is clear. There is no evidence that hairy chests cause overheating or infection. All infants should be monitored during kangaroo care, which allows safe administration of conventional mechanical ventilation and/or nasal continuous positive airway pressure during kangaroo care. A staff member is needed to attend to the ventilator tubing during transfer to the chest to prevent accidental extubation. Unless the mother is too groggy to feel safe during kangaroo care, maternal preeclampsia requiring magnesium sulfate therapy would not be a contraindication.

**References:** Gardner S.L., Goldson, E.: The neonate and the environment: Impact on development. In Gardner, S.L, Carter, B.S., Enzman-Hines M., et al. (Eds.): *Merenstein and Gardner's Handbook of Neonatal Intensive Care,* 7th ed. St. Louis, Mosby, 2011, pp 296-299.

Ludington-Hoe, S., Morgan, K., Abouelfettoh, A.: A clinical guideline for implementation of kangaroo care with premature infants of 30 or more weeks' postmenstrual age. *Advances in Neonatal Care,* 8(3):S3-S23, 2008.

6. **(C)** Long-term effects of pain include alterations in sensitivity to commonplace pain, somatic complaints, and structural changes in the brain. There are several appropriate pain assessment tools for preterm infants including the Neonatal Infant Pain Scale; the Neonatal Pain, Agitation, and Sedation Scale; and the Premature Infant Pain Profile. Short-term effects of pain exposure include decrease in oxygenation, increase in heart rate, increase in risk of intraventricular hemorrhage, and alterations in cortisol levels. The use of sucrose to reduce painful responses has been well studied in animal models as well as in humans.

**Reference:** Walden, M., Jorgensen, K.: Pain management. In Kenner, C., McGrath, J. (Eds.): *Developmental Care of Newborns and Infants.* St. Louis, Mosby, 2004, pp. 197-222.

7. **(A)** Abnormal head molding, hip adduction and external rotation, and arching posture are prevented by correct neurodevelopmental positioning. Fixed neck *extension* is an acquired positioning malformation that can be prevented by appropriate positioning. Wrist and ankle torsion are not acquired positioning malformations. Scapular *adduction* and shoulder *retraction* are acquired positioning malformations that can be prevented by appropriate positioning.

**Reference:** Carrier, C.T.: Developmental support. In Verklan, M.T., Walden, M. (Eds.): *Core Curriculum for Neonatal Intensive Care Nursing,* 4th ed. St. Louis, Saunders, 2010, pp. 209-227.

8. **(D)** Best practices include use of a procedure light to allow for a focused source instead of overhead lighting; use of acoustical tile and visual alarms; avoidance of overhead paging to reduce ambient sound level; and assessment of stress signals when providing nursing care so that the nurse can determine when to stop

providing care and let the baby recover, also known as *cue-based care timing*. Windows that allow daylight in are helpful for staff and family well-being; auditory alarms are to be avoided, because they increase ambient noise and disrupt sleep. Continuous fluorescent lighting can disrupt sleep-wake states. Day-night cycling of light can help decrease levels of stress hormones such as cortisol.

**Reference:** Carrier, C.: Caregiving and the environment. In Kenner, C., McGrath, J. (Eds.): *Developmental Care of Newborns and Infants.* St. Louis, Mosby, 2004, pp. 229-265.

9. **(A)** Feeding success can be facilitated by decreasing environmental stimuli to allow the infant to focus on the feeding and avoid overstimulating and overwhelming the infant; reducing the stress of burping by positioning and gentle handling; using paced feedings to allow for reorganization of suck, swallowing, and breath coordination; providing kangaroo care prior to feedings; and providing nonnutritive sucking. Nipple type needs to be continuously evaluated and individualized. There is no consensus on the warming of feedings, but extremes in temperature should be avoided. Use of a high-flow nipple can lead to coughing and choking. Hours of music playing increases ambient noise levels; rocking mattresses may be overstimulating.

**Reference:** McGrath, J.: Feeding. In Kenner, C., McGrath, J. (Eds.): *Developmental Care of Newborns and Infants,* St. Louis, Mosby, 2004, pp. 321-342.

10. **(C)** Gentle human touch to provide flexion and containment has a soothing effect. Additional auditory stimulation may be overwhelming. Stroking can result in decreased oxygen saturation and behavioral stress in preterm infants in unstable condition. Human touch is preferable to cloth, and flexion simulates the in utero position.

**Reference:** Gardner S.L., Goldson, E.: The neonate and the environment: Impact on development. In Gardner, S.L, Carter, B.S., Enzman-Hines M., et al. (Eds.): *Merenstein and Gardner's Handbook of Neonatal Intensive Care,* 7th ed. St. Louis, Mosby, 2011, p. 294.

11. **(A)** Major disability rates range from 20% to 50% in preterm infants, depending on gestational age, weight, and year of birth. It is estimated that 10% to 40% of preterm infants have borderline or low intelligence quotients. They are also less adaptable and more impulsive that their term counterparts. Skin-to-skin care has been shown to improve Bayley Mental Developmental Index scores at 6 and 12 months of age.

**Reference:** Pickler, R., Reyna, B., McGrath, J.: NICU and beyond benefits: Benchmarking with measurable outcomes. In Kenner, C., McGrath, J. (Eds.): *Developmental Care of Newborns and Infants,* St. Louis, Mosby, 2004, pp. 411-421.

12. **(B)** B. If at all possible, a sleeping infant should not be awakened. If it is necessary to awaken the infant, as gentle a method as possible should be used. Nurses should educate parents on their infant's behavioral states and cues. Parental involvement should never be discouraged, but if the interaction is inappropriate, parents should be given alternatives.

Because infants spend so much time asleep, parents need to be taught activities that they can do even while their infant is asleep. A goal of developmentally supportive care is to minimize external auditory stimuli. Tapping on the incubator should be avoided.

**References:** Carrier, C.T.: Developmental support. In Verklan, M.T., Walden, M. (Eds.): *Core Curriculum for Neonatal Intensive Care Nursing,* 4th ed. St. Louis, Saunders, 2010, pp. 219-220.

Gardner S.L., Goldson, E.: The neonate and the environment: Impact on development. In Gardner, S.L, Carter, B.S., Enzman-Hines M., et al. (Eds.): *Merenstein and Gardner's Handbook of Neonatal Intensive Care,* 7th ed. St. Louis, Mosby, 2011, p. 309-310.

13. **(B)** Nonnutritive sucking accelerates maturation of the sucking reflex and improves weight gain. Consideration of what has been happening to the infant and readiness for care are always important. Reduction of noxious stimuli increases physiologic stability, potentially improving blood flow to the gut. Prone or side-lying positioning improves gastric emptying and decreases regurgitation.

**Reference:** McGrath, J.: Feeding. In Kenner, C., McGrath, J. (Eds.): *Developmental Care of Newborns and Infants,* St. Louis, Mosby, 2004, pp. 321- 342.

14. **(A)** Swaddling the baby and implementing a time-out for rest and recovery provides neurodevelopmental support, promotes self-regulatory behavior, and allows return to physiologic homeostasis. Just dimming the lights may not decrease stimulation enough to allow for recovery of physiologic stability. Playing music during care to provide auditory distraction is not recommended, because the noise may add to the overstimulation and decompensation. If signs of stress are exhibited, care activities should be stopped and the baby allowed to recover physiologic stability. Continuing with the care could lead to further disorganization and physiologic and behavioral stress.

**Reference:** Pressler, J., Turnage-Carrier, C., Kenner, C.: Developmental care: An overview. In Kenner, C., McGrath, J. (Eds.): *Developmental Care of Newborns and Infants,* St. Louis, Mosby, 2004, pp. 1-29.

15. **(B)** Bright light is detrimental to the developing brain due to overstimulation of the immature central nervous system and can lead to development of physiologic and behavioral defense mechanisms, maladaptions, and poor outcomes. Reduction in visual stimuli is desirable. Monitoring may be somewhat reassuring, but does not explain the importance of a neurodevelopmentally supportive NICU environment. Cycling of day-night is beneficial for promotion of diurnal rhythms and sleep patterns.

**Reference:** Gardner S.L., Goldson, E.: The neonate and the environment: Impact on development. In Gardner, S.L, Carter, B.S., Enzman-Hines M., et al. (Eds.): *Merenstein and Gardner's Handbook of Neonatal Intensive Care,* 7th ed. St. Louis, Mosby, 2011, pp. 311-312.

16. **(D)** Nonnutritive sucking (NNS) is synergistic with sweet taste on the tip of the tongue in decreasing pain responses. NNS is consoling. Noxious oral stimuli may lead to oral aversion. NNS begins very early in

utero and does not signal feeding readiness. It does not impair, but rather is thought to improve, sucking skills if used before initiating nipple feeding.

**References:** Carrier, C.T.: Developmental support. In Verklan, M.T., Walden, M. (Eds.): *Core Curriculum for Neonatal Intensive Care Nursing,* 4th ed. St. Louis, Saunders, 2010, pp. 209-227.

Gardner S.L., Goldson, E.: The neonate and the environment: Impact on development. In Gardner, S.L, Carter, B.S., Enzman-Hines M., et al. (Eds.): *Merenstein and Gardner's Handbook of Neonatal Intensive Care,* 7th ed. St. Louis, Mosby, 2011, p. 314-318.

17. **(D)** Skin-to-skin contact provides tactile stimulation, promotes physiologic stability, and improves maternal milk production. Vestibular sensations occur with the rise and fall of the parent's chest. It is important to document the length of kangaroo care time and the infant and parent response to the activity. Standing transfer may decrease the stress of movement from incubator to parent chest.

**References:** Carrier, C.T.: Developmental support. In Verklan, M.T., Walden, M. (Eds.): *Core Curriculum for Neonatal Intensive Care Nursing,* 4th ed. St. Louis, Saunders, 2010, pp. 209-227.

Gardner S.L., Goldson, E.: The neonate and the environment: Impact on development. In Gardner, S.L, Carter, B.S., Enzman-Hines M., et al. (Eds.): *Merenstein and Gardner's Handbook of Neonatal Intensive Care,* 7th ed. St. Louis, Mosby, 2011, pp. 296-299.

18. **(B)** Intentional movement by newborns enhances neuromuscular development and stability. Muscle tone and reflex development proceeds in a caudocephalad direction: from lower to upper extremities. Nesting or containment should not restrict the movement necessary for growth and development. Regulatory efforts such as pushing against boundaries are an example of intentional movement. Restraint of movement should be limited to as short a period of time as is absolutely necessary.

**Reference:** Carrier, C.T.: Developmental support. In Verklan, M.T., Walden, M. (Eds.): *Core Curriculum for Neonatal Intensive Care Nursing,* 4th ed. St. Louis, Saunders, 2010, pp. 209-227.

19. **(C)** Early dominant states influence the reaction of a newborn to stimuli and must be taken into account when providing developmentally supportive care. Oxygen consumption is lowest during deep sleep. In the quiet alert state, the infant can maximally attend and respond to parents. Less mature infants demonstrate more drowsy than quiet alert states compared with mature infants.

**Reference:** Gardner S.L., Goldson, E.: The neonate and the environment: Impact on development. In Gardner, S.L, Carter, B.S., Enzman-Hines M., et al. (Eds.): *Merenstein and Gardner's Handbook of Neonatal Intensive Care,* 7th ed. St. Louis, Mosby, 2011, p. 275-276.

20. **(D)** Sensory integrative dysfunction is associated long term with reduction in impulse control, learning ability, ability to concentrate, capacity for abstract thought, and self-esteem. Painful stimuli are theorized to "rewire" the brain, which leads to dysfunction of sensory integration. Sensory integrative dysfunction is not expressed uniformly by infants and children—symptoms and problems may vary. The symptoms of

sensory integrative dysfunction are expressed in higher-level function.

**Reference:** Lutes, L., Graves, C., Jorgensen, K.: The NICU experience and its relationship to sensory integration: In Kenner, C., McGrath, J. (Eds.): *Developmental Care of Newborns and Infants,* St. Louis, Mosby, 2004, pp. 157-181.

21. **(C)** The brain is a chain of communication cells, and every touch, movement, and emotion affects its wiring and development. The brain triples in size during the first year of life. The quality of brain development is shaped by both genetic history and environmental factors. A very preterm infant (24 weeks' gestation) has an immature brain structure with a smooth cortex, and few sulci will form during the first year of life.

**Reference:** Lutes, L., Graves, C., Jorgensen, K.: The NICU experience and its relationship to sensory integration: In Kenner, C., McGrath, J. (Eds.): *Developmental Care of Newborns and Infants,* St. Louis, Mosby, 2004, pp. 163-164.

## CHAPTER 10: RADIOGRAPHIC EVALUATION

1. **(C)** Tetralogy of Fallot is characterized by normal pulmonary vascularity and right atrial hypertrophy, which rotates the heart. The cardiac apex appears upturned and prominent, giving the appearance of a "boot-shaped" heart. Tricuspid atresia is characterized by normal or decreased pulmonary flow, and a "rounded" cardiac apex caused by the right atrial enlargement. Ebstein anomaly is characterized by reduced pulmonary vascularity and a severely enlarged right atrium that gives the appearance of a "box-shaped" heart. Total anomalous pulmonary venous return is characterized by increased pulmonary vascularity and a normal to small heart.

**Reference:** Krishnamurthy, R., Blickman, J.G.: Heart. In Blickman, J.G., Parker, B.R., Barnes, P.D. (Eds.): *Pediatric Radiology: The Requisites,* 3rd ed. Philadelphia, Mosby, 2009, pp. 47-61.

2. **(A)** Pneumothorax is characterized by a hyperlucency between the chest wall and lung. Pneumopericardium is characterized by a hyperlucency surrounding the heart. Pneumomediastinum is characterized by an irregular gas collection, with air outlining the undersurface of the thymus gland and creating a "sail sign." Pulmonary interstitial emphysema is characterized by distinct rounded or linear thoracic lucencies that may be unilateral or bilateral.

**Reference:** Blickman, J.G., Die, L.V.: Chest. In Blickman, J.G., Parker, B.R., Barnes, P.D. (Eds.): *Pediatric Radiology: The Requisites,* 3rd ed. Philadelphia, Mosby, 2009, pp. 5-46.

3. **(D)** Necrotizing enterocolitis is characterized by bowel dilation, bowel thickening, pneumatosis that appears as a "bubbly" pattern, and branching lucencies overlying the liver. Duodenal atresia is characterized by gastric distention and a dilated duodenal bulb referred to as the *double bubble*. Meconium ileus is characterized by multiple dilated small bowel loops indicative of a low obstruction. A "soap bubble" appearance may be noted in the right side of the abdomen. Midgut malrotation radiographic findings may be variable and include duodenal obstruction secondary to Ladd

bands, or a mid small bowel obstruction. The radiograph may also have a normal appearance.

**Reference:** Sivit, C.J.: Diagnostic imaging. In Martin, R.J., Fanaroff, A.A., Walsh, M.C. (Eds.): *Neonatal-Perinatal Medicine: Diseases of the Fetus and Infant*, 8th ed. Philadelphia, Mosby, 2006, pp. 713-731.

4. **(C)** In a lateral decubitus view, the x-ray beam passes from the anterior to the posterior aspect with the cassette flat against the infant's back and the infant positioned on his or her side. In an anteroposterior view, the x-ray beam is centered on the infant's chest with the infant lying supine, and the cassette is positioned under the infant's back. In a posteroanterior view, the x-ray beam passes through the patient from back to front. The patient must be able to stand. In a cross-table lateral film, the infant is supine with the cassette placed on one side of the infant's chest and abdomen and the x-ray tube placed on the other side.

**Reference:** Novelline, R.A.: Imaging techniques. In Novelline, R.A. (Ed.): *Fundamentals of Radiology*, 6th ed. Boston, Harvard University Press, 2004, pp. 12-41.

5. **(D)** The tip of the umbilical venous catheter should be placed in the inferior vena cava just below the vena cava and the right atrium, which is T8 to T9. If the catheter tip were at T6, it would be within the heart, either in the left atrium or right ventricle. If the catheter were advanced 1 cm, the tip would be approximately at T5, which would place it in the right atrium. If the catheter were repositioned to T10, the catheter tip would be too low and could cause liver damage.

**Reference:** Bradshaw, W.T., Furdon, S.A.: A nurse's guide to early detection of umbilical venous catheter complications in infants. *Advances in Neonatal Care*, 6(3):127-138, 2006.

6. **(D)** The infant's chin should be repositioned in a neutral position. If the chin is pointing down, the endotracheal tube may appear lower than the true position. The correct position of the endotracheal tube tip is midtrachea, and it should be visible at the level of the clavicles or slightly below, which would be at approximately T1 to T2 on the radiograph. Neither suctioning nor turning the head to the left will alter the position of the tube. The chest radiograph needs to be repeated with proper chin position before the endotracheal tube is moved.

**Reference:** Kattwinkel, J., Bloom, R.S., American Heart Association, American Academy of Pediatrics: *Textbook of Neonatal Resuscitation*, 5th ed. Dallas, American Heart Association, 2006, pp. 5-1–5-42.

7. **(B)** On a radiograph, meconium aspiration is characterized by bilateral asymmetry, with areas of atelectasis and a patchy appearance, and hyperaeration with flattened hemidiaphragms. The initial intervention is to administer oxygen, because the infant is full term and the oxygen saturation is 85% after 2 hours of life. Pulmonary interstitial emphysema appears as distinct rounded or linear thoracic lucencies that may be unilateral or bilateral. Pneumonia is characterized by diffuse ground-glass opacities of variable severity (identical to respiratory distress syndrome). The radiograph may have a normal appearance or may demonstrate streaky, perihilar linear markings. An appropriate initial intervention for an infant with pneumonia is to obtain a blood specimen for culture and initiate antibiotic therapy. Transient tachypnea of the newborn is manifested as streaky, perihilar opacities and lung overinflation. The infant should not be fed because of the risk of aspiration.

**Reference:** Sivit, C.J.: Diagnostic imaging. In Martin, R.J., Fanaroff, A.A., Walsh, M.C. (Eds.): *Neonatal-Perinatal Medicine: Diseases of the Fetus and Infant*, 8th ed. Philadelphia, Mosby, 2006, pp. 713-731.

8. **(C)** Correct tip position of an upper-extremity, peripherally-inserted central line catheter is in the lower third of the superior vena cava, between T3 and T5. Leaving the catheter at T7 would cause complications. The catheter tip is too deep and should be pulled back to between T3 and T5.

**Reference:** Pettit, J., Wyckoff, M.M.: *Peripherally Inserted Central Catheters: Guidelines for Practice*, 2nd ed. Glenview, Ill., National Association of Neonatal Nurses, 2007, p. 29.

9. **(C)** Congenital diaphragmatic hernia is characterized by air-filled bowel loops in the thorax. Initially, the bowel loops may be fluid filled, which makes the diagnosis difficult. The lung on the same side of the defect is usually hypoplastic, because the mass affects its development. The initial intervention is to intubate to minimize the risk of causing a pneumothorax in the hypoplastic lung. A pneumothorax is characterized by a hyperlucency between the chest wall and lung. In pyloric stenosis, a radiograph of the abdomen may show a distended stomach with or without an air-fluid level and relatively little bowel air distally. Pyloric stenosis is not considered a surgical emergency. A midgut volvulus is characterized by a disproportionate dilatation of the stomach and duodenal loop proximal to the volvulus compared with the distal small bowel. A midgut volvulus is considered a surgical emergency.

**Reference:** Sivit, C.J.: Diagnostic imaging. In Martin, R.J., Fanaroff, A.A., Walsh, M.C. (Eds.): *Neonatal-Perinatal Medicine: Diseases of the Fetus and Infant*, 8th ed. Philadelphia, Mosby, 2006, pp. 713-731.

10. **(A)** The infant is at risk for hypoglycemia. The catheter tip would be at the origin of the superior mesenteric artery. The complications associated with a catheter tip placement between T12 and L1 include microthrombi in the intestine and the infusion of glucose near the pancreas with subsequent refractory hypoglycemia. If the catheter tip were below L5, the infant would be at risk for developing gluteal necrosis. The correct catheter tip position for a low-lying umbilical arterial catheter is considered to be below the renal arteries and above the aortic bifurcation (between L3 and L4), and below the left subclavian artery and above the diaphragm (T7 to 79) for a high catheter. The catheter should be pulled back to between L3 and L4, or, if this is the initial radiograph for UAC placement and the sterile field has not been removed, the catheter may be advanced to between T7 and T9.

**References:** Furdon, S.A., Horgan, M.J., Bradshaw, W.T., et al.: Nurse's guide to early detection of umbilical arterial catheter complications in infants. *Advances in Neonatal Care,* 6(5):242-256, 2006.

Bradshaw, W.T, Tanaka, D.T.: Physiologic monitoring. In Gardner, S.L, Carter, B.S., Enzman-Hines M., et al. (Eds.): *Merenstein and Gardner's Handbook of Neonatal Intensive Care,* 7th ed. St. Louis, Mosby, 2011, p. 140.

## CHAPTER 11: PHARMACOLOGY

1. **(B)** To prevent drug toxicity, a smaller than standard dose is expected. Most drugs are metabolized into inactive metabolites. Until the drug is metabolized, the effects of the parent drug are ongoing. Drug metabolism, which occurs in the liver, is impeded in the presence of hepatic disease. Therefore, providing a standard dose of a drug metabolized by the liver may result in drug toxicity. Both a higher than standard dose and more frequent dosing will result in toxic drug levels of hepatically metabolized drugs.

**Reference:** Capparelli, E.V.: Clinical pharmacokinetics in infants and children. In Yaffee, S.J., Aranda, J.V. (Eds.): *Neonatal and Pediatric Pharmacology: Therapeutic Principles in Practice,* 3rd ed. Philadelphia, Lippincott Williams & Wilkins, 2005, pp. 9-19.

2. **(A)** A loading or priming dose rapidly establishes a therapeutic plasma drug level. It is calculated by multiplying the volume of distribution by the desired plasma drug concentration. The loading dose establishes a desired level. Maintenance dosing is initiated after the loading dose to maintain the therapeutic level. The maintenance dose is smaller than the loading dose. With first-pass effect, the medication enters hepatic metabolism prior to entering circulation. The amount of drug available afterward may be significantly reduced. A medication without first-pass effect will achieve a higher plasma concentration but will not reach a therapeutic level until multiple doses have been administered. The ability of a medication to enter the cell does not influence the therapeutic plasma concentration.

**Reference:** Adams, P.M., Koch, R.W.: *Pharmacology: Connections to Nursing Practice,* Upper Saddle River, N.J., Pearson, 2010, pp. 40-54.

3. **(D)** Bacterial cells have a rigid cell wall to resist significant intracellular pressure. β-Lactam antibiotics weaken bacterial cell walls, which results in lysis and destruction. Sulfonamides block enzymes needed for bacterial production of folic acid. Antibiotics do not activate the immune system. They initiate bacterial death and allow the patient's immune system to complete microorganism eradication. Aminoglycosides and macrolides bind with subunits of bacterial ribosomes to prevent protein synthesis. Aminoglycosides are bacteriocidal, whereas macrolides are generally bacteriostatic.

**Reference:** Lehne, R.A.: *Pharmacology for Nursing Care,* 7th ed. St. Louis, Saunders, 2010, pp. 970-983.

4. **(B)** Antiseizure medications suppress abnormal neuronal discharges by controlling electrolyte movement or neurotransmitter balance. Glutamate is the primary stimulatory neurotransmitter in the brain. Medications potentiating the effect of glutamate increase neuronal firing. γ-Aminobutyric acid (GABA) is the primary inhibitory neurotransmitter in the brain. A reduced level of GABA permits, rather than inhibits, neuronal firing. Antiseizure medications close sodium and calcium channels, which prevents entry of those electrolytes into the neuron and reduces action potentials.

**Reference:** Adams, P.M., Koch, R.W.: *Pharmacology: Connections to Nursing Practice,* Upper Saddle River, N.J., Pearson, 2010, pp. 370-395.

5. **(C)** Although cardiovascular symptoms such as tachycardia or dysrhythmias are most indicative of methylxanthine toxicity, gastrointestinal problems commonly occur. Methylxanthines may precipitate blood glucose abnormalities, including hyperglycemia and hypoglycemia. As central nervous system stimulants, methylxanthines produced alertness. Temperature control is not affected by methylxanthines.

**References:** Adams, P.M., Koch, R.W.: *Pharmacology: Connections to Nursing Practice,* Upper Saddle River, N.J., Pearson, 2010, pp. 411-426.

Goodwin, M.: Apnea. In Verklan, M.T., Walden, M. (Eds.): *Core Curriculum for Neonatal Intensive Care Nursing,* 4th ed. St. Louis, Saunders, 2010, pp. 484-493.

6. **(D)** The positive and negative effects of fentanyl occur rapidly. The infant receiving fentanyl should be monitored for chest wall rigidity and respiratory depression. Fentanyl precipitates hypotension. Stimulation of the vagal nerve can cause a reflexive decrease in heart rate but does not cause chest wall rigidity. Anesthetic gases received in the operating room induce reactions at the time of inhalation. The infant has experienced an acute event after returning from the operating room.

**References:** Spratto, G.R., Woods, A.L.: *Delmar Nurse's Drug Handbook,* Clifton Park, N.Y.: Delmar Cengage Learning, 2010, pp. 663-667.

Walden, M.: Pain assessment and management. In Verklan, M.T., Walden, M. (Eds.): *Core Curriculum for Neonatal Intensive Care Nursing,* 4th ed. St. Louis, Saunders, 2010, pp. 333-346.

7. **(B)** Digoxin inhibits sodium–potassium–adenosine triphosphatase; this results in calcium influx into the myocardial cells, which enhances contractility (inotropy). Digoxin decreases plasma renin and aldosterone to lower afterload. It also suppresses the sinoatrial node and increases the refractory period of the atrioventricular node, which results in slow electrical conduction and a negative dromotropic effect. Digoxin increases vagal nerve tone, which results in a negative chronotropic effect.

**References:** Adams, P.M., Koch, R.W.: *Pharmacology: Connections to Nursing Practice,* Upper Saddle River, N.J., Pearson, 2010, pp. 606-621.

Spratto, G.R., Woods, A.L.: *Delmar Nurse's Drug Handbook,* Clifton Park, N.Y.: Delmar Cengage Learning, 2010, pp. 487-492.

8. **(D)** Anticholinergic drugs block acetylcholine at parasympathetic muscarinic receptors. Their actions include increased heart rate; relaxation of bronchial smooth muscle, which improves air entry into the lungs; pupil relaxation; and decreased tone and

motility of the gastrointestinal tract. Anticholinergic agents also cause mild central nervous system excitation. Ophthalmic drugs are absorbed into systemic circulation after draining into the nasopharynx via the nasolacrimal duct.

**Reference:** Lehne, R.A.: *Pharmacology for Nursing Care,* 7th ed. St. Louis, Saunders, 2010, pp. 121-130.

9. **(B)** Spironolactone is an aldosterone antagonist and mild diuretic with a slow onset of action and peak activity at 48 to 72 hours. This agent would be of limited value in acute pulmonary edema. Although allergic reactions can occur with any drug, the probability of an allergic reaction to spironolactone is small. This agent is a steroid derivative and does not contain a sulfa ring as do loop and thiazide diuretics. There is no intravenous form of spironolactone. Spironolactone prevents sodium reabsorption in the distal nephron and allows potassium reabsorption. Serum potassium levels therefore may rise with spironolactone use. Hence, the use the term *potassium sparing* is used when describing this drug's action.

**References:** Lehne, R.A.: *Pharmacology for Nursing Care,* 7th ed. St. Louis, Saunders, 2010, pp. 443-454.

Spratto, G.R., Woods, A.L.: *Delmar Nurse's Drug Handbook,* Clifton Park, N.Y.: Delmar Cengage Learning, 2010, pp. 1601-1603.

10. **(D)** Blood flow to tissues is the simplest factor determining drug distribution. Drugs are distributed via the circulatory system and reach tissues at a rate proportional to blood flow. The heart, liver, and kidneys receive a high percentage of the blood supply and thus highest exposure to drugs. *Half-life* refers to the time required for the level of a drug in the body to decrease by 50%. Half-life is a percentage, not a specific amount. Half-life determines the dosing interval of a drug. Drug interactions can affect the amount of a medication in circulation and may reduce the amount of medication available for distribution. A plateau or steady state refers to the state of equilibrium obtained when a drug is administered repeatedly at the same dose. Steady state is achieved after four half-lives.

**References:** Adams, P.M., Holland, L.N.: *Pharmacology for Nurses: A Pathophysiologic Approach,* 3rd ed. Boston, Pearson, 2011, pp. 36-44.

Lehne, R.A.: *Pharmacology for Nursing Care,* 7th ed. St. Louis, Saunders, 2010, pp. 25-45.

11. **(D)** Drugs entering the intestine in bile may be reabsorbed back into the portal venous system, which substantially prolongs a drug's presence in the body. Metabolism of a medication is also known as *biotransformation*. During this process, the structure of the original drug is altered. Most drug metabolism occurs in the liver. Oral drugs that are absorbed from the gastrointestinal tract are carried directly to the liver by the hepatic portal vein. Certain drugs are extensively inactivated on this first pass through the liver. Hepatic clearance is the ability of the liver to inactivate or biotransform a medication.

**Reference:** Lehne, R.A.: *Pharmacology for Nursing Care,* 7th ed. St. Louis, Saunders, 2010, pp. 25-45.

## CHAPTER 12: CARE OF THE EXTREMELY LOW BIRTH WEIGHT INFANT

1. **(B)** Extremely low birth weight (ELBW) infants have greater problems with transdermal fluid losses than other populations of newborns. A polyethylene wrap or bag is indicated in the delivery room to minimize these losses. Nasal continuous positive airway pressure device is not an intervention indicated specifically for the ELBW infant. There is nothing in the history to suggest the likelihood that there will be a finding of meconium at delivery. The lower the gestational age, the less likely the finding of meconium at delivery. An endotracheal tube should be prepared for all high-risk deliveries. In addition, a 3.5-mm tube is recommended for patients weighing 2000 to 3000 g and of gestational ages 28 to 34 weeks. The recommended tube size for this infant is 2.5 mm.

**References:** Kattwinkel, J., Bloom, R.S., American Heart Association, American Academy of Pediatrics: *Textbook of Neonatal Resuscitation,* 5th ed. Dallas, American Heart Association, 2006, pp. 8-6.

Vohra, S., Roberts, R.S., Zhang, B., et al.: Heat loss prevention (HeLP) in the delivery room: A randomized controlled trial of polyethylene occlusive skin wrapping in very preterm infants. *Journal of Pediatrics,* 145:750-753, 2004.

2. **(B)** Hyperoxia in the extremely low birth weight infant is associated with increased risk of retinopathy of prematurity and bronchopulmonary dysplasia. Blended oxygen should be available in any delivery room where one might anticipate the delivery of preterm infants. Infants require 100% oxygen only if they prove to be inadequately oxygenated with a lower fraction of inspired oxygen ($Fio_2$). Oxygen saturation is not normally higher than 90% during transition; thus a goal of higher than 98% would result in hyperoxia.

**References:** Chess, P.R., D'Angio, C.R., Pryhuber, G.S., et al.: Pathogenesis of bronchopulmonary dysplasia. *Seminars in Perinatology,* 30:171-178, 2006.

Coe, K.M., Butler, M., Reavis, N., et al.: Special Premie Oxygen Targeting (SPOT): A program to decrease the incidence of blindness in infants with retinopathy of prematurity. *Journal of Nursing Care Quality,* 21:230-235, 2006.

Vento, M., Moro, M., Escrig, R., et al.: Preterm resuscitation with low oxygen causes less oxidative stress, inflammation, and chronic lung disease. *Pediatrics,* 124:439-449, 2009.

3. **(C)** Each of the interventions described reduces the risk of intraventricular hemorrhage by encouraging homeostasis of cerebral blood flow. Of the interventions described, only minimizing suctioning is intended to prevent pneumothorax. None of the interventions is particularly efficacious in preventing thermal instability. Only midline head positioning is intended to prevent musculoskeletal deformities.

**References:** Hill, A., Perlman, J.M., Volpe, J.J.: Relationship of pneumothorax and occurrence of intraventricular hemorrhage in small preterm infants. *Pediatrics,* 69:144-149, 1982.

Limperopoulos, D., Gauvreau, K.K., O'Leary, H., et al.: Cerebral hemodynamic changes during intensive care of preterm infants. *Pediatrics,* 122(5):1006-1013, 2008.

Mainous, R.O., Looney, S.: A pilot study of changes in cerebral blood flow velocity, resistance, and vital signs following a painful stimulus in the preterm infant. *Advances in Neonatal Care,* 7(2):88-104, 2007.

Perlman, J.M., Volpe, J.J.: Cerebral blood flow velocity in relation to intraventricular hemorrhage in the preterm newborn infant. *Journal of Pediatrics,* 100:956-959, 1982.

Perlman, J.M., Volpe, J.J.: Suctioning in the preterm infants: effects on cerebral blood flow volume, intracranial pressure, and arterial blood pressure. *Pediatrics,* 72:329-334, 1983.

Pichler, G., van Boetzelar, M.C., Muller, W., et al.: Effect of tilting on cerebral hemodynamics in preterm and term infants. *Biology of the Neonate,* 80(3):179-185, 2001.

4. **(C)** Transdermal fluid losses in an infant of this postconceptional age may exceed 70 $g/m^2/hour$. These losses may significantly contribute to both dehydration and thermal instability. Urinary output norms in this population are usually stated as 1 to 5 ml/kg/hour. Thus, this infant's output is closer to oliguria, rather than diuresis. Although this level of fluid intake is somewhat restrictive, it is not unusual for the extremely low birth weight infant on the first day or two of life and should be adequate unless there is too much fluid loss. The evidence does not suggest that high incubator temperatures, per se, lead to dehydration.

**References:** Hammarlund, K., Sedin, G.: Transepidermal water loss in newborn infants III. Relation to gestational age. *Acta Paediatrica Scandinavia,* 68:795-801, 1979.

Kim, S.M., Lee, Y., Chen, J., et al.: Improved care and growth outcomes by using hybrid humidified incubators in very preterm infants. *Pediatrics,* 125:137-145, 2010.

5. **(A)** Caring for the infant in a humidified environment with relative humidity higher than 70% significantly reduces transdermal fluid losses, decreases the risk of dehydration associated with electrolyte imbalance, and promotes thermal stability. It is relatively safe when used per current guidelines. Higher fluid intake during the initial days of life in the extremely low birth weight (ELBW) infant may result in pulmonary edema that requires increased support of ventilation and increases the risk of later chronic lung disease. Higher fluid intake is also associated with a greater risk of clinically significant patent ductus arteriosus. Using a heated mattress may improve thermal stability, but is unlikely to affect dehydration. Adding sodium to the intravenous intake is contraindicated in the ELBW infant in the first days of life and would not likely reduce urinary output.

**Reference:** Kim, S.M., Lee, Y., Chen, J., et al.: Improved care and growth outcomes by using hybrid humidified incubators in very preterm infants. *Pediatrics,* 125:137-145, 2010.

## CHAPTER 13: CARE OF THE LATE PRETERM INFANT

1. **(C)** Late preterm infants (LPIs) are at a greater risk of acquiring respiratory syncytial virus infection than term infants due to immaturity of the immune system and respiratory system, and the incomplete transfer of maternal antibodies. Abdominal distention is not a diagnosis that is commonly seen in LPIs with feeding difficulties. Abdominal distention can be associated with obstruction or necrotizing enterocolitis (NEC). NEC predominantly affects preterm infants and

usually occurs in the first 3 to 12 days of life. Persistent patent ductus arteriosus (PDA) is inversely related to gestational age. The more premature the infant, the higher incidence of PDA.

**References:** Coffman, S.: Late preterm infants and risk for RSV. *MCN. The American Journal of Maternal Child Nursing,* 34(6):387-384, 2009.

Engle, W.A., Tomashek, K.M., Wallman, C., Committee on Fetus and Newborn: Late-preterm infants: A population at risk. *Pediatrics,* 120:1390-1401, 2007.

2. **(C)** The large size of the infant for gestational age is a result of poorly controlled maternal glucose levels during pregnancy. Fetal hyperinsulinemia contributes to delayed maturation of the lungs, which inhibits the production of surfactant and increases the risk of surfactant deficiency related to respiratory distress syndrome. Although the presenting symptoms of pneumonia are similar to those described, additional characteristics that correlate with pneumonia include a fetal monitoring tracing showing decreased variability, prolonged rupture of membranes (longer than 24 hours), and purulent or foul-smelling amniotic fluid. Bronchopulmonary dysplasia is not a disease that appears shortly after birth. Predisposing risk factors include prolonged assisted ventilation, air leaks, infection, and prematurity of less than 32 weeks' gestation. Transient tachypnea of the newborn is usually self-limiting and rarely requires supplemental oxygen at a level higher than 40%. These infants usually have mild cyanosis and may have blood gas values that reveal a mild respiratory alkalemia.

**References:** Askin, D.: Respiratory distress. In Verklan, M., Walden, M. (Eds.): *Core Curriculum for Neonatal Intensive Care Nursing,* 4th ed. St. Louis, Saunders, 2010, pp. 453-483.

Gardner, S.L., Enzman-Hines, M., Dickey, L.A.: Respiratory diseases. In Gardner, S.L., Carter, B.S., Enzman-Hines, M., et al. (Eds.): *Merenstein and Gardner's Handbook of Neonatal Intensive Care,* 7th ed. St. Louis, Mosby, 2011, pp. 581-677.

3. **(C)** Late preterm infants (LPIs) have a limited capacity to process unconjugated bilirubin compared with term infants, which places them at higher risk of developing hyperbilirubinemia. Inadequate breastfeeding resulting in an increased risk of dehydration further enhances the potential for development of severe hyperbilirubinemia, which can lead to kernicterus. LPIs are at a higher risk of developing hypothermia due to lower brown fat stores and larger body surface area compared with the term infant. LPIs are at a higher risk for developing hypoglycemia due to decreased glycogen stores and the potential for increased glucose utilization. Although LPIs can potentially develop persistent pulmonary hypertension (PPHN), there are factors other that prematurity that contribute to the development of PPHN. PPHN is a disease more prevalent in term and postterm neonates.

**References:** Bhutani, V.K., Johnson, L.: Kernicterus in late preterm infants cared for as term healthy infants. *Seminars in Perinatology,* 30:89-97, 2006.

Watchko, J.F.: Hyperbilirubinemia and bilirubin toxicity in the late preterm. *Clinics in Perinatology,* 33:839-852, 2006.

4. **(D)** The American Academy of Pediatrics recommends that infants of less than 37 weeks' gestation receive a car seat discharge test. Since late preterm infants (LPIs) often experience difficulties in breastfeeding successfully, a lactation consultation should be carried out before discharge and specific feeding education or plan and lactation recourses available after discharge. LPIs are at risk of developing dehydration when feeds are being established. Signs and symptoms of dehydration should be included in the discharge teaching of parents with LPIs. Routine newborn care focuses on hyperthermia and cord care. LPIs have problems with hypothermia. LPI education needs to focus on recognition of hypothermia. Bathing and taking a temperature are part of routine discharge teaching for all newborns. Routine hearing screening is highly recommended. Follow-up with the primary care provider after discharge should be within 1 to 3 days for LPIs.

**References:** Baker, B., McGrath, J., Lawson, R., et al.: Staff nurses working together to improve care for late-preterm infants. *Newborn and Infant Reviews*, 9(3):139-142, 2009.

Raju, T., Higgins, R., Stark, A., et al.: Optimizing care and outcome for late-preterm (near-term) infants: A summary of the workshop sponsored by the National Institute of Child Health and Human Development. *Pediatrics*, 118:1207-1214, 2006.

5. **(C)** Placing a baby under a radiant warmer can rewarm the infant too rapidly. Rapid rewarming can be associated with a sudden deterioration in the infant's clinical condition due to the sudden vasodilation. The sudden vasodilation causes the infant to become hypotensive. The increase in heart rate is a compensatory mechanism in response to the decreased cardiac output. Hypothermia and cardiovascular collapse can be a sign of sepsis. Hypothermia symptoms include bradycardia, decreased level of consciousness, decreased blood pressure, and decrease in respiratory effort. Hypoglycemia can be the result of hypothermia because of the increase in glucose metabolism.

**Reference:** Karlsen, K.: *The S.T.A.B.L.E. Program*, 5th ed. Park City, Utah, American Academy of Pediatrics, 2006, pp. 55-61.

# Section II: Pathophysiology
## System-Specific Disorders

### CHAPTER 14: CARDIOVASCULAR DISORDERS

1. **(C)** The symptoms of hepatomegaly, tachycardia, tachypnea, and gallop rhythm suggest this infant is in congestive heart failure. A classic finding in coarctation of the aorta is diminished pulses in the lower extremities. A systolic blood pressure more than 15 mm Hg higher in the upper extremities than in the lower extremities is also suggestive of coarctation of the aorta. Cardiomyopathy may present with signs and symptoms of heart failure, which can progress to poor perfusion, shock, decreased urine output, and decreased level of consciousness. Significant differences between upper and lower extremity blood pressure are not expected in cardiomyopathy. Patent ductus arteriosus classically presents with bounding pulses, hyperactive precordium, widening of the pulse pressure, low diastolic pressure, and unexplained metabolic acidosis.

Persistent pulmonary hypertension of the newborn generally presents within 12 hours of age with respiratory distress, cyanosis out of proportion to degree of distress, systolic murmur, and a single heart sound. Blood pressure may be lower than normal, but without significant differences between upper and lower extremities.

**Reference:** Sadowski, S.L.: Cardiovascular disorders. In Verklan, M.T., Walden, M. (Eds.): *Core Curriculum for Neonatal Intensive Care Nursing*, 4th ed. St. Louis, Saunders, 2010, pp. 560-561.

2. **(B)** Clinical features of Turner syndrome include webbing of the neck, low-set ears, epicanthal folds, broad nasal bridge, low posterior neckline, and marked lymphedema of the extremities. Common congenital heart defects appearing with Turner syndrome are coarctation of the aorta, bicuspid aortic valve, and valvular aortic stenosis. Clinical features of trisomy 21 include a flat occiput, eyes that slant outward, prominent epicanthal folds, flat face, Brushfield spots, flat nasal bridge, protruding tongue, loose skin around the neck, and hypotonia. Endocardial cushion defect and ventricular septal defect are commonly seen in infants with trisomy 21. Klinefelter syndrome affects males only and has clinical findings of long limbs, slim stature, elbow dysplasia, fifth finger clinodactyly, hypogonadism, cryptorchidism, hypospadias, and gynecomastia. Heart disease is not a hallmark association with Klinefelter syndrome. Clinical features of Beckwith-Wiedemann syndrome include an abdominal wall defect, large size for gestational age, large and prominent eyes, large and protruding tongue, lethargy, and poor feeding. Heart disease is not a hallmark association with Beckwith-Wiedemann syndrome.

**References:** Park, M.K.: *Pediatric Cardiology for Practitioners*, 5th ed. Philadelphia, Mosby, 2008, p. 12.

Sterk, L.: Congenital anomalies. In Verklan, M.T., Walden, M. (Eds.): *Core Curriculum for Neonatal Intensive Care Nursing*, 4th ed. St. Louis, Saunders, 2010, p. 792.

3. **(D)** Prostaglandin $E_1$ is administered to maintain patency of the ductus arteriosus. In the case of hypoplastic left heart syndrome, systemic circulation is dependent on the ductus arteriosus. As ductal patency improves, peripheral perfusion will improve. Increased oxygen saturation would be an expected finding when administering prostaglandin $E_1$ to an infant with a duct-dependent pulmonary flow defect, such as tricuspid atresia. Prostaglandin $E_1$ may cause bradycardia, which is not a desired effect of its administration. Decreased murmur intensity could signify closing of the ductus arteriosus and would not be a desired effect of prostaglandin $E_1$.

**Reference:** Sadowski, S.L.: Cardiovascular disorders. In Verklan, M.T., Walden, M. (Eds.): *Core Curriculum for Neonatal Intensive Care Nursing*, 4th ed. St. Louis, Saunders, 2010, p. 572.

4. **(A)** Prostaglandin $E_1$ is administered to maintain patency of the ductus arteriosus. In the case of tricuspid atresia, pulmonary circulation is dependent on a patent ductus arteriosus. As ductal patency improves, pulmonary blood flow will improve, as will the infant's oxygenation status. Prostaglandin $E_1$ may

cause bradycardia, which is not a desired effect of its administration. Monitoring blood pressure during prostaglandin $E_1$ administration is important, because hypotension may occur. However, changes in blood pressure are not an indication of the effectiveness of prostaglandin $E_1$ therapy in this infant. Improved capillary refill is a desired effect when administering prostaglandin $E_1$ to an infant with a duct-dependent systemic flow defect, such as hypoplastic left heart syndrome.

**Reference:** Tabbutt, S., Helfaer, M.A., Nichols, D.G.: Pharmacology of cardiovascular drugs. In Nichols, D.G., Ungerleider, R.M., Spevak, P.J., et al. (Eds.): *Critical Heart Disease in Infants and Children,* 2nd ed. Philadelphia, Mosby, 2006, p. 195.

5. **(C)** The goal of long-term management of supraventricular tachycardia (SVT) is to prevent recurrences of tachycardia episodes. Although digoxin improves cardiac contractility, it is used in SVT primarily because it slows conduction through the atrioventricular (AV) node. Digoxin is not recommended for the long-term treatment of SVT associated with Wolff-Parkinson-White syndrome because digoxin may shorten accessory pathway refractoriness, increasing conduction through the accessory pathway and thereby permitting a very rapid ventricular rate during atrial fibrillation. Other effects of digoxin include peripheral, splanchnic, and possibly pulmonary vasoconstriction. These effects do no influence the conduction system. Digoxin slows conduction through the AV node; it does not prolong the refractory period. Amiodarone is an example of a medication that increases the refractory period.

**References:** Kannankerh, P.J., Fish, F.A.: Disorders of cardiac rhythm and conduction. In Allen, H.D., Driscoll, D.T., Shaddy, R.E., et al. (Eds.): *Moss and Adams' Heart Disease in Infants, Children and Adolescents, Including the Fetus and Young Adult,* 7th ed. Philadelphia, Wolters Kluwer Health/Lippincott Williams & Wilkins, 2008, p. 311.

Kanter R.J., Carboni, M.P., Silka, M.J.: Pediatric arrhythmias. In Nichols, D.G., Ungerleider, R.M., Spevak, P.J., et al. (Eds.): *Critical Heart Disease in Infants and Children,* 2nd ed. Philadelphia, Mosby, 2006, p. 230.

Taketomo, C.K., Hodding, J.H., Krause, D.M.: *Pediatric Dosage Handbook,* 17th ed. Hudson, Ohio, Lexi-Comp, 2010, pp. 437-439.

Thomson Reuters Clinical Editorial Staff: *NeoFax 2010,* 23rd ed. Montvale, N.J., Thomson Reuters, 2010, pp. 150-151.

6. **(A)** Because of the severe reduction in left ventricular outflow, infants with hypoplastic left heart syndrome (HLHS) have diminished pulses. Their color is usually an ashen gray. A heart murmur is usually absent, however, when present, it is systolic. Profound cyanosis is not a feature of HLHS. Urine output may be decreased secondary to decreased perfusion.

**References:** Park, M.K.: *Pediatric Cardiology for Practitioners,* 5th ed. Philadelphia, Mosby, 2008, p. 270.

Sadowski, S.L.: Cardiovascular disorders. In Verklan, M.T., Walden, M. (Eds.): *Core Curriculum for Neonatal Intensive Care Nursing,* 4th ed. St. Louis, Saunders, 2010, p. 572.

7. **(D)** Indomethacin can cause a temporary decrease in renal function; thus, urine output must be carefully monitored. Other adverse effects of indomethacin include platelet dysfunction, hypoglycemia, and gastrointestinal bleeding. The nurse should monitor the following for a patient receiving indomethacin: urine output; levels of serum electrolytes, glucose, creatinine, and blood urea nitrogen; and platelet count. Indomethacin does not cause an increase or decrease in white blood cell count, nor does it have a significant effect on systemic circulation. Thrombocytopenia, not thrombocytosis, is a side effect of indomethacin.

**References:** Sadowski, S.L.: Cardiovascular disorders. In Verklan, M.T., Walden, M. (Eds.): *Core Curriculum for Neonatal Intensive Care Nursing,* 4th ed. St. Louis, Saunders, 2010, pp. 555-556.

Thomson Reuters Clinical Editorial Staff: *NeoFax 2010,* 23rd ed. Montvale, N.J., Thomson Reuters, 2010, pp. 180-181.

8. **(D)** Providing a balance of the systemic and pulmonary circulations is the overall goal in the preoperative management of the infant with hypoplastic left heart syndrome (HLHS). A large systemic-to-pulmonary communication, such as a ductus arteriosus, is required for systemic circulation. Pulmonary vascular resistance (PVR) is the major factor determining the amount of circulation that goes to the pulmonary or systemic circuits. High systemic saturations can lead to lowered PVR and decreased systemic circulation. High systemic blood pressures can increase left-to-right shunting, which decreases the amount of blood flow in the systemic circulation.

**Reference:** Steven, J.M., Marino, B.S., Jobes, D.R.: Hypoplastic left heart syndrome. In Nichols, D.G., Ungerleider, R.M., Spevak, P.J., et al. (Eds.): *Critical Heart Disease in Infants and Children,* 2nd ed. Philadelphia, Mosby, 2006, pp. 826-827.

9. **(A)** Hyperkalemia often occurs in acute renal failure. Abnormalities on the electrocardiogram (ECG) can be seen once serum potassium levels exceed 6 mEq/L. The earliest ECG abnormality seen in hyperkalemia is tall, peaked, symmetrical T waves. As serum potassium levels increase, additional abnormalities are seen in the following sequence: prolongation of the QRS complex; prolongation of the PR interval; disappearance of the P wave; wide, bizarre biphasic QRS complex (sine wave); asystole. Laboratory values indicate hyponatremia and hypoglycemia; however, neither of these conditions is associated with abnormalities on the ECG. The hallmark ECG abnormality associated with hypocalcemia is a prolonged QT interval.

**Reference:** Park, M.K.: *Pediatric Cardiology for Practitioners,* 5th ed. Philadelphia, Mosby, 2008, p. 65.

10. **(D)** During a balloon septostomy, a balloon-tipped catheter is threaded from the inferior vena cava into the right atrium. The tip is then passed across the foramen ovale to the left atrium, the tip is inflated, and the catheter is quickly pulled back, tearing a hole in the atrial septum. This hole will allow mixing of blood at the atrial level. The balloon atrial septostomy can be a lifesaving procedure in infants with transposition of the great vessels and poor intercirculatory mixing. Balloon septostomy does not affect cardiac output.

Pharmacologic measures, such as the administration of inotropes, are used to increase cardiac output. A procedure to increase pulmonary blood flow is the Blalock-Taussig shunt. Balloon dilation or valvotomy may be performed to relieve pulmonary valve stenosis.

**Reference:** Park, M.K.: *Pediatric Cardiology for Practitioners*, 5th ed. Philadelphia, Mosby, 2008, pp. 222-223.

11. **(D)** Supplemental oxygen is often given to infants with suspected heart disease without a full understanding of its potential adverse effects. In single-ventricle conditions (e.g., hypoplastic left heart syndrome [HLHS]), supplemental oxygen can produce pulmonary vasodilation, which results in increased blood flow to the lungs and decreased blood flow to the systemic circulation. The resulting clinical signs include a fall in urine output, diminished pulses, prolonged capillary refill, and metabolic acidosis. Although supplemental oxygen is associated with the development of retinopathy of prematurity, the primary reason oxygen should be used with caution in infants with HLHS is its effect on the pulmonary arteries and pulmonary vascular resistance. Increased $Po_2$ levels encourage constriction of the ductus arteriosus, an undesired effect in HLHS. Supplemental oxygen can increase oxygen levels in patients with cyanotic heart lesions, producing undesired changes in ductal patency and pulmonary vascular resistance.

**Reference:** Steven, J.M., Marino B.S., Jobes, D.R.: Hypoplastic left heart syndrome. In Nichols, D.G., Ungerleider, R.M., Spevak, P.J., et al. (Eds.): *Critical Heart Disease in Infants and Children*, 2nd ed. Philadelphia, Mosby, 2006, pp. 826-827.

12. **(D)** The four determinants of cardiac output are preload, afterload, heart rate, and contractility. Increasing contractility increases cardiac output, and decreasing contractility decreases cardiac output. Factors that decrease contractility include acidosis, hypoxia, electrolyte disturbances, and hypoglycemia. Preload is affected primarily by intravascular fluid volume. Afterload is the resistance against which the heart must pump and is affected by pulmonary and systemic vascular resistance. Hypoglycemia does not affect pulmonary and systemic vascular resistance. Heart rate is not usually affected by hypoglycemia.

**Reference:** Sadowski, S.L.: Cardiovascular disorders. In Verklan, M.T., Walden, M. (Eds.): *Core Curriculum for Neonatal Intensive Care Nursing*, 4th ed. St. Louis, Saunders, 2010, p. 541.

13. **(C)** Cyanosis is the bluish discoloration of the skin that occurs when 5 g/dl of hemoglobin is desaturated. The appearance of cyanosis depends on the hemoglobin level. Infants with high hemoglobin levels may appear cyanotic despite having sufficient amounts of oxygen-saturated hemoglobin. Infants with low hemoglobin levels may appear pink despite systemic arterial desaturation. Cyanosis due to a congenital heart defect is related to critically decreased pulmonary blood flow, abnormal mixing of systemic and venous blood before delivery to the systemic circulation, or increased pulmonary blood flow and pulmonary edema leading to alveolar hypoxia. A congenital heart defect classified as a cyanotic lesion may not produce

cyanosis if there is adequate pulmonary blood flow or mixing of oxygenated and deoxygenated blood. Anemia decreases the visibility of cyanosis. Depending on the degree of shunting, infants with cyanotic heart lesions may not be cyanotic. A congenital heart defect with increased pulmonary blood flow can lead to pulmonary edema, alveolar hypoxia, and eventually cyanosis.

**References:** Park, M.K.: *Pediatric Cardiology for Practitioners*, 5th ed. Philadelphia, Mosby, 2008, p. 140.

Sadowski, S.L.: Cardiovascular disorders. In Verklan, M.T., Walden, M. (Eds.): *Core Curriculum for Neonatal Intensive Care Nursing*, 4th ed. St. Louis, Saunders, 2010, p. 545.

Zahka, K.G., Gruenstin, D.H.: Approach to the neonate with cardiovascular disease. In Martin, R.J., Fanaroff, A.A., Walsh, M.C.: *Fanaroff and Martin's Neonatal-Perinatal Medicine: Diseases of the Fetus and Infant*, 8th ed. St. Louis, Mosby, 2006, p. 1215.

14. **(D)** The rhythm strip demonstrates supraventricular tachycardia (SVT). The heart rate is approximately 250 beats/minute (as calculated by dividing 60 by the RR interval, or 60/0.24). The RR interval is regular. The characteristic electrocardiogram features of SVT include a fixed rate higher than 200 beats/minute, a fixed RR interval, and a regular narrow QRS complex with a 1:1 relationship between the P wave and QRS complex. Occasionally, aberrancy can produce a widened QRS complex. P waves may come before or after the QRS, or be obscured. Infants with SVT often present with heart rates higher than 220 to 240 beats/minute. The heart rate rarely goes over 200 beats/minute in sinus tachycardia. Normal sinus rhythm is characterized by a rate normal for age. The normal heart rate for a newborn is 120 to 180 beats/minute and may drop as low as 90 beats/minute. Ventricular tachycardia is characterized by a ventricular rate of 120 to 200 beats/minute, wide, bizarre QRS complexes, with T waves pointing in the opposite direction.

**Reference:** Kenney, P.M., Hoover, D., Williams, L.C., et al.: Cardiovascular diseases and surgical interventions. In Gardner, S.L., Carter, B.S., Enzman-Hines, M., et al. (Eds.): *Merenstein and Gardner's Handbook of Neonatal Intensive Care*, 7th ed. St. Louis, Mosby, 2011, pp. 710-711.

15. **(D)** The PR interval in the tracing (measured from the beginning of the P wave to the beginning of the QRS complex) is 77 milliseconds, which is below the lower limit of normal. There is an initial slurring of the upstroke of the QRS, referred to as a *delta wave*. The QRS duration is 80 milliseconds, which is above the upper limit of normal. Wolff-Parkinson-White (WPW) syndrome is characterized by a short PR interval, a delta wave, and a wide QRS complex. Ebstein anomaly is characterized by a downward displacement of the tricuspid valve into the right ventricle. Infants with Ebstein anomaly are at risk for WPW. Patients with WPW are prone to attacks of supraventricular tachycardia. Complete atrioventricular block is characterized by a ventricular rate slower than the atrial rate and no association between the ventricular and atrial rates. These features are not evident in the rhythm strip. First-degree heart block is characterized by a prolonged PR interval, not seen in this rhythm strip. A premature atrial contraction (PAC) is a beat

that occurs before the next beat is due. The P-wave morphology depends on the site from which the beat originated. The RR interval following the PAC is usually normal. There is no slurring of QRS morphology associated with a PAC.

References: Delhaas, T., Marchie Sarvaas, G.J.D., Rijlaarsdam, M.E., et al.: A multicenter, long-term study on arrhythmias in children with Ebstein anomaly. *Pediatric Cardiology*, 31:229-233, 2010.

Park, M.K.: *Pediatric Cardiology for Practitioners*, 5th ed. Philadelphia, Mosby, 2008, p. 59.

16. **(D)** Propranolol, a β-blocker, increases the refractory period through the atrioventricular (AV) node and is useful for preventing recurrent supraventricular tachycardias (SVTs) that use the AV node as part of the reentry circuit. Propranolol is a preferred drug to prevent SVT in Wolff-Parkinson-White (WPW) syndrome. Digoxin should not be used in WPW syndrome because it may increase conduction through the accessory pathway, thereby permitting a very rapid ventricular rate during atrial fibrillation. Atropine is an anticholinergic agent and is used primarily to increase heart rate. Adenosine is indicated for the conversion of SVT to normal sinus rhythm.

References: Kanter R.J., Carboni, M.P., Silka, M.J.: Pediatric arrhythmias. In Nichols, D.G., Ungerleider, R.M., Spevak, P.J., et al. (Eds.): *Critical Heart Disease in Infants and Children*, 2nd ed. Philadelphia, Mosby, 2006, pp. 229-230.

Park, M.K.: *Pediatric Cardiology for Practitioners*, 5th ed. Philadelphia, Mosby, 2008, p. 427.

17. **(D)** Pulmonary atresia is characterized by the absence of the pulmonary valve and the inability to send blood out of the right ventricle to the lungs. Venous blood returning to the right side of the heart crosses the foramen ovale to the left atrium, passes into the left ventricle, then passes out the aorta. Prostaglandin $E_1$ is indicated to maintain ductal patency and shunting of deoxygenated blood to the lungs. Although digoxin improves cardiac output, the primary concern in the management of pulmonary atresia is maintenance of pulmonary blood flow. This goal can be accomplished with the use of a drug that maintains the patency of the ductus arteriosus. Furosemide is a diuretic and is not indicated in this case. Propranolol is a β-adrenergic receptor blocking agent and is used in the treatment of tachyarrhythmias and hypertension.

References: Park, M.K.: *Pediatric Cardiology for Practitioners*, 5th ed. Philadelphia, Mosby, 2008, p. 59.

Sadowski, S.L.: Cardiovascular disorders. In Verklan, M.T., Walden, M. (Eds.): *Core Curriculum for Neonatal Intensive Care Nursing*, 4th ed. St. Louis, Saunders, 2010, p. 566.

18. **(D)** The narrow QRS complex and rapid heart rate suggest that this infant is in supraventricular tachycardia (SVT). The infant's immediate condition is stable. Synchronized cardioversion at 0.5 to 1 J/kg is recommended for SVT unresponsive to initial measures. Synchronized cardioversion is the delivery of an electrical shock to the heart that is synchronized to the QRS complex. Defibrillation is the delivery of an electrical shock to the heart that is not synchronized to the QRS complex. If the patient has an R wave, as is present in SVT, and defibrillation is performed, the electrical shock may be delivered during the vulnerable repolarization period (T wave), triggering ventricular fibrillation. Overdrive pacing can be effective in converting SVT to normal sinus rhythm; however, other interventions should be tried first. Atropine increases heart rate and is used to treat bradycardia caused by increased vagal tone, cholinergic drug toxicity, or atrioventricular block.

Reference: Ralston, M., Hazinski, M.F., Zaritsky, A.L., et al.: *PALS Provider Manual*, Dallas, American Heart Association, 2006, pp. 136-137.

19. **(C)** The purpose of zero referencing a hemodynamic monitoring system is to negate the effects of atmospheric and hydrostatic pressure on physiologic measurements. During zero referencing, the air-fluid interface of the zeroing stopcock is aligned with the phlebostatic axis. By aligning these two points, hydrostatic pressure caused by fluid in the tubing is eliminated. By exposing the transducer to air, atmospheric pressure is read as zero. The technique for monitor calibration varies by manufacturer and model. Often, the monitor has a calibration button that, when pushed, sends a known electrical signal to the amplifier. The monitor then displays the output and the nurse compares the output value with the expected output stated by the manufacturer. A transducer can be calibrated only by applying a known amount of pressure to the transducer and observing the pressure displayed by the monitor. Each component of a hemodynamic monitoring system must be assessed for proper functioning using a method specific to the monitoring component.

Reference: Nohrenberg, J.L., Moseley, M.J., Sole, M.L.: Hemodynamic monitoring. In Sole, M.L., Klein, D.G., Moseley, M.J. (Eds.): *Introduction to Critical Care Nursing*, 5th ed. St. Louis, Saunders, 2009, p. 154.

20. **(C)** When the air-fluid interface of the zeroing stopcock is placed level with the phlebostatic axis, the effects of hydrostatic pressure are eliminated from the monitoring system. The transducer may be placed at any level. If the transducer is at midchest level but the air-fluid interface is not, hydrostatic pressure between the transducer and stopcock will not be eliminated during zeroing, which will lead to false readings. Placement of the intraflow/fast-flush device has no influence on the accuracy of zero balancing. During zero balancing, the stopcock used to open the system to air is the important stopcock to level with the patient's phlebostatic axis.

Reference: Shaffer, R.B.: Arterial catheter insertion (assist), care, and removal. In Wiegland, D.L. (Ed.): *AACN Procedure Manual for Critical Care*, 6th ed. St. Louis, Saunders, 2011, pp. 535-547.

21. **(B)** Steady-state levels of digoxin more accurately reflect efficacy and toxicity than peak levels; thus, samples for measurement of serum digoxin levels should be obtained during steady-state conditions. Digoxin levels achieve equilibrium 6 to 8 hours after administration.

**Reference:** Lott, J.W.: Cardiovascular system. In Kenner, C., Lott, J.W. (Eds.): *Comprehensive Neonatal Care: An Interdisciplinary Approach,* 4th ed. St. Louis, Saunders, 2007, p. 36.

22. **(C)** Cardiac output is determined by heart rate, preload, contractility, and afterload. The neonatal myocardium has fewer contractile elements, and the structure of the contractile elements is less organized. Consequently, the neonatal myocardium is relatively noncompliant (stiff). As a result, response to preload is diminished. After birth, the newborn heart has a limited ability to increase cardiac output in response to alterations in preload or afterload. Cardiac output in neonates is primarily dependent on heart rate. The myocyte is the contractile unit of the myocardium. Myocytes are arranged in bundles and are held together by connective tissue. These bundles are arranged more loosely and in a less organized alignment in the newborn. These differences may account for the fact that the neonatal myocardium is relatively stiff and less compliant.

**References:** Epstein, D., Wetzel, R.: Cardiovascular physiology and shock. In Nichols, D.G., Ungerleider, R.M., Spevak, P.J., et al. (Eds.): *Critical Heart Disease in Infants and Children,* 2nd ed. Philadelphia, Mosby, 2006, pp. 21-22.

Mahony, L.: Development of myocardial structure and function. In Allen, H.D., Driscoll, D.T., Shaddy, R.E., et al. (Eds.): *Moss and Adams' Heart Disease in Infants, Children and Adolescents, Including the Fetus and Young Adult,* 7th ed. Philadelphia, Wolters Kluwer Health/Lippincott Williams & Wilkins, 2008, pp. 573-587.

23. **(D)** This infant is exhibiting signs of a hypercyanotic episode ("tet spell"). Hypercyanotic spells are characterized by intense cyanosis with deep and fast respirations. During the episode, the murmur of pulmonic stenosis becomes very soft and may even disappear. During a hypercyanotic episode, there is a relative decrease in resistance to left ventricular outflow compared with right ventricular outflow, which causes an increase in right-to-left shunting. Initial treatment includes placing the infant in a knee-chest position to increase systemic vascular resistance; administering oxygen to improve oxygen saturation (although this response is limited); and administering morphine sulfate to calm the infant and suppress the respiratory center, which eliminates hyperpnea, a contributing factor in the maintenance of a hypercyanotic episode. Sodium bicarbonate may be necessary to treat metabolic acidosis. Sodium nitroprusside would make the situation worse because it would decrease systemic vascular resistance and thus increase right-to-left shunting.

**Reference:** Park, M.K.: *Pediatric Cardiology for Practitioners,* 5th ed. Philadelphia, Mosby, 2008, pp. 151-152.

24. **(A)** Preload is the stretch on myocardial fibers just before contraction. In the clinical setting, preload is evaluated by assessing the pressure in the ventricles at end diastole. In the absence of tricuspid valve disease, right ventricular end-diastolic pressure is the same as right atrial pressure. In the absence of central venous obstruction, central venous pressure is the same as right atrial pressure. Central venous pressure

monitoring can be done in the neonate through an umbilical venous catheter placed with the tip close to the right atrium. Arterial systolic pressure can be used as an indirect measure of afterload of the left side of the heart; however, it is best evaluated with the use of a pulmonary artery catheter. Arterial diastolic pressure can be used as an indirect measure of the afterload of the left side of the heart; however, it is best evaluated with the use of a pulmonary artery catheter. Pulmonary artery systolic pressure can be used as an indirect measure of the afterload of the right side of the heart.

**References:** Kluckow, M.: Hypotension in the newborn infant. In Polin, R.A., Yoder, M.C. (Eds.): *Workbook in Practical Neonatology,* 4th ed. Philadelphia, Saunders, 2007, p. 279.

Preuss, T., Wiegland, D.L.: Central venous/right atrial pressure monitoring. In Wiegland, D.L. (Ed.): *AACN Procedure Manual for Critical Care,* 6th ed. St. Louis, Saunders, 2011, p. 603.

25. **(C)** During fetal life, the alveoli are fluid filled and hypoxic, which leads to pulmonary artery vasoconstriction and increased pulmonary vascular resistance and pressure. Systemic vascular pressure and resistance are low, because a majority of the fetal systemic circulation flows to the placenta, which is a low-resistance organ. With initial respiratory efforts following birth, pulmonary vascular resistance drops primarily in response to increasing $Po_2$ and increases in pulmonary vasodilators (e.g., prostaglandin $E_2$ and nitric oxide). Systemic vascular resistance rises with cord clamping, which increases the volume of blood that must be accommodated in the systemic circulation. A further increase in pulmonary vascular resistance or decrease in systemic vascular resistance after birth would be detrimental to the infant.

**References:** Blackburn, S.: Placental, fetal, and transitional circulation revisited. *Journal of Perinatal and Neonatal Nursing,* 20(4):290-294, 2006.

Kenney, P.M., Hoover, D., Williams, L.C., et al.: Cardiovascular diseases and surgical interventions. In Gardner, S.L., Carter, B.S., Enzman-Hines, M., et al. (Eds.): *Merenstein and Gardner's Handbook of Neonatal Intensive Care,* 7th ed. St. Louis, Mosby, 2011, p. 680.

26. **(C)** The ductus arteriosus is a channel connecting the pulmonary artery and the aorta. The direction of blood flow across the ductus is determined by the resistance in the pulmonary and systemic circuits. In the fetus, the pulmonary circuit is a higher-resistance circuit. Consequently, in the fetus, blood flows from the pulmonary artery to the aorta across the ductus arteriosus. The foramen ovale allows for mixing of blood at the atrial level. There is no fetal shunt that allows mixing of blood between the ventricles. The ductus venosus shunts blood from the umbilical vein to the inferior vena cava.

**Reference:** Verklan, M.T.: Adaptation to extrauterine life. In Verklan, M.T., Walden, M. (Eds.): *Core Curriculum for Neonatal Intensive Care Nursing,* 4th ed. St. Louis, Saunders, 2010, p. 72.

27. **(D)** Echocardiography is a noninvasive tool that uses sound waves to visualize cardiac structures and measure cardiac function. The electrocardiogram measures the electrical activity of the heart. Cardiovascular

magnetic resonance imaging can be used to assess myocardial perfusion as well as cardiac anatomy and function and provide measurements of blood flow. Cardiac catheterization can be used to measure intracardiac pressures and oxygen saturation.

**References:** Geva, T., Powell, A.J.: In Allen, H.D., Driscoll, D.T., Shaddy, R.E., et al. (Eds.): *Moss and Adams' Heart Disease in Infants, Children and Adolescents, Including the Fetus and Young Adult,* 7th ed. Philadelphia, Wolters Kluwer Health/Lippincott Williams & Wilkins, 2008, p. 163.

Lane, L.: Radiologic evaluation. In Verklan, M.T., Walden, M. (Eds.): *Core Curriculum for Neonatal Intensive Care Nursing,* 4th ed. St. Louis, Saunders, 2010, p. 297.

28. **(D)** Transient ischemia due to vasospasm is a frequent complication of umbilical artery catheterization. The ischemia is characterized by blue toes. Warming the opposite foot causes a reflex vasodilation and improved blood flow to the extremity. Ischemia that is recurrent or does not go away should prompt removal of the catheter. Blanching of the toes or buttocks can indicate emboli, and the catheter should be removed immediately. In transient ischemia due to vasospasm, neither administering oxygen nor massaging the affected foot is helpful.

**Reference:** Bradshaw, W.T., Tanaka, D.T.: Physiologic monitoring. In Gardner, S.L., Carter, B.S., Enzman-Hines, M., et al. (Eds.): *Merenstein and Gardner's Handbook of Neonatal Intensive Care,* 7th ed. St. Louis, Mosby, 2011, pp. 148-149.

29. **(D)** A dampened waveform indicates that the waveform is not being effectively transmitted to the transducer. Possible causes include blood clots in the monitoring system, loose connections, kinked tubing, compliant tubing, and location of the catheter tip against a vessel wall. The pulsatile energy that distends the tubing with each heartbeat (systole) is diminished by increasing the length of the monitoring system. Thus, adding more tubing to the system increases the length the pressure pulse has to travel and can dampen the waveform further. Because debris in the catheter can result in a dampened waveform, flushing the catheter, after attempting to aspirate, would be an appropriate troubleshooting intervention.

**References:** Nohrenberg, J.L., Moseley, M.J., Sole, M.L.: Hemodynamic monitoring. In Sole, M.L., Klein, D.G., Moseley, M.J. (Eds.): *Introduction to Critical Care Nursing,* 5th ed. St. Louis, Saunders, 2009, pp. 154-155.

Shaffer, R.B.: Arterial catheter insertion (assist), care, and removal. In Wiegland, D.L. (Ed.): *AACN Procedure Manual for Critical Care,* 6th ed. St. Louis, Saunders, 2011, pp. 535-547.

30. **(B)** In an infant with congestive heart failure (CHF), cardiac output is unable to meet the demands of the body. CHF results in systemic and venous congestion. The goals of therapy are to improve the functioning of the heart and minimize the work that it has to do. Therapy often includes the use of digoxin to improve cardiac contractility and a diuretic to eliminate excess intravascular fluid. Maximizing blood pressure will increase afterload. The heart will have to work harder to overcome the increased afterload. Although decreasing systemic vascular resistance may be helpful in the management of CHF, interventions to decrease preload are frequently employed to decrease the volume of blood the heart must handle.

**Reference:** Lott, J.W.: In Kenner, C., Lott, J.W. (Eds.): *Comprehensive Neonatal Care: An Interdisciplinary Approach,* 4th ed. St. Louis, Saunders, 2007, pp. 57-59.

31. **(D)** Common signs of congestive heart failure (CHF) are tachycardia, tachypnea, hepatomegaly, and rales. Given the history of atrioventricular (AV) canal defect, CHF is the most likely problem. It is common for an infant with an AV canal defect to develop CHF at this age because of the decreasing pulmonary vascular resistance and increasing left-to-right shunting of blood. An infant with dehydration would not demonstrate the pulmonary and venous congestion symptoms of rales and hepatomegaly. A septic infant may be tachycardic and tachypneic, but is unlikely to have hepatomegaly. An infant with pneumonia may have tachycardia, tachypnea, and rales, but is unlikely to have hepatomegaly. One would also expect a lower oxygen saturation in an infant with pneumonia. An infant with dehydration would not demonstrate the pulmonary and venous congestion symptoms of rales and hepatomegaly.

**Reference:** Sadowski, S.L.: Cardiovascular disorders. In Verklan, M.T., Walden, M. (Eds.): *Core Curriculum for Neonatal Intensive Care Nursing,* 4th ed. St. Louis, Saunders, 2010, p. 574.

32. **(B)** The mainstay of therapy for congestive heart failure is diuretics, inotropes (e.g., dobutamine, digoxin), and afterload-reducing agents. Prostaglandin $E_1$ is used to maintain patency of the ductus arteriosus. Maintaining patency of the ductus arteriosus in the atrioventricular canal would lead to even more overloading of the pulmonary circuit. There is no indication for administering either adenosine or ibuprofen.

**Reference:** Park, M.K.: *Pediatric Cardiology for Practitioners,* 5th ed. Philadelphia, Mosby, 2008, p. 466.

33. **(B)** Cyanosis that is caused by a congenital heart lesion results from the shunting of unoxygenated systemic venous blood into the systemic arterial system (right-to-left shunt), bypassing the lungs. In pulmonary atresia, there is a complete absence of a pulmonic valve. Blood cannot flow from the right ventricle to the pulmonary arteries. There must be an intraatrial or intraventricular communication for the blood in the right atrium to exit, resulting in a right-to-left shunt and circulation of deoxygenated blood in the systemic circuit and cyanosis. Aortic stenosis is a narrowing of the left ventricular outflow tract and is not usually associated with cyanosis. Atrial septal defect (ASD) is associated with a left-to-right shunt. Cyanosis is not a feature of ASD. Ventricular septal defect (VSD) is associated with a left-to-right shunt. Cyanosis is not usually a feature of VSD. Cyanosis may develop if pulmonary vascular resistance increases to a point that shunting at the ventricular level becomes right to left.

**Reference:** Lott, J.W.: In Kenner, C., Lott, J.W. (Eds.): *Comprehensive Neonatal Care: An Interdisciplinary Approach,* 4th ed. St. Louis, Saunders, 2007, pp. 47-48.

34. **(C)** Signs and symptoms of a patent ductus arteriosus (PDA) are related to the degree of left-to-right shunting across the ductus and left ventricular volume overload. Infants may be asymptomatic in the absence of these findings. Infants with PDA will often present with an increased need for ventilatory support and hypercarbia due to pulmonary edema. Additional clinical features of PDA include a murmur heard best at the left sternal border in the second and third intercostal spaces, an active precordium, and widened pulse pressure. Because of the lower pulmonary vascular resistance, blood shunts from left to right across the ductus. As the left-to-right shunt increases, the peripheral pulses become more prominent, and there is an increase in pulmonary blood flow with a consequential steal of blood that would normally perfuse the body. The incidence of PDA is inversely proportional to gestational age, close to 80% in infants weighing less than 1200 g. Signs of sepsis are generally nonspecific and nonlocalizing. Signs of sepsis may include temperature instability, respiratory distress, lethargy, jaundice, tachycardia, and tachypnea. The infant with pneumonia often demonstrates tachypnea, decreased oxygen saturation, apnea, retractions, grunting, and temperature instability. Signs of intraventricular hemorrhage vary, but include sudden deterioration, oxygen desaturation, bradycardia, metabolic acidosis, hypotonia, full fontanelles, and seizure activity.

**References:** Park, M.K.: *Pediatric Cardiology for Practitioners*, 5th ed. Philadelphia, Mosby, 2008, p. 466.

Sadowski, S.L.: Cardiovascular disorders. In Verklan, M.T., Walden, M. (Eds.): *Core Curriculum for Neonatal Intensive Care Nursing*, 4th ed. St. Louis, Saunders, 2010, p. 554.

35. **(D)** The effectiveness of adenosine is dependent on the dose, injection speed, site of injection, and circulation time from the vein to the heart. Adenosine should not be administered via the umbilical artery catheter, because the drug will be metabolized by the time it reaches the heart. Adenosine has a half-life of 10 to 15 seconds and must be administered rapidly and at the site most proximal to the heart. Adenosine administration should be followed immediately with a normal saline flush. Adenosine is never given via an endotracheal tube.

**References:** Ralston, M., Hazinski, M.F., Zaritsky, A.L., et al.: *PALS Provider Manual*, Dallas, American Heart Association, 2006, p. 137.

Taketomo, C.K., Hodding, J.H., Krause, D.M.: *Pediatric Dosage Handbook*, 17th ed. Hudson, Ohio, Lexi-Comp, 2010, p. 52.

Thomson Reuters Clinical Editorial Staff: *NeoFax 2010*, 23rd ed. Montvale, N.J., Thomson Reuters, 2010, p. 136.

36. **(C)** Dobutamine is a synthetic catecholamine with primarily $\beta_1$-adrenergic activity. Although it may decrease systemic and pulmonary vascular resistance in adults, it improves cardiac output mostly by improving cardiac contractility. Dobutamine is not a venodilator and thus does not decrease preload. Medications that decrease preload include sodium nitroprusside and diuretics. Dobutamine has little effect on heart rate. Cardiac medications that increase heart rate include epinephrine, norepinephrine, atropine, and isoproterenol.

**References:** Tabbutt, S., Helfaer, M.A., Nichols, D.G.: Pharmacology of cardiovascular drugs. In Nichols, D.G., Ungerleider, R.M., Spevak, P.J., et al. (Eds.): *Critical Heart Disease in Infants and Children*, 2nd ed. Philadelphia, Mosby, 2006, pp. 180-181.

Thomson Reuters Clinical Editorial Staff: *NeoFax 2010*, 23rd ed. Montvale, N.J., Thomson Reuters, 2010, p. 153.

37. **(A)** The cardiac troponins are polypeptides that regulate muscle contraction. Cardiac troponins (troponin I and troponin T) are markers of myocardial injury and may be elevated in myocarditis. Tetralogy of Fallot does not affect troponin levels. The diagnosis of infective endocarditis is made according to the modified Duke criteria, which includes pathologic evidence of microorganism invasion and clinical criteria such as positive blood culture results, evidence of endocardial involvement, fever, and vascular phenomena. Wolff-Parkinson-White (WPW) syndrome does not affect troponin levels. WPW syndrome is best diagnosed with electrocardiography.

**References:** Daniels, C.J.: Myocardial ischemia. In Allen, H.D., Driscoll, D.T., Shaddy, R.E., et al. (Eds.): *Moss and Adams' Heart Disease in Infants, Children and Adolescents, Including the Fetus and Young Adult*, 7th ed. Philadelphia, Wolters Kluwer Health/Lippincott Williams & Wilkins, 2008, p. 1314.

Park, M.K.: *Pediatric Cardiology for Practitioners*, 5th ed. Philadelphia, Mosby, 2008, p. 466.

38. **(D)** Complete heart block may be congenital or acquired. Maternal collagen diseases, such as lupus erythematosus, are highly associated with the congenital form. Maternal autoimmune antibodies cross the placenta and damage the atrioventricular node or bundle of His. Sinus bradycardia may occur with vagal stimulation, hypoxia, increased intracranial pressure, hypothermia, hypothyroidism, hyperkalemia, and administration of drugs such as digitalis and $\beta$-adrenergic blocking agents. Long QT syndrome (LQTS) may be congenital or acquired. Congenital types of LQTS are associated with Romano-Ward syndrome, an autosomal dominant disorder, and Jervell and Lange-Nielsen syndrome, an autosomal recessive condition. Supraventricular tachycardia is associated with Wolff-Parkinson-White syndrome and some congenital heart defects (e.g., Ebstein anomaly, single ventricle), and may occur following cardiac surgery.

**References:** Kannankerh, P.J., Fish, F.A.: Disorders of cardiac rhythm and conduction. In Allen, H.D., Driscoll, D.T., Shaddy, R.E., et al. (Eds.): *Moss and Adams' Heart Disease in Infants, Children and Adolescents, Including the Fetus and Young Adult*, 7th ed. Philadelphia, Wolters Kluwer Health/Lippincott Williams & Wilkins, 2008, p. 304.

Kenney, P.M., Hoover, D., Williams, L.C., et al.: Cardiovascular diseases and surgical interventions. In Gardner, S.L., Carter, B.S., Enzman-Hines, M., et al. (Eds.): *Merenstein and Gardner's Handbook of Neonatal Intensive Care*, 7th ed. St. Louis, Mosby, 2011, p. 712.

39. **(D)** The test used to determine the percentage of glucose unable to get into cells is the percentage of glycosylated hemoglobin, or hemoglobin $A_{1c}$. An $A_{1c}$ level of up to 5% is normal. A level between 5.1%

and 7% is called a *prediabetic state* and is a precursor to diabetes because it indicates insulin resistance. At a level of 7%, diabetes is diagnosed, according to the National Institutes of Health. It is well known that pregestational and early gestational glucose control greatly influence the rate of miscarriage and fetal anomalies. The hemoglobin $A_{1c}$ level at 14 weeks, which reflects glycemic control 3 to 4 weeks prior to measurement, is predictive of the rate of fetal anomalies. A hemoglobin $A_{1c}$ level higher than 8.5% confers a risk of birth defects of approximately 22%, versus 3.4% in women with $A_{1c}$ levels less than 8.5%. The pattern of anomalies secondary to diabetes is characteristic. Infants of diabetic mothers are particularly prone to defects in the cardiovascular system, central nervous system, and skeletal system. Cardiac anomalies that are commonly associated with maternal hyperglycemia include ventricular septal defect, transposition of the great vessels, patent ductus arteriosus, and endocardial cushion defect. Aortic stenosis, Ebstein anomaly, and tetralogy of Fallot are not associated with maternal hyperglycemia or maternal diabetes.

**References:** Abu-Sulaiman, R.M., Subaih, B.: Congenital heart disease in infants of diabetic mothers: Echographic study. *Pediatric Cardiology*, 25(2):137-140, 2004.

American Diabetes Association: Standards of medical care in diabetes: Detection and diagnosis of gestational diabetes mellitus (GDM). *Diabetes Care*, 31(1):S12-S54, 2008.

Guerin, A., Nisenbaum, R., Ray, J.: Use of maternal GHb concentration to estimate the risk of congenital anomalies in the offspring of women with prepregnancy diabetes. *Diabetes Care*, 30(7):1920-1925, 2007.

Nold, J.L., Georgieff, M.K.: Infants of diabetic mothers. *Pediatric Clinics of North America*, 51:619-637, 2004.

40. **(B)** Infants born to women taking phenytoin have a greater than usual number of major birth defects like cleft lip, cleft palate, and heart malformations. The hydantoin (phenytoin) syndrome, consisting of the constellation of growth and performance delays, craniofacial abnormalities, and hypoplasia of the nails and distal phalanges, has been well recognized. Insulin is not known to be associated with congenital heart defects. Labetalol, used to treat maternal hypertension, is not associated with cardiac defects. Tetracycline is not known to be associated with congenital heart defects. However, tetracyclines cross the placenta readily and are category D drugs, because they are known teratogens. Tetracyclines exert their adverse effects by inhibiting protein synthesis and by competing with calcium for incorporation into bone. Thus, tetracycline can deposit in growing bones and may disturb longitudinal growth. These agents can also cause dental effects, including yellow-brown discoloration of the teeth, hypoplasia, and enamel defects.

**Reference:** Glickstein, J.S.: Cardiology. In Polin, R.A., Spitzer, A.R. (Eds.): *Fetal and Neonatal Secrets*, 2nd ed. Philadelphia, Mosby, 2007, p. 83.

41. **(C)** The apical impulse represents the forward thrust of the left ventricle during systole. The apical impulse is usually seen in the neonate in the fourth intercostal space, left of the midclavicular line. An apical impulse located downward or to the left

suggests cardiac enlargement. The second heart sound ($S_2$) is produced by closure of the aortic and pulmonic valves. The first heart sound ($S_1$) is produced by closure of the mitral and tricuspid valves. Continuous systolic or crescendo murmurs with a grade I-II intensity, auscultated over the left sternal border and heard within the first 8 hours of life, are typically suggestive of transient left-to-right flow through the ductus arteriosus during the period when pulmonary vascular resistance is falling but ductal closure has not yet occurred.

**Reference:** Lott, J.W.: Cardiovascular system. In Kenner, C., Lott, J.W. (Eds.): *Comprehensive Neonatal Care: An Interdisciplinary Approach*, 4th ed. St. Louis, Saunders, 2007, p. 36.

42. **(D)** Murmur at the upper left sternal edge, bounding peripheral pulses, and increased precordial cardiac impulse are consistent clinical findings associated with patent ductus arteriosus (PDA). Cardiac arrhythmias, weak peripheral pulses, and hypertension are not typical findings of PDA. Diaphoresis and poor feeding are not typical findings of PDA, especially in a 28-week-gestational-age infant. However, in the presence of large left-to-right shunting across the ductus and increased left ventricular volume overload, congestive heart failure can develop, in which case the infant may present with diaphoresis and poor feeding.

**Reference:** Glickstein, J.S.: Cardiology. In Polin, R.A., Spitzer, A.R. (Eds.): *Fetal and Neonatal Secrets*, 2nd ed. Philadelphia, Mosby, 2007, pp. 80-114.

43. **(C)** The clinical signs and symptoms of a patent ductus arteriosus most typically manifest at 3 to 4 days of life.

**Reference:** Glickstein, J.S.: Cardiology. In Polin, R.A., Spitzer, A.R. (Eds.): *Fetal and Neonatal Secrets*, 2nd ed. Philadelphia, Mosby, 2007, pp. 80-114.

44. **(D)** Ventricular septal defects (VSDs) rank highest in frequency of all cardiac defects. VSDs account for 15% to 20% of all cardiac malformations, not including those occurring as part of cyanotic congenital heart defects. VSDs occur in approximately 1 in 3000 live births. Pulmonic stenosis occurs in 8% to 12% of all congenital heart defects. Atrial septal defect occurs in approximately 1 in 5000 live births. Coarctation of the aorta accounts for approximately 8% to 10% of congenital heart defects.

**References:** Park, M.K.: *Pediatric Cardiology for Practitioners*, 5th ed. Philadelphia, Mosby, 2008, p. 166.

Sadowski, S.L.: Cardiovascular disorders. In Verklan, M.T., Walden, M. (Eds.): *Core Curriculum for Neonatal Intensive Care Nursing*, 4th ed. St. Louis, Saunders, 2010, p. 556.

45. **(B)** Tetralogy of Fallot occurs in approximately 1 in 5000 live births, accounts for approximately 5% to 10% of all congenital heart defects, and is the most common cyanotic congenital heart defect. Pulmonary atresia is a relatively rare congenital heart defect, occurring in 1 in 14,000 live births and accounting for fewer than 1% of cardiac defects. The incidence of hypoplastic left heart syndrome (HLHS) is 0.16 to 0.36 in 1000 live births. HLHS comprises 1.2% to 1.5% of all congenital heart defects. The rate of occurrence is increased in patients with Turner syndrome, Noonan

syndrome, Smith-Lemli-Opitz syndrome, and Holt-Oram syndrome. Certain chromosomal duplications, translocations, and deletions are also associated with HLHS. Transposition of the great arteries accounts for approximately 5% to 7% of all congenital heart defects. Transposition of the great arteries is the second most common cyanotic congenital heart defect.

**References:** Park, M.K.: *Pediatric Cardiology for Practitioners,* 5th ed. Philadelphia, Mosby, 2008, pp. 215-302.

Sadowski, S.L.: Cardiovascular disorders. In Verklan, M.T., Walden, M. (Eds.): *Core Curriculum for Neonatal Intensive Care Nursing,* 4th ed. St. Louis, Saunders, 2010, pp. 534-568.

46. **(C)** DiGeorge syndrome (DGS) is also known as *velocardiofacial, CATCH 22* (*c*ardiac defects, *a*bnormal facies, *t*hymic hypoplasia, *c*left palate, *h*ypocalcemia), *Shprintzen,* or *conotruncal anomaly-face syndrome.* Characteristic craniofacial findings of DGS include secondary cleft palate, prominent nose with squared nasal root and narrow alar base, narrow palpebral fissures, abundant scalp hair, deficient malar area, vertical maxillary excess with a long face, retruded mandible with chin deficiency, minor auricular anomalies, and microcephaly. Affected individuals may have slender and hyperextensible hands and fingers. Patients with DGS may have aplasia or hypoplasia of the thymus leading to abnormal T-cell function. Transient neonatal hypocalcemia resulting from primary hypoparathyroidism may occur in 70% to 80% of infants with DGS. Eighty-five percent of affected individuals have conotruncal defects, including tetralogy of Fallot, truncus arteriosus, interrupted aortic arch, or perimembranous ventricular septal defects. The pattern of organ malformations involving the heart, thymus gland, and parathyroid gland coincides with an abnormal migration of neural crest cells leading to abnormal development of the fourth branchial arch and third and fourth pharyngeal pouches. DGS is an autosomal dominant disorder and is the most common chromosomal deletion syndrome in humans, occurring in 1 in 4000 live births. The deletion associated with DGS has been identified on chromosome 22 at q11.2. The characteristic clinical features of trisomy 21 include small head (brachycephaly); flat facies with increased interocular distance (hypertelorism); depressed nasal bridge; flat occiput, broad short neck; relatively small mouth with protrusion of the tongue (macroglossia); short stature (below normal height); broad, short hands, feet, and digits; short curved fifth finger (dysplasia of the midphalanx); and clinodactyly of the fifth finger. Congenital heart defects occur in 40% to 60% of patients with trisomy 21 and include complete atrioventricular canal defects, ventricular septal defects, and tetralogy of Fallot. Gilbert syndrome is the most common hereditary cause of increased bilirubin level and is found in up to 5% of the population. The main symptom is otherwise harmless jaundice that does not require treatment, caused by elevated levels of unconjugated bilirubin in the bloodstream (hyperbilirubinemia). Cornelia de Lange syndrome is a rare genetic disorder. Associated symptoms and findings typically include delays in physical development before and after birth; characteristic abnormalities of the head and facial area, resulting in a distinctive facial appearance; malformations of the hands and arms; and mild to severe mental retardation. Many infants and children with the disorder have an unusually small, short head (microbrachycephaly); an abnormally long vertical groove between the upper lip and nose (philtrum); a depressed nasal bridge; upturned nostrils (anteverted nares); and a protruding upper jaw (maxillary prognathism). Additional characteristic facial abnormalities may include thin, down-turned lips; low-set ears; arched, well-defined eyebrows that grow together across the bridge of the nose (synophrys); an unusually low hairline on the forehead and the back of the neck; and abnormally curly, long eyelashes. Affected individuals may also have distinctive malformations of the limbs, such as unusually small hands and feet, inward deviation (clinodactyly) of the fifth fingers, or webbing (syndactyly) of certain toes. Infants with Cornelia de Lange syndrome may also have feeding and breathing difficulties, an increased susceptibility to respiratory infections, a low-pitched "growling" cry, heart defects, delayed skeletal maturation, hearing loss, and other physical abnormalities. The range and severity of associated symptoms and findings may be extremely variable from case to case.

**References:** Bishara, N., Clericuzio, C.L.: Common dysmorphic syndromes in the NICU. *NeoReviews,* 9:e29. 2008.

Jones, K.L.: DiGeorge syndrome. In *Smith's Recognizable Patterns of Human Malformation,* 6th ed. Philadelphia, Saunders, 2006, pp. 298-301.

Leong, F.T., Freeman, L.J., Keavney, B.D.: Fresh fields and pathways new: Recent genetic insights into cardiac malformation. *Heart,* 85:442-447, 2009.

47. **(C)** Noonan syndrome is the second most common genetic syndrome associated with congenital heart defects. Phenotypic features that together tend to distinguish Noonan syndrome from other known disorders are webbing of the neck, pectus excavatum, cryptorchidism, and pulmonary stenosis (commonly valvular). Other heart problems reported to be associated with Noonan syndrome are hypertrophic cardiomyopathy, atrial septal defect, tetralogy of Fallot, coarctation of the aorta, mitral valve anomalies, and atrioventricular canal. Ebstein anomaly is a rare congenital heart defect, with most cases occurring sporadically. Associated cardiac lesions are common and include patent foramen ovale, atrial septal defect, ventricular septal defect, and pulmonary stenosis. Ebstein anomaly involves tricuspid stenosis and insufficiency. Ventricular septal defect (VSD) is the most common lesion in most chromosomal syndromes. VSD is associated with trisomy 13, trisomy 18, and trisomy 21. Hypoplastic left heart syndrome appears in infants with deletion of chromosome arms 11q (Jacobsen syndrome) and 4p (Wolf-Hirschhorn syndrome), Turner syndrome, trisomy 13, and trisomy 18.

**References:** Jones, K.L.: Noonan syndrome. In *Smith's Recognizable Pattern of Human Malformation,* 6th ed. Philadelphia, Saunders, 2006, p. 124.

Tartaglia, M., Gelb, B.D.: Noonan syndrome and related disorders: Genetics and pathogenesis. *Annual Review of Genomics and Human Genetics,* 6:45-68, 2005.

48. **(D)** Transposition of the great arteries consists of a reversal of the normal anatomic position of the great vessels so that the aorta represents the outflow of the right ventricle and the pulmonary artery serves as the left ventricular outflow. A single arterial outflow from both ventricles (supplying the systemic, coronary, and pulmonary circulations) in association with a ventricular septal defect is the primary abnormality of truncus arteriosus. Narrowing of the descending aorta adjacent to insertion of the ductus arteriosus describes coarctation of the aorta. When the pulmonary veins drain into the right atrium directly or through connection with the systemic veins, the condition is known as *total anomalous pulmonary venous return*.

**Reference:** Davies, R., Chen, J.M., Quagebeur, J.M., et al.: Cardiac surgery in the neonate with congenital heart disease. In Kleinman, C.S., Seri, I. (Eds.): *Hemodynamics and Cardiology: Neonatal Questions and Controversies.* Philadelphia, Saunders, 2008, pp. 355-375.

49. **(C)** Hyperdynamic precordial activity is a consistent finding that reflects right ventricular volume and pressure overload in infants with hypoplastic left heart syndrome (HLHS). Even though infants with HLHS have complete admixture of systemic and pulmonary venous return, pulmonary blood flow relative to marginal systemic blood flow is increased, which may result in oxygen saturations as high as 85% to 88%. Cyanosis is difficult to recognize at this level. The second heart sound is single if aortic atresia is present. Decrease in the amplitude of peripheral pulses often is cited, but is evident only after ductal constriction in a symptomatic infant.

**Reference:** Fricker, J.: Hypoplastic left heart syndrome: Diagnosis and early management. *NeoReviews,* 9:e253-e259, 2008.

50. **(D)** Infants with supraventricular tachycardia (SVT) often present with heart rates higher than 220 to 240 beats/minute. As the heart rate increases, the ventricles have less time to fill. Subsequently, cardiac output decreases. Left untreated, otherwise healthy infants with SVT can develop congestive heart failure within 24 to 48 hours. SVT results in a decrease in preload. Ventricular size and shape, aortic and pulmonary vascular impedance, and systemic and pulmonary vascular resistance are factors that oppose myocardial muscle fiber shortening, thereby affecting afterload. Factors that increase end-diastolic volume (preload) increase afterload and threaten cardiac output. SVT results in decreased end-diastolic volume. Although cardiac contractility can decrease with higher heart rates, this phenomenon is not the primary reason cardiac output decreases in SVT.

**Reference:** Hermosura, T., Bradshaw, W.T.: Wolff-Parkinson-White syndrome in infants. *Neonatal Network,* 29(4):215-223, 2010.

51. **(B)** Pompe disease (glycogen storage disease type II) is an autosomal recessive glycogen storage disease. The hallmark of infant-onset Pompe disease is marked cardiomyopathy. Electrocardiographic findings include short PR interval, prominent P waves, and massive QRS voltage. These infants typically present rapidly with initial observations of profound hypotonia, muscle weakness, and a "floppy baby" appearance, as well as hepatomegaly, feeding difficulties, and respiratory distress. Galactosemia is an inherited disorder of carbohydrate metabolism. Most infants with galactosemia are identified in the first few weeks of life due to feeding intolerance, vomiting, diarrhea, poor weight gain, jaundice, hepatomegaly, and hypoglycemia. Cardiomyopathy is not associated with galactosemia. Niemann-Pick disease type C is a disorder of intracellular cholesterol transport. Neonatal-onset Niemann-Pick type C is characterized by direct hyperbilirubinemia, hepatosplenomegaly, ascites, and hypotonia. Congenital adrenal hyperplasia (CAH) is a group of disorders resulting from deficient activity of an enzyme necessary to synthesize cortisol from cholesterol. The hallmark phenotype of CAH is genital virilization. Cardiomyopathy is not associated with CAH.

**Reference:** Stokowski, L.: Metabolic system. In Kenner, C., Lott, J.W. (Eds.): *Comprehensive Neonatal Care: An Interdisciplinary Approach,* 4th ed. St. Louis, Saunders, pp. 134-151.

52. **(D)** Prostaglandin $E_1$ is used to promote dilation of the ductus arteriosus in infants with duct-dependent congenital heart lesions. In infants with hypoplastic left heart syndrome, reestablishment of ductus arteriosus patency will reestablish systemic blood flow. Blood supply to the descending aorta and to the aortic arch and coronary arteries is dependent on a patent ductus arteriosus. Prostaglandin $E_1$ is administered at 0.05 to 0.1 mcg/kg/minute. Sildenafil is used in neonates with persistent pulmonary hypertension refractory to inhaled nitric oxide and other conventional therapies and in those who are persistently unable to be weaned off inhaled nitric oxide. Lidocaine is used for short-term control of ventricular arrhythmias, including ventricular tachycardia, premature ventricular contractions, and arrhythmias resulting from digitalis intoxication. Indomethacin is used to close the ductus arteriosus.

**Reference:** Thomson Reuters Clinical Editorial Staff: *NeoFax 2010,* 23rd ed. Montvale, N.J., Thomson Reuters, 2010, p. 138.

53. **(C)** The correct blood pressure cuff width is 40% to 50% of the circumference of the extremity. In addition, the cuff's inflatable bladder should entirely circle the extremity without overlapping. The most frequent reason for a hypertensive blood pressure measurement in the newborn is use of a cuff that is too small.

**Reference:** Park, M.K.: *Pediatric Cardiology for Practitioners,* 5th ed. Philadelphia, Mosby, 2008, p. 18.

54. **(A)** For accuracy, blood pressure measurements in this neonate were taken on at least three separate occasions, using a cuff that has a cuff width–to–arm circumference ratio between 0.45 and 0.55, while the infant was asleep. In addition, the blood pressure was consistently taken in the same extremity to avoid differences in measurements. The most common cause of neonatal hypertension is renovascular or renal parenchymal disease. The renovascular cause is strongly associated with the use of umbilical arterial catheters. The mechanism of hypertension is believed to be

disruption of vascular endothelium by the catheter, embolization of the renal artery, renal hypoperfusion, and release of renin. Since neonatal hypertension is rarely caused by endocrine disorders, a thyroid scan would not be beneficial. An endocrine workup would be indicated if the infant had abnormal metabolic screen results or fluid-electrolyte abnormalities. Neurologic causes of neonatal hypertension include seizures, intracranial hemorrhage, intracranial hypertension, pain, and prolonged sedation or analgesia. Since the infant described in the case did not have a history of intraventricular hemorrhage or sedation, results of a head sonogram will probably be normal and not helpful in determining the cause of the hypertension. Although this infant had a history of respiratory distress syndrome requiring mechanical ventilation, he was weaned to room air by 21 days of life and received no supplemental oxygen at 34 weeks' postmenstrual age. Hence, his clinical course precludes the diagnosis of bronchopulmonary dysplasia, which can be associated with neonatal hypertension. The chest radiograph is unlikely to help determine the cause of the infant's hypertension.

**References:** Andreoli, S.P.: Renal failure in the newborn infant. In Polin, R.A., Yoder, M.C. (Eds.): *Workbook in Practical Neonatology,* 4th ed. Philadelphia, Saunders, 2007, pp. 341-343.

Jones, J.E., Jose, P.A.: Neonatal blood pressure regulation. *Seminars in Perinatology,* 28:141-148, 2004.

55. **(C)** Hydralazine has been used extensively to treat mild to moderate hypertension in newborn infants. Hydralazine directly relaxes arteriolar smooth muscle tone to decrease vascular resistance, which results in improved cardiac output. Digoxin is used to treat heart failure caused by decreased myocardial contractility. It can also be used to treat supraventricular tachycardia (SVT), atrial flutter, and atrial fibrillation. Amiodarone is used to treat life-threatening or drug-resistant SVT, ventricular tachycardia, and postoperative junctional ectopic tachycardia. Procainamide is used in the treatment of SVT that is refractory to vagal maneuvers and adenosine.

**References:** Andreoli, S.P. Renal failure in the newborn infant. In Polin, R.A., Yoder, M.C. (Eds.). *Workbook in Practical Neonatology,* 4th ed. Philadelphia, Saunders, 2007, pp. 341-343.

Thomson Reuters Clinical Editorial Staff: *NeoFax 2010,* 23rd ed. Montvale, N.J., Thomson Reuters, 2010, p. 176.

## CHAPTER 15: PULMONARY DISORDERS

1. **(D)** The canalicular phase of fetal lung development (16-26 weeks' gestation) is characterized by the formation of gas-exchanging acini. The development of respiratory bronchioles and pulmonary capillaries occurs. The degree of acinus-capillary coupling has a direct effect on the gas exchange that occurs. Surfactant secretion from type II cells is detectable between 24 and 25 weeks' gestation, very late in the canalicular phase. The alveolar stage begins around 36 weeks' gestation. The capillary network increases significantly at 30 weeks' gestation during the saccular stage.

**Reference:** Blackburn, S.T.: *Maternal, Fetal, and Neonatal Physiology: A Clinical Perspective,* 3rd ed. St. Louis, Saunders, 2007, pp. 315-374.

2. **(D)** The terminal sac stage of fetal lung development is characterized by the refinement of the acini. Primary saccules continue to divide. The development of the surfactant system occurs. An increase in the alveolar–blood barrier surface area increases secondary to capillary invasion. The respiratory system continues to mature through childhood, with the greatest growth in the first 1 to 2 years. Alveoli number and width increase until approximately 8 years of age, when 300 million alveoli are present. Afterward, further growth of the lung is proportional to the growth of the body. Pulmonary vascularization begins in the pseudoglandular period and continues until full lung growth is obtained around 8 years of age. Lecithin is a pulmonary phospholipid first detected with the initiation of surfactant production at 24 to 25 weeks' gestation during the late canalicular stage.

**Reference:** Blackburn, S.T.: *Maternal, Fetal, and Neonatal Physiology: A Clinical Perspective,* 3rd ed. St. Louis, Saunders, 2007, pp. 315-374.

3. **(C)** Pleural fluid draining from a chylothorax contains a high number of lymphocytes. Removal of these cells, which play a significant role in the immune system, places the infant at risk for infection due to lymphopenia. Continuous drainage of a chylothorax via a tube thoracotomy relieves dyspnea, which may evolve to apnea. A chylothorax results from leakage of fluid from a lymphatic vessel. It does not involve air leakage as seen in a pneumothorax. *Subcutaneous emphysema* denotes an air leak from pleural tissue.

**References:** Kosar, R., Adams, S.D.: Chylothorax. 2009. Available at: http://emedicine.medscape.com/article/172527-overview. Retrieved 05/31/10.

Machin, G.A.: Hydrops, cystic hygroma, hydrothorax, pericardial effusions, and fetal ascites. In Gilbert-Barness, E. (Ed.): *Potter's Pathology of the Fetus, Infant and Child,* 2nd ed. Philadelphia, 2007, pp. 333-354.

4. **(D)** Maturation occurs around 19 years of age with final vascular growth, decreased number of mucus glands, and adult shape of the thorax. Approximately 15 percent of alveoli are developed at term. Alveoli continue to develop and the diaphragm continues to mature after 12 to 15 months of age. The alveolar number is approximately 300 million. Further maturation of the pulmonary vasculature occurs after 6 to 8 years of age.

**Reference:** Blackburn, S.T.: *Maternal, Fetal, and Neonatal Physiology: A Clinical Perspective,* 3rd ed. St. Louis, Saunders, 2007, pp. 315-374.

5. **(D)** Establishing an air-liquid interface in the alveolus is one of two transitional events required for extrauterine functioning. The other is a rhythmic respiration pattern. Alveolar opening pressure is reduced in the presence of active surfactant. Lung fluid production slows in late pregnancy. Absorption commences with labor. Lung aeration, which is possible with surfactant, replaces lung fluid, and 80% to 90% of functional residual capacity is established within 1 hour of birth. Structural maturation is a stepwise process occurring over several years.

**Reference:** Blackburn, S.T.: *Maternal, Fetal, and Neonatal Physiology: A Clinical Perspective,* 3rd ed. St. Louis, Saunders, 2007, pp. 315-374.

6. **(C)** Hyperglycemia and hyperinsulinemia present in diabetes inhibit surfactant C (phosphatidylcholine) protein synthesis. Heroin induces fetal hypoxia and stress; stress accelerates lung maturation. Maternal hypertension and intrauterine growth restriction both stress the fetus, promoting lung maturation.

**References:** Blackburn, S.T.: *Maternal, Fetal, and Neonatal Physiology: A Clinical Perspective,* 3rd ed. St. Louis, Saunders, 2007, pp. 315-374.

Rodriguez, R.C.: Respiratory distress syndrome and its management. In Martin, R.J., Fanaroff, A.A., Walsh, M.C. (Eds.): *Fanaroff and Martin's Neonatal-Perinatal Medicine: Diseases of the Fetus and Infant,* 8th ed. Philadelphia, Mosby, 2006, pp. 1097-1107.

7. **(C)** Surfactant is produced and secreted by the lamellar bodies of the type II cells of the lungs. Acini are the gas-exchanging portion of lung tissue. Type I pneumocytes are thin cells of the alveoli and are responsible for gas exchange. Surfactant protein A is one of the four protein components of surfactant.

**Reference:** Blackburn, S.T.: *Maternal, Fetal, and Neonatal Physiology: A Clinical Perspective,* 3rd ed. St. Louis, Saunders, 2007, pp. 315-374.

8. **(A)** Retractions are the result of increased chest wall compliance, immature intercostal muscles, and increased inspiratory pressure. Retractions worsen with increasing disease. Hypotension frequently occurs with respiratory disease as a late finding due to hypoxia and acidosis caused by poor respiratory effort. Acrocyanosis is a peripheral blueness of the extremities and is normal within the first 24 hours of life. The normal respiratory rate in a newborn is 30 to 60 breaths/minute.

**Reference:** Gardner, S.L., Enzman-Hines, M., Dickey, L.A.: Respiratory diseases. In Gardner, S.L., Carter, B.S., Enzman-Hines, M., et al. (Eds.): *Merenstein and Gardner's Handbook of Neonatal Intensive Care,* 7th ed. St. Louis, Mosby, 2011, pp. 581-677.

9. **(C)** Hypocapnia induces cerebral ischemia leading to neuronal cell injury and death. Tachypnea increases minute ventilation and lowers carbon dioxide levels in the blood. The nephron responds to low carbon dioxide blood levels by loss of bicarbonate in the urine filtrate in an attempt to normalize acid-base status. Gastroesophageal reflux disease is a pathologic response to an incompetent lower esophageal sphincter.

**Reference:** Curley, G., Kavanagh, B.P., Laffey, J.G.: Hypocapnia and the injured brain: More harm than benefit. *Critical Care Medicine,* 38(5):1348-1359, 2010.

10. **(B)** Respiratory distress syndrome (RDS) is the result of surfactant deficiency. The incidence of RDS is inversely proportional to the gestational age of the infant, and RDS is the most common pulmonary problem in the preterm infant. At 30 weeks' gestational age, surfactant production is minimal, which leads to atelectasis, hypoxia, and acidosis. The infant's attempt to increase ventilation is characterized by grunting, nasal flaring, and retractions. Preterm infants with surfactant deficiency may develop an air leak syndrome, which is usually iatrogenic resulting from the therapies given. Presence of an air leak at birth before the infant has undergone positive pressure ventilation is less likely. Although meconium aspiration syndrome can lead to these signs, the passage of meconium was not present in this scenario. Transient tachypnea of the newborn is due to retained fetal lung fluid and is most likely to be experienced by full-term infants who are born by cesarean section or have experienced perinatal hypoxia.

**References:** Blackburn, S.T.: *Maternal, Fetal, and Neonatal Physiology: A Clinical Perspective,* 3rd ed. St. Louis, Saunders, 2007, pp. 315-374.

Gardner, S.L., Enzman-Hines, M., Dickey, L.A.: Respiratory diseases. In Gardner, S.L., Carter, B.S., Enzman-Hines, M., et al. (Eds.): *Merenstein and Gardner's Handbook of Neonatal Intensive Care,* 7th ed. St. Louis, Mosby, 2011, pp. 581-677.

11. **(D)** Expiratory grunting is an attempt to slow expiratory flow rates, prevent alveolar atelectasis, and maintain functional residual capacity. Energy conservation is important for the sick neonate. The sick neonate typically demonstrates decreased tone and activity. Upper airway resistance is a function of nasal resistance and the cartilage and supporting structures of the pharyngeal airway. Large airway obstruction is caused by mucus or congenital defects and is not relieved by expiratory grunting.

**Reference:** Blackburn, S.T.: *Maternal, Fetal, and Neonatal Physiology: A Clinical Perspective,* 3rd ed. St. Louis, Saunders, 2007, pp. 315-374.

12. **(B)** The diagnosis of sepsis is hard to make based on clinical findings alone. A positive finding on cultures of the blood, cerebrospinal fluid, or urine is the gold standard. Ocular contamination acquired during passage through the birth canal would be eradicated by application of antibiotic ointment after delivery. Culture of nasal secretions is a surveillance method typically used to detect methicillin-resistant *Staphylococcus aureus.* Culture of surface specimens is a surveillance method and not a definitive diagnostic method.

**Reference:** Lott, J.W.: Immunology and infectious disease. In Verklan, M.T., Walden, W. (Eds.): *Core Curriculum for Neonatal Intensive Care Nursing,* 4th ed. St. Louis, Saunders, 2010, pp. 694-723.

13. **(D)** Air bronchograms are air in the bronchial tree visualized against a background of generalized alveolar atelectasis and are characteristic of respiratory distress syndrome. In pneumonia, the chest radiograph demonstrates patchy, occasionally asymmetric, radiating, bilateral interstitial infiltrates. The radiographic appearance of pulmonary edema varies from a diffuse haziness to a whiteout. Pulmonary interstitial emphysema is seen as multiple small, cystlike radiolucencies with a varying pattern. A pneumothorax appears as an air collection in the pleural space. A pneumomediastinum appears as an air collection in the mediastinum. A pneumopericardium is demonstrated by a halo of free air in the pericardial space.

**Reference:** Lane, L.: Radiologic evaluation. In Verklan, M.T., Walden, M. (Eds.): *Core Curriculum for Neonatal Intensive Care Nursing,* 4th ed. St. Louis, Saunders, 2010, pp. 270-298.

14. **(C)** The pH of 7.25 indicates acidosis. The $Paco_2$ is indicative of a respiratory component. The $HCO_3$ of 21 is normal. Therefore, the cause of the acidosis is respiratory, not metabolic. The hallmark of metabolic acidosis is a low $HCO_3$. Metabolic alkalosis demonstrates an elevated pH due to a high $HCO_3$. The pH would be elevated (alkalotic) if $Paco_2$ were low.

**Reference:** Wood, A.M., Jones, M.D. Jr.: Acid-base homeostasis and oxygenation. In Gardner, S.L., Carter, B.S., Enzman-Hines, M., et al. (Eds.): *Merenstein and Gardner's Handbook of Neonatal Intensive Care,* 7th ed. St. Louis, Mosby, 2011, pp. 153-163.

15. **(D)** Criteria for endotracheal suctioning include visible secretions in the tube, coarse breath sounds, increased agitation, and changes in arterial blood gas values. After suctioning, the infant is reassessed to determine the effectiveness of the procedure. Repositioning of the infant is necessary to prevent localization of secretions in the dependent pulmonary structures. Pain management is used to improve ventilator synchrony and pulmonary function, decrease stress, and prevent complications. However, provision of an adequate airway take precedence over either of these interventions. Equipment alarms are present to notify care providers that predetermined limits have been exceeded. Alarms require an action response to determine the cause of the alarm and return the infant to an acceptable range of response.

**References:** Gardner, S.L., Enzman-Hines, M., Dickey, L.A.: Pain and pain relief. In Gardner, S.L., Carter, B.S., Enzman-Hines, M., et al. (Eds.): *Merenstein and Gardner's Handbook of Neonatal Intensive Care,* 7th ed. St. Louis, Mosby, 2011, pp. 223-269.

Gardner, S.L., Enzman-Hines, M., Dickey, L.A.: Respiratory diseases. In Gardner, S.L., Carter, B.S., Enzman-Hines, M., et al. (Eds.): *Merenstein and Gardner's Handbook of Neonatal Intensive Care,* 7th ed. St. Louis, Mosby, 2011, pp. 581-677.

16. **(D)** Patent ductus arteriosus is an outcome of surfactant usage. Clinical findings include bounding peripheral pulses, widening pulse pressure, diminished left ventricular output with decreased renal and mesenteric blood flow, and metabolic acidosis. A murmur is typically, though not always, present. The initial signs of sepsis are nonspecific and nonlocalizing, and include vital sign abnormalities, respiratory distress, lethargy, and feeding problems. Signs of a gradual air leak include restlessness, tachypnea, and increased work of breathing. An acute air leak manifests with bradycardia and muffled heart sounds, air hunger, and cyanosis, and cardiopulmonary arrest can result. Signs and symptoms of pneumonia are nonspecific and include respiratory distress and temperature instability.

**References:** Gardner, S.L., Enzman-Hines, M., Dickey, L.A.: Respiratory diseases. In Gardner, S.L., Carter, B.S., Enzman-Hines, M., et al. (Eds.): *Merenstein and Gardner's Handbook of Neonatal Intensive Care,* 7th ed. St. Louis, Mosby, 2011, pp. 581-677.

Sadowski, S.L.: Cardiovascular disorders. In Verklan, M.T., Walden, M. (Eds.): *Core Curriculum for Neonatal Intensive Care Nursing,* 4th ed. St. Louis, Saunders, 2010, pp. 534-588.

Venkatesh, M.P., Adams, K.M., Weisman, L.E.: Infection in the neonate. In Gardner, S.L., Carter, B.S., Enzman-Hines, M., et al. (Eds.): *Merenstein and Gardner's Handbook of Neonatal Intensive Care,* 7th ed. St. Louis, Mosby, 2011, pp. 553-580.

17. **(B)** The inhibition of cyclooxygenase by the nonsteroidal antiinflammatory agent indomethacin (Indocin) results in decreased prostaglandin synthesis and contributes to ductus arteriosus closure. A left-to-right shunt through the ductus arteriosus results in pulmonary edema and respiratory compromise. Restriction of fluids and diuretic use are interventions implemented to reduce pulmonary symptoms. Acetaminophen (Tylenol) has minimal effects on peripheral prostaglandin synthesis. Prostaglandin $E_1$ (Alprostadil) is a vasodilator used to provide patency of the ductus arteriosus.

**References:** Blackburn, S.T.: *Maternal, Fetal, and Neonatal Physiology: A Clinical Perspective,* 3rd ed. St. Louis, Saunders, 2007, pp. 267-314.

Spratto, G.R., Woods, A.L.: *Delmar Nurse's Drug Handbook.* Clifton Park, N.Y., Delmar Cengage Learning, 2010, pp. 12-16, 856-859, 2003-2007.

18. **(D)** Blood flow through a patent ductus arteriosus (PDA) is pressure dependent. In a preterm infant, as pulmonary vascular resistance decreases, blood leaves the aorta and enters the pulmonary artery, which results in a left-to-right shunt, pulmonary edema, and diminished gas exchange at the alveolar level. Systemic blood flow is reduced, which leads to hypotension with diminished peripheral pulses, slower capillary refill, and decreased distal organ perfusion. The left-to-right shunting of blood from the aorta to the pulmonary artery results in hyperperfusion, not hypoperfusion, of the pulmonary circuit. Right-to-left shunting of blood occurs through the PDA when right-sided pressure exceeds systemic pressure, as in persistent pulmonary hypertension.

**Reference:** Blackburn, S.T.: *Maternal, Fetal, and Neonatal Physiology: A Clinical Perspective,* 3rd ed. St. Louis, Saunders, 2007, pp. 267-314.

19. **(D)** The preterm infant has less pulmonary arterial muscle and immature pulmonary parenchyma. The left-to-right shunting in patent ductus arteriosus (PDA) results in increased pulmonary blood flow and increases the chance of pulmonary hemorrhage. Because this left-to-right shunting steals blood from the systemic circulation, hypoperfusion of the tissues occurs and metabolic acidosis develops. Preterm infants with surfactant deficiency may develop an air leak syndrome, which is usually iatrogenic resulting from the therapies given. The administration of surfactant rapidly increases alveolar recruitment and improves alveolar gas exchange. Attention to ventilatory management is required to prevent air leak. Pulmonary hypoplasia results from intrinsic abnormalities in lung development, from compression as in congenital diaphragmatic hernia, or from oligohydramnios as occurs with renal agenesis.

References: Blackburn, S.T.: *Maternal, Fetal, and Neonatal Physiology: A Clinical Perspective,* 3rd ed. St. Louis, Saunders, 2007, pp. 267-314, 315-374.

Gardner, S.L., Enzman-Hines, M., Dickey, L.A.: Respiratory diseases. In Gardner, S.L., Carter, B.S., Enzman-Hines, M., et al. (Eds.): *Merenstein and Gardner's Handbook of Neonatal Intensive Care,* 7th ed. St. Louis, Mosby, 2011, pp. 581-677.

20. **(C)** A neutral thermal environment maintains normal body temperature, the temperature at which an individual's oxygen consumption is minimized. Although adequate fluid intake is necessary to meet the body's demands, excessive fluid contributes to volume overload and patency of the ductus arteriosus, which can lead to pulmonary function abnormalities. For an acutely ill infant, minimal stimulation limits stressors that interfere with physiologic stability. Maintaining an oxygen saturation level at 90% to 92% keeps the infant in a normoxemic state under most conditions.

References: Bradshaw, W.T., Tanaka, D.T.: Physiologic monitoring. In Gardner, S.L., Carter, B.S., Enzman-Hines, M., et al. (Eds.): *Merenstein and Gardner's Handbook of Neonatal Intensive Care,* 7th ed. St. Louis, Mosby, 2011, pp. 134-152.

Brown, V.D., Landers, S.: Heat balance. In Gardner, S.L., Carter, B.S., Enzman-Hines, M., et al. (Eds.): *Merenstein and Gardner's Handbook of Neonatal Intensive Care,* 7th ed. St. Louis, Mosby, 2011, pp. 113-133.

Gardner, S.L., Goldson, E.: The neonate and the environment: Impact on development. In Gardner, S.L., Carter, B.S., Enzman-Hines, M., et al. (Eds.): *Merenstein and Gardner's Handbook of Neonatal Intensive Care,* 7th ed. St. Louis, Mosby, 2011, pp. 270-331.

21. **(D)** An infant with respiratory distress syndrome may exhibit oliguria, especially if the infant is hypoxic or renal perfusion is diminished. A natural diuresis occurs at 48 to 72 hours of age and precedes the onset of the recovery phase. Renal failure results in body fluid excess. Removal of excess lung fluid and pulmonary edema heralds improving pulmonary status. An infant with chronic lung disease exhibits fluid intolerance, including growth failure, weight gain, edema, and decreased urine output.

References: Askin, D.F.: Respiratory distress. In Verklan, M.T., Walden, M. (Eds.): *Core Curriculum for Neonatal Intensive Care Nursing,* 4th ed. St. Louis, Saunders, 2010, pp. 453-483.

Halbardier, B.H.: Fluid and electrolyte management. In Verklan, M.T., Walden, M. (Eds.): *Core Curriculum for Neonatal Intensive Care Nursing,* 4th ed. St. Louis, Saunders, 2010, pp. 156-171.

22. **(A)** Pathogens responsible for early-onset pneumonia are acquired transplacentally and from the birth canal before or during delivery. Maternal fever indicates infection; premature rupture of membranes, prolonged labor, and excessive obstetric manipulations predispose to ascending infection. The cause of respiratory distress syndrome is surfactant deficiency. Meconium aspiration syndrome occurs predominately in term or postterm infants who have experienced hypoxia with relaxation of the anal sphincter and the expulsion of meconium into the amniotic fluid followed by fetal gasping. Transient tachypnea of the newborn generally occurs in term or late-preterm infants with a history of cesarean section or precipitous delivery. Fetal interstitial lung fluid results in collapse of the bronchioli.

References: Gardner, S.L., Enzman-Hines, M., Dickey, L.A.: Respiratory diseases. In Gardner, S.L., Carter, B.S., Enzman-Hines, M., et al. (Eds.): *Merenstein and Gardner's Handbook of Neonatal Intensive Care,* 7th ed. St. Louis, Mosby, 2011, pp. 581-677.

Venkatesh, M.P., Adams, K.M., Weisman L.E.: Infection in the neonate. In Gardner, S.L., Carter, B.S., Enzman-Hines, M., et al. (Eds.): *Merenstein and Gardner's Handbook of Neonatal Intensive Care,* 7th ed. St. Louis, Mosby, 2011, pp. 554-580.

23. **(D)** Supplemental oxygen administration has relieved this infant's hypoxemia and is readily available as therapy. Supplemental oxygen will treat the diagnosed problem of hypoxemia. An infant who is large for gestational age as a result of maternal diabetes is at increased risk for surfactant deficiency, because the hyperglycemia and hyperinsulinemia present in diabetes inhibit surfactant C (phosphatidylcholine) protein synthesis. Surfactant replacement therapy is given after surfactant deficiency is diagnosed from the history, clinical presentation, and chest radiograph. Nitric oxide is a vasodilating agent used in the treatment of persistent pulmonary hypertension to relax pulmonary vasculature and enhance pulmonary blood flow. Intubation and mechanical ventilation are strategies used in pulmonary failure or apnea. The infant's blood gas results show hypoxia, not respiratory failure. The infant is not apneic.

Reference: Gardner, S.L., Enzman-Hines, M., Dickey, L.A.: Respiratory diseases. In Gardner, S.L., Carter, B.S., Enzman-Hines, M., et al. (Eds.): *Merenstein and Gardner's Handbook of Neonatal Intensive Care,* 7th ed. St. Louis, Mosby, 2011, pp. 581-677.

24. **(D)** Transient tachypnea of the newborn manifests on chest radiograph as bilateral, symmetric, perihilar streakiness caused by increased interstitial and alveolar fluid. Respiratory distress syndrome appears on chest radiograph as bilateral diffuse alveolar infiltrates and a reticulogranular appearance due to alveolar atelectasis. Meconium aspiration syndrome manifests on chest radiograph as bilateral, asymmetric areas of atelectasis and hyperaeration of the lungs with flattened hemidiaphragms. Pulmonary interstitial emphysema appears on chest radiograph as multiple, small, cyst-like radiolucencies caused by alveolar overdistention secondary to assisted ventilation.

References: Gardner, S.L., Enzman-Hines, M., Dickey, L.A.: Respiratory diseases. In Gardner, S.L., Carter, B.S., Enzman-Hines, M., et al. (Eds.): *Merenstein and Gardner's Handbook of Neonatal Intensive Care,* 7th ed. St. Louis, Mosby, 2011, pp. 581-677.

Lane, L.: Radiologic evaluation. In Verklan, M.T., Walden, M. (Eds.): *Core Curriculum for Neonatal Intensive Care Nursing,* 4th ed. St. Louis, Saunders, 2010, pp. 270-298.

25. **(B)** Transient tachypnea of the newborn generally occurs in term or late-preterm infants with a history of cesarean section or precipitous delivery. Lack of compression of the fetal chest results in retained fetal interstitial lung fluid, which leads to collapse of the

bronchioli. Chest radiographic findings include prominent perihilar streaking, hyperaeration, and mild to moderate cardiomegaly. The perihilar streaking represents engorgement of the periarterial lymphatics that participate in the clearance of alveolar fluid. Aspiration of amniotic fluid and debris as well as meconium typically occurs in term or postterm infants who have experienced hypoxia. Hypoxia results in in utero fetal gasping and inhalation of substances into the airways. Pulmonary hypoplasia results when normal lung development is interrupted early in gestation. Causes include space-occupying lesions and oligohydramnios due to renal agenesis. Progressive atelectasis is seen with surfactant deficiency.

**Reference:** Gardner, S.L., Enzman-Hines, M., Dickey, L.A.: Respiratory diseases. In Gardner, S.L., Carter, B.S., Enzman-Hines, M., et al. (Eds.): *Merenstein and Gardner's Handbook of Neonatal Intensive Care,* 7th ed. St. Louis, Mosby, 2011, pp. 581-677.

26. **(A)** Pneumonia can be congenital or acquired. Clinical signs are similar to those of transient tachypnea of the newborn, including tachypnea, oxygen desaturation, and decreased lung compliance. A pneumothorax is an emergent event that results when alveoli rupture, usually as the result of assisted ventilation. Clinical presentation includes respiratory problems (decreased breath sounds on the affected side, tachypnea or increased work of breathing, and oxygen desaturation), and cardiovascular manifestations (hypotension, diminished peripheral pulses, and poor capillary refill). A pleural effusion is not a disease but is the result of another disease process such as heart or renal failure, or chylothorax. Pulmonary interstitial emphysema results from alveolar overdistention and rupture secondary to assisted ventilation. Interstitial air dissects into nonventilated tissues around blood or lymphatic vessels and appears on chest radiographs as multiple small, cystlike radiolucencies.

**References:** Askin, D.F.: Respiratory distress. In Verklan, M.T., Walden, M. (Eds.): *Core Curriculum for Neonatal Intensive Care Nursing,* 4th ed. St. Louis, Saunders, 2010, pp. 453-483.

Schumann, L.: Respiratory function and alterations in gas exchange. In Copstead, L.C., Banasik, J.L. (Eds.): *Pathophysiology,* 4th ed. St. Louis, Saunders, 2010, pp. 510-537.

27. **(D)** Hypoxia and acidosis are endogenous mediators that increase pulmonary vascular resistance and lead to persistent pulmonary hypertension and hypoperfusion of the lungs. Pneumonia results from bacterial, viral, or mycoplasmal organisms acquired transplacentally, during delivery, or postnatally. Pneumonia is due to an immature immune system, colonization of the mother's genital and vaginal tracts with pathogens, amnionitis, prolonged rupture of membranes, and nosocomial infections acquired in the NICU. Transient tachypnea of the newborn generally occurs in term or late-preterm infants with a history of cesarean section or precipitous delivery. Lack of compression of the fetal chest results in retained fetal interstitial lung fluid, which leads to collapse of the bronchioli. Asphyxia prevents a decrease in pulmonary vascular resistance, which leads to pulmonary artery pressure equal to or higher than systemic

pressure. This results in a right-to-left shunt through either the foramen ovale, ductus arteriosus, or both.

**Reference:** Gardner, S.L., Enzman-Hines, M., Dickey, L.A.: Respiratory diseases. In Gardner, S.L., Carter, B.S., Enzman-Hines, M., et al. (Eds.): *Merenstein and Gardner's Handbook of Neonatal Intensive Care,* 7th ed. St. Louis, Mosby, 2011, pp. 581-677.

28. **(A)** Central apnea is the absence of breathing effort. Without respiratory effort, airflow is zero. In obstructive apnea, breathing efforts are present but airflow is blocked. Mixed apnea is characterized by an initial central apneic episode followed by obstruction of the airway. A pattern of cyclic respirations of breathing for 10 to 15 seconds, followed by apnea for 5 to 10 seconds, occurring at least three times in succession, is referred to as *periodic breathing.*

**Reference:** Gardner, S.L., Enzman-Hines, M., Dickey, L.A.: Respiratory diseases. In Gardner, S.L., Carter, B.S., Enzman-Hines, M., et al. (Eds.): *Merenstein and Gardner's Handbook of Neonatal Intensive Care,* 7th ed. St. Louis, Mosby, 2011, pp. 581-677.

29. **(C)** Responses to hypoxemia and changes in $Paco_2$ are different in the adult and in the neonate. The adult responds with sustained increased ventilation. The neonate, however, demonstrates a brief period of increased ventilation as chemoreceptors in the medulla and carotid and aortic vessels sense an abnormal $Paco_2$ level, followed by respiratory depression as the sensitivity of peripheral and central chemoreceptors diminishes. Disturbances in rate and rhythm develop.

**Reference:** Gardner, S.L., Enzman-Hines, M., Dickey, L.A.: Respiratory diseases. In Gardner, S.L., Carter, B.S., Enzman-Hines, M., et al. (Eds.): *Merenstein and Gardner's Handbook of Neonatal Intensive Care,* 7th ed. St. Louis, Mosby, 2011, pp. 581-677.

30. **(B)** Weighing on a cold scale is one example of environmental stress, which has been shown to precipitate apneic episodes. Limiting loud noises reduces noxious stimuli and apneic events. Abrupt changes in temperature, especially hyperthermia, trigger apnea. Maintaining the environmental temperature in the lower-normal range reduces apneic events. Small rolls or other positioning aids may to used to prevent airway obstruction.

**Reference:** Gardner, S.L., Enzman-Hines, M., Dickey, L.A.: Respiratory diseases. In Gardner, S.L., Carter, B.S., Enzman-Hines, M., et al. (Eds.): *Merenstein and Gardner's Handbook of Neonatal Intensive Care,* 7th ed. St. Louis, Mosby, 2011, pp. 581-677.

31. **(C)** Tachycardia is an adverse effect of caffeine. Therefore, the dose should not be administered and the physician or neonatal nurse practitioner should be notified immediately. Serum drug level will be measured to check for caffeine toxicity. The nurse should monitor the infant for additional adverse effects, including ventricular ectopy, gastrointestinal upset, and central nervous system manifestations of restlessness, irritability, and agitation.

**References:** Gardner, S.L., Enzman-Hines, M., Dickey, L.A.: Respiratory diseases. In Gardner, S.L., Carter, B.S., Enzman-Hines, M., et al. (Eds.): *Merenstein and Gardner's Handbook of*

*Neonatal Intensive Care,* 7th ed. St. Louis, Mosby, 2011, pp. 581-677.

Goodwin, M.: Apnea. In Verklan, M.T., Walden, M. (Eds.): *Core Curriculum for Neonatal Intensive Care Nursing,* 4th ed. St. Louis, Saunders, 2010, pp. 484- 493.

**32. (C)** The need for subsequent arterial blood gas (ABG) measurements is reduced but not eliminated. The monitor must be calibrated before use and then correlated with ABG results. The placement site must be changed frequently based on the probe temperature and the condition of infant's skin to prevent skin burns. When the site is changed, the monitor must be recalibrated and another ABG analysis performed to determine the correlation between the monitor values and the ABG results. A transcutaneous monitor is very useful when obtaining specimens for ABG analysis is difficult or when rapid changes in oxygen and ventilation provision are occurring. However, arterial and transcutaneous oxygen values are not identical because of local oxygen consumption by the skin, heating of the skin, oxygen diffusion time, and the response time of the electrode. An umbilical artery catheter is removed when it is no longer required for patient care. Although the $Po_2$ and $Pco_2$ monitors are used as one method of assessment, they do not replace ABG analysis, and therefore the umbilical catheter cannot yet be removed. Transcutaneous $Po_2$ and $Pco_2$ monitors can show blood value trends but are subject to drift when left in place for longer than 4 hours or when the infant is not well perfused or has a low temperature. The range of accuracy of transcutaneous $Po_2$ monitors is limited. Values lower than 40 mm Hg and higher than 120 mm Hg are not accurately reflected.

**References:** Bradshaw, W.T., Tanaka, D.T.: Physiologic monitoring. In Gardner, S.L., Carter, B.S., Enzman-Hines, M., et al. (Eds.): *Merenstein and Gardner's Handbook of Neonatal Intensive Care,* 7th ed. St. Louis, Mosby, 2011, pp. 134-152.

Truog, W.E., Golombek, S.G.: Principles of management of respiratory problems. In MacDonald, M.G., Mullett, M.D., Seshia, M.M. (Eds.): *Avery's Neonatology: Pathophysiology and Management of the Newborn,* 6th ed. Philadelphia, Lippincott Williams & Wilkins, 2005, pp. 600-621.

**33. (C)** The most common bacterial organisms causing pneumonia in the newborn period are group B streptococci and gram-negative organisms. Although *Chlamydia trachomatis* can be acquired at birth, it is not among the most common etiologic agents of pneumonia. Respiratory syncytial virus is a nosocomial cause of pneumonia. Infections caused by *Candida* fungal species occur most often in neonates requiring prolonged hospitalization. These organisms are another nosocomial cause of pneumonia.

**References:** Askin, D.F.: Respiratory distress. In Verklan, M.T., Walden, M. (Eds.): *Core Curriculum for Neonatal Intensive Care Nursing,* 4th ed. St. Louis, Saunders, 2010, pp. 453-483.

Gardner, S.L., Enzman-Hines, M., Dickey, L.A.: Respiratory diseases. In Gardner, S.L., Carter, B.S., Enzman-Hines, M., et al. (Eds.): *Merenstein and Gardner's Handbook of Neonatal Intensive Care,* 7th ed. St. Louis, Mosby, 2011, pp. 581-677.

**34. (C)** Fetuses with in utero hypoxemia and acidosis often pass meconium and initiate respiratory efforts.

Respiratory efforts increase the risk of meconium aspiration. If meconium is retrieved from the trachea during neonatal resuscitation after birth, vigilance is required for the development of meconium aspiration syndrome (MAS), frequently with persistent pulmonary hypertension. Mild MAS can show a normal lung pattern on chest radiograph. Pulmonary edema is associated with a high fluid intake and significant patent ductus arteriosus, congenital heart defects that increase pulmonary blood flow, and lung injury. It rarely manifests at birth unless the infant has experienced heart failure in utero. Although respiratory distress has multiple causes, the risk of meconium aspiration syndrome (MAS) is primary due to the history and presentation at birth. In the absence of indications for MAS, the care provider would proceed with differential diagnosis. Transient tachypnea of the newborn is caused by retained fetal lung fluid and is most likely to be experienced by full-term infants who are born by cesarean section or have experienced perinatal hypoxia. Tachypnea is present. The chest radiograph shows perihilar streaking secondary to retained lung fluid.

**References:** American Heart Association, American Academy of Pediatrics: American Heart Association guidelines for cardiopulmonary resuscitation and emergency cardiovascular care of pediatric and neonatal patients: Neonatal resuscitation guidelines. *Pediatrics,* 117(5):e1029-e1038, 2006.

International Liaison Committee on Resuscitation (ILCOR): Consensus on science with treatment recommendations for pediatric and neonatal patients: neonatal resuscitation. *Pediatrics,* 117(5):e978-e988, 2006.

Lane, L.: Radiologic evaluation. In Verklan, M.T., Walden, M. (Eds.): *Core Curriculum for Neonatal Intensive Care Nursing,* 4th ed. St. Louis, Saunders, 2010, pp. 270-298.

**35. (B)** Meconium aspiration syndrome (MAS) places the infant at risk for air leak due to the ball-valve phenomenon: air enters the alveoli but cannot escape. Distended alveoli rupture, which results in air leak. Air leak is a major risk factor associated with assisted ventilation in infants with MAS. A tension pneumothorax occurs as air builds up under pressure in the pleural space. The affected lung collapses and forces the mediastinum toward the contralateral side. Signs and symptoms of tension pneumothorax are acute respiratory decompensation with cyanosis, apnea, and bradycardia. On examination, the affected lung will exhibit diminished breath sounds. Increased anteroposterior diameter of the chest will be noted on visualization. Serous fluid is produced from the parietal pleural capillaries and enters the pleural space. It is reabsorbed into the parietal pleural lymphatics. Production and absorption of serous fluid are constant. In disease states, production may increase, which results in a pleural effusion. A pleural effusion is not an acute event but rather occurs over time. A pulmonary hemorrhage manifests with sudden, severe respiratory distress accompanied by bright red blood or frothy pink secretions from the trachea. It is usually due to increased pulmonary capillary hydrostatic pressure resulting in capillary rupture. Pulmonary interstitial emphysema (PIE) is an air leak syndrome that can occur following vigorous resuscitation efforts or accompany assisted ventilation. Air dissects around blood vessels or along lymphatics. PIE manifests with hypoxia and hypercapnia. It may progress to pneumothorax or pneumomediastinum.

**References:** Askin, D.F.: Respiratory distress. In Verklan, M.T., Walden, M. (Eds.): *Core Curriculum for Neonatal Intensive Care Nursing*, 4th ed. St. Louis, Saunders, 2010, pp. 453-483.

Schumann, L.: Restrictive pulmonary disorders. In Copstead, L.C., Banasik, J.L. (Eds.): *Pathophysiology*, 4th ed. St. Louis, Saunders, 2010, pp. 563-588.

36. **(C)** Congenital diaphragmatic hernia (CDH) is a herniation of abdominal organs into the thoracic cavity through a diaphragmatic defect. Clinical signs include respiratory distress and cyanosis at birth or shortly thereafter. The infant deteriorates, rather than improves, with bag-and-mask ventilation because the intestines distend with air and further compromise lung function. Breath sounds are diminished, point of maximal impulse may be shifted, the chest is barrel shaped, and the abdomen is scaphoid. A radiograph taken immediately after birth may not demonstrate intestine in the thorax, but later images will clearly demonstrate air-filled bowel. Survival rate is 50%. A tension pneumothorax occurs as air builds up under pressure in the pleural space. The affected lung collapses and forces the mediastinum toward the contralateral side, which results in decompensation. Assisted ventilation generally precedes pneumothorax. In this situation, the infant exhibited acute distress prior to any resuscitation efforts. Pneumomediastinum occurs after positive pressure ventilation and with meconium aspiration syndrome (MAS). Air travels via vascular sheaths to the lining of the lung and moves into the mediastinum, which results in pneumomediastinum. Signs include increased anteroposterior diameter of the chest and indistinct heart sounds. Cystic adenomatoid malformation is a primary pulmonary tissue dysplasia in which terminal bronchioles fail to canalize, which leads to multiple small pulmonary cysts. Respiratory symptoms vary from none to distress at birth. It can be distinguished from CDH by radiograph. Survival rate is 90%.

**References:** Askin, D.F.: Respiratory distress. In Verklan, M.T., Walden, M. (Eds.): *Core Curriculum for Neonatal Intensive Care Nursing*, 4th ed. St. Louis, Saunders, 2010, pp. 453-483.

Bradshaw, W.T.: Gastrointestinal disorders. In Verklan, M.T., Walden, M. (Eds.): *Core Curriculum for Neonatal Intensive Care Nursing*, 4th ed. St. Louis, Saunders, 2010, pp. 589-637.

37. **(C)** In bronchopulmonary dysplasia (BPD), the lung is injured in the canalicular period by an inflammatory reaction. Causes include immaturity, infection, volutrauma or barotrauma, and oxidative stress. Excessive fluid intake and hypervolemia contribute to the development of a patent ductus arteriosus with left-to-right shunting and pulmonary vascular volume overload. Pulmonary capillary leak creates a barrier to gas diffusion necessitating increased respiratory support and higher oxygen concentration. The incidence of BPD is inversely proportional to gestational age, and it occurs predominately in more preterm infants. Transient tachypnea of the newborn is retained

fetal lung fluid and is predominately seen in term or near-term infants born by cesarean section. Tachypnea is present, but these infants seldom require mechanical ventilation, recover rapidly, and have no residual effects.

**References:** Askin, D.F.: Respiratory distress. In Verklan, M.T., Walden, M. (Eds.): *Core Curriculum for Neonatal Intensive Care Nursing*, 4th ed. St. Louis, Saunders, 2010, pp. 453-483.

Blackburn, S.T.: *Maternal, Fetal, and Neonatal Physiology: A Clinical Perspective*, 3rd ed. St. Louis, Saunders, 2007, pp. 315-374.

38. **(D)** In bronchopulmonary dysplasia, by the end of the first or second week of life, the chest radiograph shows haziness of vessel margins progressing to linear densities representing alveolar collapse. This is followed by a bubbly appearance with hyperaeration, especially at the lung bases. Serous fluid is produced from the parietal pleural capillaries and enters the pleural space. It is reabsorbed into the parietal pleural lymphatics. Production and absorption of serous fluid are constant. In disease states, production may increase, which results in a pleural effusion. A pleural effusion is not an acute event but rather occurs over time. A pleural effusion is not a disease itself but is the result of another disease process, such as heart or renal failure, or chylothorax. Patchy alveolar infiltrates are present in pneumonia. Absence of parenchymal markings denotes diminished pulmonary blood flow and is consistent with right-sided heart and outflow tract obstruction or persistent pulmonary hypertension.

**References:** Lane, L.: Radiologic evaluation. In Verklan, M.T., Walden, M. (Eds.): *Core Curriculum for Neonatal Intensive Care Nursing*, 4th ed. St. Louis, Saunders, 2010, pp. 270-298.

Schumann, L.: Respiratory function and alterations in gas exchange. In Copstead, L.C., Banasik, J.L. (Eds.): *Pathophysiology*, 4th ed. St. Louis, Saunders, 2010, pp. 510-537.

39. **(B)** The ventilatory rate and tidal volume directly affect $Paco_2$ values. When the ventilatory rate, and thus the minute ventilation, is decreased, $Paco_2$ level will rise to help correct respiratory alkalosis. An increase in minute ventilation as seen with an increased ventilator rate will further reduce $Paco_2$ levels, contributing to worsening respiratory alkalosis. Increasing the peak inspiratory pressure (PIP) will increase tidal volume and further reduce the $Paco_2$ value. Decreasing the positive end-expiratory pressure (PEEP) without decreasing the PIP will produce a larger tidal volume, which will result in further carbon dioxide elimination. Decreasing the PEEP beyond compliance may result in alveolar collapse.

**Reference:** Carlo, W.A., Martin, R.J., Fanaroff, A.A.: Assisted ventilation and complications of respiratory distress. In Martin, R.J., Fanaroff, A.A., Walsh, M.C. (Eds.): *Fanaroff and Martin's Neonatal-Perinatal Medicine: Diseases of the Fetus and Infant*, 8th ed. Philadelphia, Mosby, 2006, pp. 1108-1122.

40. **(C)** Gas remaining in the lungs after a normal expiration is known as *functional residual capacity* (FRC). FRC is approximately 30 ml/kg. Tidal volume is the amount of air that moves in and out of the lungs with a normal breath. The volume of air maximally inhaled and forcefully exhaled is the vital capacity. The

volume of gas not involved in gas exchange is physiologic dead space. This volume includes gas in conducting airways and gas in nonperfused alveoli.

**Reference:** Askin, D.F., Diehl-Jones, W.: Assisted ventilation. In Verklan, M.T., Walden, M. (Eds.): *Core Curriculum for Neonatal Intensive Care Nursing,* 4th ed., St. Louis, Saunders, 2010, pp. 494-520.

**41. (D)** An important aspect of chest tube care is the frequent monitoring and documentation of tube patency, oscillation of fluid within the drainage system, and presence or absence of bubbling in the water seal chamber. Continuous bubbling in the water seal chamber indicates an air leak; the source may be either the patient or the system. Developmentally appropriate positioning is not contraindicated in the infant with a chest tube. The infant should be maintained in a tucked midline position with care taken not to kink or dislodge the chest tube. Milking and stripping of the chest tube is not necessary. If visible clots and debris are seen in the chest tube and are not free flowing, gentle kneading, not stripping, of the chest tube may be indicated.

**References:** Carrier, C.T.: Developmental support. In Verklan, M.T., Walden, M. (Eds.): *Core Curriculum for Neonatal Care Nursing,* 4th ed. St. Louis, Saunders, 2010, pp. 208-232.

Gardner, S.L., Enzman-Hines, M., Dickey, L.A.: Respiratory diseases. In Gardner, S.L., Carter, B.S., Enzman-Hines, M., et al. (Eds.): *Merenstein and Gardner's Handbook of Neonatal Intensive Care,* 7th ed. St. Louis, Mosby, 2011, pp. 581-677.

**42. (B)** Pneumopericardium is characterized by cyanosis, muffled heart sounds, hypotension, and bradycardia. The chest radiograph reveals a "halo" around the heart. In pneumothorax the chest radiograph reveals accumulation of air in the pleural space. A collection of air in the mediastinum with air frequently outlining the undersurface of the thymus (sail sign) indicates a pneumomediastinum. Pulmonary interstitial emphysema is characterized by overdistended alveoli that appear as cystlike radiolucencies. With ruptured alveoli, air intravasates into interstitial lung tissue.

**References:** Gardner, S.L., Enzman-Hines, M., Dickey, L.A.: Respiratory diseases. In Gardner, S.L., Carter, B.S., Enzman-Hines, M., et al. (Eds.): *Merenstein and Gardner's Handbook of Neonatal Intensive Care,* 7th ed. St. Louis, Mosby, 2011, pp. 581-677.

Lane, L.: Radiologic evaluation. In Verklan, M.T., Walden, M. (Eds.): *Core Curriculum for Neonatal Intensive Care Nursing,* 4th ed. St. Louis, Saunders, 2010, pp. 270-298.

**43. (D)** Inhaled nitric oxide (iNO) has been proven to be a selective and potent pulmonary vasodilator. iNO prolongs clotting time but has no known myocardial effects. Although iNO plays a role in bronchodilation, its primary use is as a major mediator of endothelial function resulting in vascular dilation. iNO is rapidly inactivated with a half-life of 3 to 5 seconds. For this reason, it exerts no effect on systemic blood pressure.

**References:** Askin, D.F.: Respiratory distress. In Verklan, M.T., Walden, M. (Eds.): *Core Curriculum for Neonatal Intensive Care Nursing,* 4th ed. St. Louis, Saunders, 2010, pp. 453-483.

Giles, T.D.: Aspects of nitric oxide in health and disease: A focus on hypertension and cardiovascular disease. *Journal of Clinical Hypertension,* 8(12 suppl 4):2-16, 2006.

**44. (D)** Surgical repair of a congenital diaphragmatic hernia is performed once pulmonary and cardiovascular stabilization has been achieved. Early management includes mechanical ventilation, sedation and chemical paralysis, frequent monitoring of arterial blood gas values, inotropic support for systemic hypotension, and correction of metabolic acidosis. Extracorporeal membrane oxygenation (ECMO) and inhaled nitric oxide (iNO) may be indicated in severe cases. Immediate surgical repair is associated with a higher mortality rate. An immediate repair precludes stabilization and evaluation for associated conditions that may preclude ECMO or surgery. Use of surfactant is controversial, with some research showing a benefit and other studies indicating no benefit. Overall stability of the patient's condition contributes to a successful outcome. iNO may be given to promote pulmonary vasculature relaxation and help to increase pulmonary blood flow and gas exchange. This therapy is used to stabilize the infant's condition prior to and following surgery.

**References:** Bradshaw, W.T.: Gastrointestinal disorders. In Verklan, M.T., Walden, M. (Eds.): *Core Curriculum for Neonatal Intensive Care Nursing,* 4th ed. St. Louis, Saunders, 2010, pp. 589-637.

Hartnett, K.S.: Congenital diaphragmatic hernia: Advanced physiology and care concepts. *Advances in Neonatal Care,* 8(2):107-115, 2008.

**45. (C)** Long-term complications associated with congenital diaphragmatic hernia (CDH) repair include chronic lung disease, recurrent diaphragmatic hernia, gastroesophageal reflux, growth restriction, and neurodevelopmental delay. A chylothorax may be a complication of thoracic surgery evidenced shortly after surgery. Potter syndrome is characterized by bilateral renal agenesis. The syndrome is present before birth, not after CDH repair. Necrotizing enterocolitis (NEC) is predominately a disease of prematurity. CDH is primarily a disease of the term infant. Hypoxemia and acidosis accompanying CDH may contribute to the development of NEC shortly after an insult, rather than over the long term. Following CDH repair, all infants have intestinal malrotation. Further surgery may be necessary if midgut volvulus develops.

**References:** Botwinski, C.: Renal and genitourinary disorders. In Verklan, M.T., Walden, M. (Eds.): *Core Curriculum for Neonatal Intensive Care Nursing,* 4th ed. St. Louis, Saunders, 2010, pp. 724-747.

Hartnett, K.S.: Congenital diaphragmatic hernia: Advanced physiology and care concepts. *Advances in Neonatal Care,* 8(2), 2008, 107-115.

Lovvorn, H.N. III, Gleen, J.B., Pacetti, A.S., et al.: Neonatal surgery. In Gardner, S.L., Carter, B.S., Enzman-Hines, M., et al. (Eds.): *Merenstein and Gardner's Handbook of Neonatal Intensive Care,* 7th ed. St. Louis, Mosby, 2011, pp. 812-847.

**46. (A)** The development of vascular structures to supply air spaces occurs during the canalicular phase. The end of the embryonic stage is characterized by evidence of the trachea and the segmental and subsegmental bronchi. The pseudoglandular phase, extending from 7 to 16 weeks, is characterized by the completion of 16 bronchial divisions. Alveolar expansion is the completion of alveolarization.

**Reference:** Ballard, R.: Respiratory system. In Taeusch, H.W., Ballard, R.A., Gleason, C.A. (Eds.): *Avery's Diseases of the Newborn*, 8th ed. Philadelphia, Saunders, 2005, pp. 601-607.

47. **(D)** Adenosine inhibits heart rate by blocking electrical conduction at the atrioventricular node and inhibits respirations. Hyperglycemia is associated with increased respiratory rate. Caffeine increases breathing by stimulating the central nervous system. Isoproterenol enhances respirations.

**Reference:** Ballard, R.: Respiratory system. In Taeusch, H.W., Ballard, R.A., Gleason, C.A. (Eds.): *Avery's Diseases of the Newborn*, 8th ed. Philadelphia, Saunders, 2005, p. 616.

48. **(C)** Increasing peak inspiratory pressure will increase tidal volume, thereby decreasing $Paco_2$. $Paco_2$ is inversely proportional to respiratory rate. If the ventilator rate is decreased, $Paco_2$ will increase. Tidal volume is directly proportional to $Paco_2$. Decreasing the inspiratory time will decrease tidal volume, thereby increasing $Paco_2$. Increasing positive end-expiratory pressure will decrease the tidal volume, thereby increasing $Paco_2$.

**Reference:** Ballard, R.: Respiratory system. In Taeusch, H.W., Ballard, R.A., Gleason, C.A. (Eds.): *Avery's Diseases of the Newborn*, 8th ed. Philadelphia, Saunders, 2005, p. 654.

49. **(B)** On the chest radiograph, pulmonary interstitial emphysema is characterized by hyperinflated lungs with coarse radiolucencies extending from the pleura to the hilum. Respiratory distress syndrome is characterized by air bronchograms and hypoinflated lungs. Transient tachypnea of the newborn is characterized by a large cardiovascular silhouette with air bronchograms and streaky lung fields. The radiograph findings will generally clear by 24 hours of age. Persistent pulmonary hypertension of the newborn is characterized by hyperlucent lung fields with decreased vascularity.

**References:** Ballard, R.: Respiratory system. In Taeusch, H.W., Ballard, R.A., Gleason, C.A. (Eds.): *Avery's Diseases of the Newborn*, 8th ed. Philadelphia, Saunders, 2005, pp. 660, 691, 698, 709.

Lane, L.: Radiologic evaluation. In Verklan, M.T., Walden, M. (Eds.): *Core Curriculum for Neonatal Intensive Care Nursing*, 4th ed. St. Louis, Saunders, 2010, pp. 270-298.

50. **(B)** Cyanosis with vigorous respirations is indicative of an obstructed endotracheal tube. Once obstruction of the endotracheal tube has been excluded, chest radiography would be indicated. Although pancuronium could be administered, cyanosis with vigorous respirations is indicative of an obstructed endotracheal tube. The nurse should determine the underlying cause of the agitation and cyanosis and intervene appropriately. Various modes of ventilation can be considered with asynchronous respirations. However, an obstructed endotracheal tube must be excluded first.

**Reference:** Carlo, W.A.: Assisted ventilation. In Klaus, M.H., Fanaroff, A.A., (Eds.): *Care of the High-Risk Neonate*, 5th ed. Philadelphia, Saunders, 2001, pp. 277-299.

51. **(C)** Adenosine triphosphate is a purine receptor agonist that is a potent stimulator of surfactant secretion. Surfactant secretion is stimulated by hyperventilation. Hypoventilation decreases surfactant production. Surfactant stimulation is enhanced by mechanical stretch and lung hyperinflation. β-Adrenergic agonists stimulate surfactant secretion.

**Reference:** Jobe, A.H.: The respiratory system. In Martin, R.J., Fanaroff, A.A., Walsh, M.C. (Eds.): *Fanaroff and Martin's Neonatal-Perinatal Medicine: Diseases of the Fetus and Infant*, 8th ed. Philadelphia, Mosby, 2006, pp. 1069-1078.

52. **(A)** An increase in pH causes a shift to the left in the oxygen dissociation curve. An increase in $Paco_2$, an increase in temperature, and an increase in diphosphoglycerate level all cause a shift to the right in the oxygen dissociation curve.

**Reference:** Jobe, A.H.: The respiratory system. In Martin, R.J., Fanaroff, A.A., Walsh, M.C. (Eds.): *Fanaroff and Martin's Neonatal-Perinatal Medicine: Diseases of the Fetus and Infant*, 8th ed. Philadelphia, Mosby, 2006, pp. 1069-1078.

53. **(A)** A pathologic condition in the mother or infant should be highly suspected when an infant has apnea in the first 24 hours of life. Sepsis is an example of a pathologic state. Placing infants on the back to sleep has led to a 40% reduction in cases of sudden infant death syndrome. Hypoglycemia can lead to apnea in an infant. Apnea after the first 24 hours of life not associated with another pathologic condition in a preterm infant can be classified as apnea of prematurity.

**References:** Gardner, S.L., Enzman-Hines, M., Dickey, L.A.: Respiratory diseases. In Gardner, S.L., Carter, B.S., Enzman-Hines, M., et al. (Eds.): *Merenstein and Gardner's Handbook of Neonatal Intensive Care*, 7th ed. St. Louis, Mosby, 2011, pp. 581-677.

Gomella, T.L., Cunningham, M.D., Eyal, F.G., and Tuttle, D.: *Neonatology Management, Procedures, On-Call Problems, Diseases, and Drugs*, 6th ed. New York: McGraw-Hill, 2009, pp. 412-413.

54. **(A)** Bronchopulmonary dysplasia is characterized by right ventricular hypertrophy and right axis deviation on EKG, respiratory wheezing, hepatomegaly from heart failure, and cystic lesions on chest radiograph. Respiratory distress syndrome is characterized by radiographic findings of hypoinflation with air bronchograms. Meconium aspiration syndrome is characterized by hyperinflated lungs with coarse patchy infiltrates, increased anteroposterior diameter, and respiratory distress. Pulmonary interstitial emphysema is characterized by radiographic findings of linear lucencies, accompanied by progressive deterioration of blood gas values.

**References:** Askin, D.F.: Respiratory distress. In Verklan, M.T., Walden, M. (Eds.): *Core Curriculum for Neonatal Intensive Care Nursing*, 4th ed. St. Louis, Saunders, 2010, pp. 453-483.

Gomella, T.L., Cunningham, M.D., Eyal, F.G., and Tuttle, D.: *Neonatology Management, Procedures, On-Call Problems, Diseases, and Drugs*, 6th ed. New York: McGraw-Hill, 2009, p. 417.

55. **(B)** The history and clinical findings suggest that this infant has meconium aspiration syndrome (MAS). Hyperinflation occurs due to ball-valve air trapping. Lower inspiratory time will allow adequate exhalation time to prevent air trapping. Infants with MAS require higher respiratory rates than those with respiratory distress syndrome. Because of the resulting atelectasis, higher peak inspiratory pressure is indicated for adequate lung expansion. Lower positive end-expiratory pressure is indicated to prevent air trapping.

**References:** Askin, D.F.: Respiratory distress. In Verklan, M.T., Walden, M. (Eds.): *Core Curriculum for Neonatal Intensive Care Nursing*, 4th ed. St. Louis, Saunders, 2010, pp. 453-483.

Gardner, S.L., Enzman-Hines, M., Dickey, L.A.: Respiratory diseases. In Gardner, S.L., Carter, B.S., Enzman-Hines, M., et al. (Eds.): *Merenstein and Gardner's Handbook of Neonatal Intensive Care*, 7th ed., St. Louis, Mosby, 2011, pp. 581-677.

Gomella, T.L., Cunningham, M.D., Eyal, F.G., and Tuttle, D.: *Neonatology Management, Procedures, On-Call Problems, Diseases, and Drugs*, 6th ed. New York: McGraw-Hill, 2009, pp. 574-578.

56. **(D)** Clinical signs and symptoms of respiratory distress in the newborn include grunting (to keep alveoli open), flaring (to increase air intake), and retractions (reflecting increased work of breathing). Hypotension, although associated with respiratory distress, is a late finding in a term infant. Premature infants frequently have hypotension at or shortly after birth. Central cyanosis is associated with respiratory distress. Acrocyanosis is a normal finding within the first 24 hours of life. Periodic breathing does not occur in the first 2 days of life.

**References:** Brodsky, D., Martin, C.: *Neonatology Review.* Philadelphia, Hanley & Belfus, 2003, p. 72.

Welty, S., Hansen, T., Corbet, A.: Respiratory distress in the preterm infant. In Tausch, H.W., Ballard, R.A., Gleason, C.A. (Eds.): *Avery's Diseases of the Newborn*, 8th ed. Philadelphia, Saunders, 2005, pp. 619, 687-697.

57. **(C)** Preterm infants are expected to lose 10% of their birth weight. This weight loss is the result of excretion of extracellular fluid. If weight loss does not occur, then there is a normal total body sodium level in the presence of extra body water, which causes hyponatremia. Excessive evaporative losses leads to hypernatremia. Increased urine output would result in either normal serum sodium values or hypernatremia. Increased urine output would also result in documented weight loss.

**Reference:** Welty, S., Hansen, T., Corbet, A.: Respiratory distress in the preterm infant. In Tausch, H.W., Ballard, R.A., Gleason, C.A. (Eds.): *Avery's Diseases of the Newborn*, 8th ed. Philadelphia, Saunders, 2005, pp. 687-697.

58. **(D)** Placing a transparent plastic covering over an infant on an open warmer will help to maintain a neutral thermal environment and thereby decrease oxygen consumption. The preferable way to obtain laboratory specimens in an infant with respiratory distress syndrome is via central umbilical arterial or venous access. If central access is unattainable, laboratory draws should be clustered. After 3 to 5 days of life, normal fluid intake is 150 to 175 ml/kg/day. Fluid restriction has been found to decrease the incidence of

patent ductus arteriosus, necrotizing enterocolitis, and death. Suctioning has been shown to increase oxygen consumption and raise arterial blood pressure, thus placing the infant at risk for intraventricular hemorrhage. Suctioning is performed when indicated based on physical assessment; it is not scheduled.

**Reference:** Welty, S., Hansen, T., Corbet, A.: Respiratory distress in the preterm infant. In Tausch, H.W., Ballard, R.A., Gleason, C.A. (Eds.): *Avery's Diseases of the Newborn*, 8th ed. Philadelphia, Saunders, 2005, pp. 693-694.

59. **(A)** Nitric oxide in the circulation reacts with the iron-containing molecules in hemoglobin. Nitric oxide reduces oxyhemoglobin, producing methemoglobin. Inhaled nitric oxide (iNO) has a half-life of 3 to 5 seconds. The exact dosage of iNO has not been established. However, research supports initiation at 20 ppm with specific decreases over the next few days. Weaning from iNO should be regulated in a stepwise fashion. Abrupt cessation can result in rebound elevated pulmonary vascular resistance.

**References:** Askin, D.F.: Respiratory distress. In Verklan, M.T., Walden, M. (Eds.): *Core Curriculum for Neonatal Intensive Care Nursing*, 4th ed. St. Louis, Saunders, 2010, pp. 453-483.

Hamon, I., Gauthier-Moulinier, H., Grelet-Dessioux, E., et al. (2010): Methaemoglobinaemia risk factors with inhaled nitric oxide therapy in newborn infants. *Acta Paediatrics* 99(10), 1467-1473.

60. **(C)** Prophylactic administration of surfactant occurs soon after birth, following the initial resuscitation and endotracheal intubation. Rescue therapy is administered to infants with progressive oxygen requirements in the first day of life and may consist of multiple doses. Assisted ventilation is any pulmonary support that fosters alveolar gas exchange and normal pulmonary function. It ranges from oxygen supplementation to mechanical ventilation. Medications used in resuscitative efforts are termed *resuscitation drugs.* These chemical agents increase the rate and strength of cardiac contractions and cause peripheral vasoconstriction, channeling circulatory volume centrally.

**References:** Askin, D.F.: Respiratory distress. In Verklan, M.T., Walden, M. (Eds.): *Core Curriculum for Neonatal Intensive Care Nursing*, 4th ed. St. Louis, Saunders, 2010, pp. 453-483.

Askin, D.F., Diehl-Jones, W.: Assisted ventilation. In Verklan, M.T., Walden, M. (Eds.): *Core Curriculum for Neonatal Intensive Care Nursing*, 4th ed. St. Louis, Saunders, 2010, pp. 494-520.

Niermeyer, S., Clarke, S.B.: Delivery room care. In Gardner, S.L., Carter, B.S., Enzman-Hines, M., et al. (Eds.): *Merenstein and Gardner's Handbook of Neonatal Intensive Care*, 7th ed. St. Louis, Mosby, 2011, pp. 52-77.

61. **(C)** Indomethacin inhibits platelet aggregation. Platelet count must be normal prior to administration of indomethacin to prevent unintended blood loss. The minimum acceptable platelet count is 60,000/mm³. A serum creatinine level of 2.0 mg/dl is a contraindication to the administration of indomethacin because it indicates impaired renal function. Indomethacin has vasoconstrictive effects on the renal artery. Decreased renal blood flow due to indomethacin administration would further compromise renal function. A low urine output can be symptomatic of

decreased renal function. Indomethacin administration is contraindicated in a patient with urine output of less than 0.6 ml/kg/hour, because its administration would further compromise renal function. Radiographic evidence of necrotizing enterocolitis is a contraindication to indomethacin administration because indomethacin impairs blood flow to the mesentery and intestines.

**Reference:** Lucus, V.W., Ginsberg, H.G.: Cardiovascular aspects. In Goldsmith, J.P., Karotin, E.K. (Eds.): *Assisted Ventilation of the Neonate,* 4th ed. Philadelphia, Saunders, 2003, p. 406.

62. **(B)** Laryngomalacia is the leading cause of stridor in the infant. An infant with choanal atresia will have varying degrees of cyanosis at rest and with sucking based on the severity of the lesion. Symptoms improve with crying. Clinically, the infant with vocal cord paralysis has a weak cry, but may develop stridor when stressed. Vocal cord paralysis is second to laryngomalacia as the cause of stridor in the infant. Congenital subglottic stenosis is characterized by crouplike episodes.

**Reference:** Miller, M.J., Fanaroff, A.A., Martin, R.J.: Respiratory disorders in the preterm and term infants. In Martin, R.J., Fanaroff, A.A., Walsh, M.C. (Eds.): *Fanaroff and Martin's Neonatal-Perinatal Medicine: Diseases of the Fetus and Infant,* 8th ed. Philadelphia, Mosby, 2006, pp. 1147-1154.

63. **(D)** Secondary apnea is a result of prolonged asphyxia. It is marked by gasping respirations and a decrease in blood pressure and heart rate that is not responsive to stimulation and/or oxygen supplementation. Idiopathic apnea is also known as *apnea of prematurity.* This particular infant had a gestational age of 38 weeks at birth. In obstructive apnea, the infant has spontaneous respiratory effort, but airflow is absent. Primary apnea is the absence of respirations after a period of rapid respiratory effort that is associated with asphyxia during the delivery process. Oxygen supplementation and/or stimulation will help to initiate spontaneous respirations.

**Reference:** Goodwin, M.: Apnea. In Verklan, M.T., Walden, M. (Eds.): *Core Curriculum for Neonatal Intensive Care Nursing,* 4th ed. St. Louis, Saunders, 2010, pp. 484- 493.

64. **(D)** The immediate initial step after determining the absence of respirations (as has been done in this scenario) is to provide gentle tactile stimulation. This is all the infant may require to resume spontaneous respirations. If apnea persists despite tactile stimulation, supplemental oxygen can be administered. Although assessing breath sounds is important, the initiation of respirations must take precedence. Physical assessment of breath sounds can be completed after spontaneous respirations have been achieved. If oxygen supplementation and tactile stimulation have not produced spontaneous respirations, positive pressure ventilation is indicated.

**Reference:** Gardner, S.L., Enzman-Hines, M., Dickey, L.A.: Respiratory diseases. In Gardner, S.L., Carter, B.S., Enzman-Hines, M., et al. (Eds.): *Merenstein and Gardner's Handbook of Neonatal Intensive Care,* 7th ed. St. Louis, Mosby, 2011, pp. 581-677.

65. **(B)** Doxapram is a respiratory stimulant used to treat apnea that is refractory to methylxanthine therapy. Caffeine, theophylline, and aminophylline are methylxanthines used to treat apnea.

**Reference:** Lehne, R.A.: *Pharmacology for Nursing Care,* 7th ed. St. Louis, Saunders, 2010, pp. 391-402.

66. **(C)** Maintaining the environmental temperature in a neutral thermal range can help to alleviate temperature stress, which can lead to iatrogenic apnea. Apnea can be induced by a multitude of causes, including iatrogenic factors. A vagal response secondary to procedures such as suctioning stimulates apnea. Sudden environmental changes, such as the change from a warm incubator to a cold scale, also can induce apnea. Tapping on the outside of the incubator is an example of a noxious stimulus that can lead to apnea.

**Reference:** Gardner, S.L., Enzman-Hines, M., Dickey, L.A.: Respiratory diseases. In Gardner, S.L., Carter, B.S., Enzman-Hines, M., et al. (Eds.): *Merenstein and Gardner's Handbook of Neonatal Intensive Care,* 7th ed. St. Louis, Mosby, 2011, pp. 581-677.

67. **(D)** Caffeine has a longer half-life than theophylline, which results in smaller changes in plasma concentration. Caffeine is formulated for oral or parenteral administration. It is administered once a day to neonates. Caffeine is not known to be excreted more rapidly by the kidneys.

**Reference:** Goodwin, M.: Apnea. In Verklan, M.T., Walden, M. (Eds.): *Core Curriculum for Neonatal Intensive Care Nursing,* 4th ed. St. Louis, Saunders, 2010, pp. 484- 493.

68. **(C)** Continuous positive airway pressure (CPAP) ventilation is therapeutic in the treatment of an infant with laryngomalacia because it prevents collapse of poorly formed cartilage structures. CPAP ventilation is not used in an infant with a cleft palate because of the inability to secure a seal that allows delivery of airway pressure. Nasal CPAP will not be effective in an infant with choanal atresia because of blockage of the posterior nares. CPAP ventilation is contraindicated in an infant with tracheoesophageal fistula because distending pressure would cause tracheal air to take the path of least resistance and enter the distal esophagus; this would cause gastric distention and possible rupture.

**Reference:** Wiswell, T.E., Srinivasan, P.: Continuous positive airway pressure. In Goldsmith, J.P., Karotkin, E.K. (Eds.): *Assisted Ventilation of the Neonate,* 4th ed. Philadelphia, Saunders, 2003, pp. 141-143.

69. **(D)** The nasogastric tube should receive the least consideration. Infants are obligate nose breathers, and maximum continuous positive airway pressure (CPAP) needs to be maintained. Gastric overdistention can be managed by using a larger-bore orogastric tube. $Paco_2$ retention at increased levels of CPAP has been documented due to alveolar overdistention. Monitoring of $Paco_2$ levels is thus warranted. Decreased glomerular filtration rate has been documented in infants undergoing CPAP ventilation. Urine output should be monitored carefully. Vital signs and pulse oximetry readings must be monitored to determine oxygen saturation and detect complications early.

**Reference:** Wiswell, T.E., Srinivasan, P.: Continuous positive airway pressure. In Goldsmith, J.P., Karotkin, E.K. (Eds.): *Assisted Ventilation of the Neonate,* 4th ed. Philadelphia, Saunders, 2003, pp. 141-143.

70. **(D)** Full-term infants with a small congenital diaphragmatic hernia without liver herniation have a good prognosis and therefore meet the criteria for management using extracorporeal membrane oxygenation (ECMO). Infants with severe lung hypoplasia are excluded from treatment with ECMO because the disease is irreversible. The gestational age requirement for ECMO is 34 weeks or longer. Normal findings on cranial ultrasonography are required for treatment with ECMO. Some centers have been able to manage infants with bilateral grade I intracranial hemorrhage with lower dosages of heparin; however, infants with bilateral grade IV intracranial hemorrhages are excluded from ECMO at all centers.

**Reference:** Stork, E.K.: Therapy for cardiorespiratory failure. In Martin, R.J., Fanaroff, A.A., Walsh, M.C. (Eds.): *Fanaroff and Martin's Neonatal-Perinatal Medicine: Diseases of the Fetus and Infant,* 8th ed. Philadelphia, Mosby, 2006, pp. 1170-1172.

71. **(A)** In vascular ring, the aortic arch and anomalous vessels form a partial or complete ring around either the trachea, the esophagus, or both, resulting in compression of those structures. They occur outside the pulmonary system. Choanal atresia is an anatomic blockage of the posterior nares by bone or tissue resulting in airway obstruction in the nose. Bronchomalacia is an airway obstruction caused by a deficiency of cartilage in the trachea or bronchi. Pierre Robin sequence is characterized by micrognathia with glossoptosis, resulting in upper airway obstruction.

**Reference:** Miller, M.J., Fanaroff, A.A., Martin, R.J.: Respiratory disorders in preterm and term Infants. In Martin, R.J., Fanaroff, A.A., Walsh, M.C. (Eds.): *Fanaroff and Martin's Neonatal-Perinatal Medicine: Diseases of the Fetus and Infant,* 8th ed. Philadelphia, Mosby, 2006, p. 1143.

72. **(A)** The oxygen index (OI) is a measure used to assess refractory hypoxemia. One of the criteria for initiating extracorporeal membrane oxygenation (ECMO) treatment is an OI of 35 to 60 for 0.5 to 6 hours. A $Pao_2$ of 40 for 2 hours is an inclusion criterion for ECMO. A pH that is lower than 7.25 for more than 2 hours or is accompanied by hypotension is an inclusion criterion. ECMO has been considered as a treatment of last resort for infants with life-threatening cardiorespiratory disease that is unresponsive to maximum medical management. ECMO is extremely expensive and invasive. Alternative therapies, such as inhaled nitric oxide, are very effective in treating persistent pulmonary hypertension by vasodilating the pulmonary vasculature and enhancing pulmonary blood flow and thus gas exchange at the alveolar level.

**Reference:** Stork, E.K.: Therapy for cardiorespiratory failure. In Martin, R.J., Fanaroff, A.A., Walsh, M.C. (Eds.): *Fanaroff and Martin's Neonatal-Perinatal Medicine: Diseases of the Fetus and Infant,* 8th ed. Philadelphia, Mosby, 2006, pp. 1170-1174.

73. **(C)** Bronchopulmonary dysplasia (BPD) is more common in infants who have undergone mechanical ventilation. This is due to the associated barotrauma and oxygen toxicity. The incidence of BPD is inversely proportional to gestational age. Excessive fluid administration places an infant at high risk for BPD. Excessive fluid contributes to patent ductus arteriosus with left-to-right shunt, pulmonary edema, and impaired alveolar gas exchange. Mechanical ventilation and oxygen supplementation provided to overcome impaired alveolar gas exchange result in damage to the lung and the development of BPD. Twenty-one percent oxygen is room air and would not cause oxygen toxicity.

**Reference:** Bancalari, E.H.: Bronchopulmonary dysplasia and neonatal chronic lung disease. In Martin, R.J., Fanaroff, A.A., Walsh, M.C. (Eds.): *Fanaroff and Martin's Neonatal-Perinatal Medicine: Diseases of the Fetus and Infant,* 8th ed. Philadelphia, Mosby, 2006, pp. 1155-1158.

74. **(A)** Lymphatic drainage is impaired in infants with bronchopulmonary dysplasia (BPD), which predisposes them to pulmonary edema. Infants with BPD have increased capillary permeability and decreased oncotic pressure, both of which also increase the risk of pulmonary edema. Pulmonary vascular resistance is increased in infants with BPD.

**Reference:** Bancalari, E.H.: Bronchopulmonary dysplasia and neonatal chronic lung disease. In Martin, R.J., Fanaroff, A.A., Walsh, M.C. (Eds.): *Fanaroff and Martin's Neonatal-Perinatal Medicine: Diseases of the Fetus and Infant,* 8th ed. Philadelphia, Mosby, 2006, pp. 1160-1161.

75. **(A)** Furosemide can damage the stria vascularis, part of the cochlear duct. Hearing impairment may be temporary or permanent. Furosemide blocks tubular reabsorption of potassium through a direct interaction with transport systems located in the luminal surface of the renal tubule, thereby leading to hypokalemia. The reabsorption of chloride in the ascending loop of Henle is blocked by furosemide, which leads to hypochloremia. Metabolic alkalosis is associated with furosemide use. Loss of fluid volume creates a relative elevated bicarbonate level.

**References:** Baldwin, K.A., Budzinski, C.E., Shapiro, C.J.: Acute sensorineural hearing loss: Furosemide ototoxicity revisited. *Hospital Pharmacy,* 43(12)-982-988, 2008.

Bancalari, E.H.: Bronchopulmonary dysplasia and neonatal chronic lung disease. In Martin, R.J., Fanaroff, A.A., Walsh, M.C. (Eds.): *Fanaroff and Martin's Neonatal-Perinatal Medicine: Diseases of the Fetus and Infant,* 8th ed. Philadelphia, Mosby, 2006, pp. 1164-1165.

76. **(D)** Infants with bronchopulmonary dysplasia (BPD) have a caloric requirement of 150 to 180 kcal/kg/day to compensate for the increased metabolic demands of respiratory effort and the fluid restriction that is required. Growth failure is common if fewer calories are provided.

**References:** Askin, D.F.: Respiratory distress. In Verklan, M.T., Walden, M. (Eds.): *Core Curriculum for Neonatal Intensive Care Nursing,* 4th ed. St. Louis, Saunders, 2010, pp. 453-483.

Halbardier, B.H.: Fluid and electrolyte management. In Verklan, M.T., Walden, M. (Eds.): *Core Curriculum for Neonatal Intensive Care Nursing,* 4th ed. St. Louis, Saunders, 2010, pp. 156-171.

77. **(C)** An increased incidence of neurodevelopmental dysfunction, including cerebral palsy, has been widely associated with dexamethasone use. Dexamethasone use has not been associated with an increased incidence of pulmonary air leak, necrotizing enterocolitis, or severe retinopathy of prematurity.

**Reference:** Askin, D.F., Diehl-Jones, W.: Assisted ventilation. In Verklan, M.T., Walden, M. (Eds.): *Core Curriculum for Neonatal Intensive Care Nursing*, 4th ed. St. Louis, Saunders, 2010, pp. 494-520.

78. **(A)** Short inspiratory times allow for longer expiratory times. In bronchopulmonary dysplasia (BPD), expiration is prolonged. Lung compliance decreases at higher inspiratory rates in infants with BPD. Therefore, a high rate such as 50 breaths/minute would not be tolerated. Oxygen is a potent vasodilator. Higher levels of oxygen are often required in infants with BPD to overcome pulmonary vascular resistance. A peak end-expiratory pressure (PEEP) of 5 to 8 cm $H_2O$ is often required in infants who have severe BPD with subsequent bronchomalacia. The higher PEEP helps to improve alveolar ventilation.

**Reference:** Bancalari, E.H.: Bronchopulmonary dysplasia and neonatal chronic lung disease. In Martin, R.J., Fanaroff, A.A., Walsh, M.C. (Eds.): *Fanaroff and Martin's Neonatal-Perinatal Medicine: Diseases of the Fetus and Infant*, 8th ed. Philadelphia, Mosby, 2006, pp. 1164-1165.

79. **(D)** When acid-base status is being assessed, the pH and the two acid-base determinants ($Paco_2$ and $HCO_3$) are examined. In this case, the blood gas values reflect partial compensation in which both acid-base components remain abnormal in opposite directions as the pH approaches a normal value. A near-normal pH and base excess of +2 do not support metabolic acidosis. The $Paco_2$ of 67 indicates respiratory acidosis, not alkalosis.

**Reference:** Wood, A.M., Jones, M.D. Jr.: Acid-base homeostasis and oxygenation. In Gardner, S.L., Carter, B.S., Enzman-Hines, M., et al. (Eds.): *Merenstein and Gardner's Handbook of Neonatal Intensive Care*, 7th ed. St. Louis, Mosby, 2011, pp. 153-163.

80. **(A)** Corticosteroids have been shown to decrease the permeability of the pulmonary vasculature, which minimizes pulmonary edema. Dexamethasone has also been shown to increase diuresis. A urine output of 5 ml/kg/hr is indicative of increased diuresis. Corticosteroid use has been shown to promote rapid ventilatory weaning, not increase the need for ventilator support. Corticosteroids improve lung compliance, dilate airways, and enhance the synthesis of surfactant. The mean arterial pressure for this patient should be around that for the corrected gestational age, which is 56 mm Hg. A common side effect of dexamethasone is hypertension. Therefore, the nurse should expect the blood pressure to be higher than 56 mm Hg. Biventricular hypertrophy, not atrophy, has been associated with dexamethasone use.

**Reference:** Spratto, G.R., Woods, A.L. *2010 Edition Delmar Nurse's Drug Handbook.* Clifton Park, NY, Delmar Cengage Learning, 2010, pp. 459-462.

81. **(C)** Albuterol is a bronchodilator—specifically, a $\beta_2$-adrenergic agent—that within minutes effectively increases compliance and decreases resistance. Caffeine is a methylxanthine used to maintain decreased airway resistance. Furosemide is a loop diuretic used to treat pulmonary edema in infants with bronchopulmonary dysplasia. It does not relieve bronchospasm. Theophylline is a methylxanthine that is used in patients with bronchopulmonary dysplasia to decrease airway resistance. It is not used as a first-line treatment for an acute bronchospastic episode due to its relatively slow onset of action.

**References:** Gardner, S.L., Enzman-Hines, M., Dickey, L.A.: Respiratory diseases. In Gardner, S.L., Carter, B.S., Enzman-Hines, M., et al. (Eds.): *Merenstein and Gardner's Handbook of Neonatal Intensive Care*, 7th ed. St. Louis, Mosby, 2011, pp. 581-677.

Spratto, G.R., Woods, A.L. *2010 Edition Delmar Nurse's Drug Handbook.* Clifton Park, NY, Delmar Cengage Learning, 2010, pp. 459-462.

82. **(D)** Pink-tinged secretions are indicative of a pulmonary hemorrhage with minimal bleeding. Treatment of a pulmonary hemorrhage in an intubated patient is to increase the peak end-expiratory pressure to tamponade the bleeding at the site. Suctioning should be limited in infants with pulmonary hemorrhage. A platelet transfusion is not indicated. A red blood cell transfusion is not warranted.

**Reference:** Lewis, F.C., Reynolds, M.R., Arensman, R.M.: Extracorporeal membrane oxygenation. In Goldsmith, J.P., Karotkin, E.K. (Eds.): *Assisted Ventilation of the Neonate*, 4th ed. Philadelphia, Saunders, 2003, p. 270.

83. **(D)** Patient selection criteria for extracorporeal membrane oxygenation (ECMO) include gestational age of longer than 34 weeks, birth weight of more than 2 kg, presence of grade II or less intracranial hemorrhage, absence of complex congenital heart disease or lethal malformations, and reversible lung disease. Persistent pulmonary hypertension of the newborn (PPHN) is an acute and reversible cardiorespiratory disease. ECMO is warranted if standard therapies fail to reverse PPHN. Pulmonary hypoplasia is an irreversible condition. Use of ECMO would not change the outcome. ECMO would not be indicated in infants with bronchopulmonary dysplasia. The initial pulmonary damage is irreversible, and maintaining the patient on ECMO until new lung growth occurs is not feasible. Transient tachypnea of the newborn is a mild, self-limiting disease that does not warrant invasive ECMO therapy.

**References:** Bancalari, E.H.: Bronchopulmonary dysplasia and neonatal chronic lung disease. In Martin, R.J., Fanaroff, A.A., Walsh, M.C. (Eds.): *Fanaroff and Martin's Neonatal-Perinatal Medicine: Diseases of the Fetus and Infant*, 8th ed. Philadelphia, Mosby, 2006, pp. 1155-1194.

Lund, C.H.: Extracorporeal membrane oxygenation. In Verklan, M.T., Walden, M. (Eds.): *Core Curriculum for Neonatal Intensive Care Nursing*, 4th ed. St. Louis, Saunders, 2010, pp. 521-533.

84. **(B)** In congenital lobar emphysema (CLE), air is trapped in one or more lung lobes at birth due to a

defect in bronchial cartilage; obstructive emphysema occurs because air enters but cannot leave the lobe due to collapse of the poorly structured airway. CLE is generally limited to the upper lobes and is the most common cystic lung defect. In bronchopulmonary dysplasia, the chest radiograph shows a bubbly appearance with hyperaeration more pronounced at the lung bases. In congenital diaphragmatic hernia, the intestine herniates into the thoracic cavity. As air enters the gastrointestinal tract and proceeds to the intestine, intraluminal bowel gas is visible in the chest on the radiograph. Cystic adenomatoid malformation appears on the chest radiograph as a single or multiple air-filled cysts. It is a primary pulmonary development disorder of terminal bronchiole canalization failure.

**References:** Askin, D.F.: Respiratory distress. In Verklan, M.T., Walden, M. (Eds.): *Core Curriculum for Neonatal Intensive Care Nursing,* 4th ed. St. Louis, Saunders, 2010, pp. 453-483.

Lane, L.: Radiologic evaluation. In Verklan, M.T., Walden, M. (Eds.): *Core Curriculum for Neonatal Intensive Care Nursing,* 4th ed. St. Louis, Saunders, 2010, pp. 270-298.

85. **(D)** In esophageal atresia with tracheoesophageal fistula, the esophagus ends in a blind pouch in 85% of cases. Attempts to feed and the accumulation of oropharyngeal secretions results in respiratory distress and the need for suctioning. Polyhydramnios suggests a condition in which the fetus does not swallow amniotic fluid normally, as with an upper gastrointestinal obstruction. Choanal atresia is a membranous or bony obstruction of one or both nares. Presentation is characterized by noisy breathing, cyanosis, and apnea if the mouth is closed. A crying infant will be pink. Pulmonary hypoplasia results from lung compression due to congenital anomalies or oligohydramnios. The infant usually shows severe respiratory distress, not intermittent distress, and acid-base disturbances. Mortality rate is high. Infants with congenital heart disease may show cyanosis. Most infants with congenital heart disease do not have respiratory distress.

**References:** Askin, D.F.: Respiratory distress. In Verklan, M.T., Walden, M. (Eds.): *Core Curriculum for Neonatal Intensive Care Nursing,* 4th ed. St. Louis, Saunders, 2010, pp. 453-483.

Gardner, S.L., Hernandez, J.A.: Initial nursery care. In Gardner, S.L., Carter, B.S., Enzman-Hines, M., et al. (Eds.): *Merenstein and Gardner's Handbook of Neonatal Intensive Care,* 7th ed. St. Louis, Mosby, 2011, pp. 78-112.

Kenney, P.M., Hoover, D., Williams, L.C., et al.: Cardiovascular diseases and surgical interventions. In Gardner, S.L., Carter, B.S., Enzman-Hines, M., et al. (Eds.): *Merenstein and Gardner's Handbook of Neonatal Intensive Care,* 7th ed. St. Louis, Mosby, 2011, pp. 678-716.

Lovvorn, H.N. III, Gleen, J.B., Pacetti, A.S., et al.: Neonatal surgery. In Gardner, S.L., Carter, B.S., Enzman-Hines, M., et al. (Eds.): *Merenstein and Gardner's Handbook of Neonatal Intensive Care,* 7th ed. St. Louis, Mosby, 2011, pp. 812-847.

86. **(C)** The oxygen-hemoglobin dissociation curve reflects oxygen tension—the partial pressure of oxygen bound to hemoglobin. Cyanosis is a late sign of respiratory insufficiency and indicates the presence of 3 to 5 g of desaturated hemoglobin. Cyanosis may not be present in severe anemic states. A shift to the right on the hemoglobin-oxygen dissociation curve indicates decreased affinity of hemoglobin for oxygen. Hemoglobin's affinity for oxygen is primarily affected by the type of hemoglobin (fetal vs. adult), temperature, pH, $Paco_2$, and level of 2,3-diphosphoglycerate.

**Reference:** Carlo, W.A., DiFiore J.M.: Assessment of pulmonary function. In Martin, R.J., Fanaroff, A.A., Walsh, M.C. (Eds.): *Fanaroff and Martin's Neonatal-Perinatal Medicine: Diseases of the Fetus and Infant,* 8th ed. Philadelphia, Mosby, 2006, pp. 1087-1097.

87. **(D)** Obtaining accurate pulse oximetry readings depends on adequate perfusion of the monitoring site, probe position, and the ability of the equipment to detect arterial pulsations. Gestational age does not affect the accuracy of saturation readings. Pulse oximetry is the most common noninvasive method of measuring hemoglobin saturation in infants, including preterm infants. The use of vasodilating drugs, particularly those that dilate the peripheral vasculature, enhances pulse oximetry accuracy, because adequate perfusion of the probe site is vital to the use of this equipment. A low oxygen saturation value may be present with congenital heart anomalies. The low value is the result of poor alveolar gas exchange or a cardiac defect that results in mixing of oxygenated and deoxygenated blood. The low value is an accurate reflection of hemoglobin saturation.

**Reference:** Bradshaw, W.T., Tanaka, D.T.: Physiologic monitoring. In Gardner, S.L., Carter, B.S., Enzman-Hines, M., et al. (Eds.): *Merenstein and Gardner's Handbook of Neonatal Intensive Care,* 7th ed. St. Louis, Mosby, 2011, pp. 134-152.

88. **(C)** The flow rate through an oxygen hood must be sufficient to prevent the retention of carbon dioxide. This requires a flow meter and oxygen blender so that adequate flow is provided and the prescribed oxygen concentration is delivered. Oxygen administration requires some form of continuous monitoring. A nasal cannula is used to administer oxygen to an infant who is developing social and motor skills. Exact oxygen concentration is unknown when a nasal cannula is used because of entrainment of room air when the mouth is open. Nasal continuous positive airway pressure is not warranted if the infant demonstrates sufficient ventilation to maintain a normal $Paco_2$ value.

**Reference:** Gardner, S.L., Enzman-Hines, M., Dickey, L.A.: Respiratory diseases. In Gardner, S.L., Carter, B.S., Enzman-Hines, M., et al. (Eds.): *Merenstein and Gardner's Handbook of Neonatal Intensive Care,* 7th ed. St. Louis, Mosby, 2011, pp. 581-677.

89. **(D)** Research has demonstrated that the use of heliox reduces the length of time mechanical ventilation is required in infants with obstructive pulmonary diseases such as reactive airway, bronchiolitis secondary to respiratory syncytial virus infection, and pulmonary interstitial emphysema. A nontension pneumothorax may be treated by oxygen supplementation at an inspired oxygen fraction ($Fio_2$) of 1.0 to increase sixfold the rate of absorption of the pneumothorax by means of the nitrogen washout method. In

this method oxygen replaces nitrogen in the extrapulmonary space, which results in reduction or resolution of the pneumothorax. Intracranial hemorrhage varies from mild to severe and is not associated with the use of heliox. Necrotizing enterocolitis is an inflammatory intestinal process. Heliox is used in the treatment of pulmonary disease.

**References:** Gardner, S.L., Enzman-Hines, M., Dickey, L.A.: Respiratory diseases. In Gardner, S.L., Carter, B.S., Enzman-Hines, M., et al. (Eds.): *Merenstein and Gardner's Handbook of Neonatal Intensive Care*, 7th ed. St. Louis, Mosby, 2011, pp. 581-677.

Migliori, C., Gancia, P., Garzoli, E., et al.: The effects of helium/oxygen mixture (heliox) before and after extubation in long-term mechanically ventilated very low birth weight infants. *Pediatrics*, 123:1524-1528, 2009.

90. **(B)** Infants with Pierre Robin sequence, which is characterized by micrognathia and glossoptosis, are at increased risk of posterior airway obstruction resulting in obstructive apnea. Cor pulmonale is also known as *right ventricular failure*. It occurs with right-sided outflow tract obstruction and prolonged pulmonary vasoconstriction and remodeling as seen in bronchopulmonary dysplasia. Subglottic stenosis is a complication of long-term endotracheal intubation. Reactive airway disease is a pulmonary response to an antigen or substance not normally present in the tracheobronchial tree. Aspiration of formula or gastric contents is a common precipitating event.

**References:** Heiss-Harria, G.M., Bailey, T.: Common invasive procedures. In Verklan, M.T., Walden, W. (Eds.): *Core Curriculum for Neonatal Intensive Care Nursing*, 4th ed. St. Louis, Saunders, 2010, pp. 299-332.

Miller, M.J., Fanaroff, A.A., Martin, R.J.: Respiratory disorders in preterm and term Infants. In Martin, R.J., Fanaroff, A.A., Walsh, M.C. (Eds.): *Fanaroff and Martin's Neonatal-Perinatal Medicine: Diseases of the Fetus and Infant*, 8th ed. Philadelphia, Mosby, 2006, p. 1143.

## CHAPTER 16: GASTROINTESTINAL DISORDERS

1. **(D)** Neonates with unrepaired esophageal atresia and tracheoesophageal fistula are at risk for aspiration of pooled secretions in the proximal pouch. An immediate intervention in these infants should be placing a sump tube (Replogle) into the proximal pouch and raising the head of the bed to more than 30 degrees. Enteral feeds should not be initiated due to risk of aspiration and impending surgery. Although antibiotics will most likely be indicated, maintaining a safe airway is the immediate priority for this neonate. Positive pressure ventilation should be avoided if possible because of the risk of abdominal distention due to the flow of air from the trachea into the esophagus and remaining gastrointestinal tract.

**References:** Bradshaw, W.: Gastrointestinal disorders. In Verklan, M., Walden, M. (Eds.): *Core Curriculum for Neonatal Intensive Care Nursing*, 4th ed. St. Louis, Saunders, 2010, p. 601.

Hansen, A.R., Lillehei, C.: Respiratory disorders. Part 1: Esophageal atresia and tracheoesophageal fistula. In Hansen, A.R., Puder, M. (Eds.): *Manual of Neonatal Surgical Intensive Care*, 2nd ed. Shelton, Conn., B.C. Decker/People's Medical Publishing House, 2009, pp. 159-167.

2. **(B)** Associated anomalies are seen in more that half of neonates with esophageal atresia and tracheoesophageal fistula (EA/TEF). The most common are cardiac defects, which occur in approximately 20% to 37% of these neonates. Another common defect is VACTERL association (*v*ertebral, *a*nal, *c*ardiac, *tra*cheal, *e*sophageal, *r*enal, and *l*imb), which is seen in 5% to 10% of neonates with EA/TEF. Omphalocele, cardiomegaly, and macroglossia are associated with Beckwith-Wiedemann syndrome. Short stature, micrognathia, hearing loss, and low-set ears are associated findings in infants with Cornelia de Lange syndrome. Cardiac defects, hypoplasia of the thymus, hypocalcemia, and microcephaly are associated with DiGeorge syndrome.

**References:** Bradshaw, W.: Gastrointestinal disorders. In Verklan, M., Walden, M. (Eds.): *Core Curriculum for Neonatal Intensive Care Nursing*, 4th ed. St. Louis, Saunders, 2010, p. 600.

Hansen, A.R., Lillehei, C.: Respiratory disorders. Part 1: Esophageal atresia and tracheoesophageal fistula. In Hansen, A.R., Puder, M. (Eds.): *Manual of Neonatal Surgical Intensive Care*, 2nd ed. Shelton, Conn., B.C. Decker/People's Medical Publishing House, 2009, pp. 159-167.

3. **(B)** Primary repair of esophageal atresia and tracheoesophageal fistula (EA/TEF) includes a ligation of the TEF and anastomosis of the proximal and distal segments of the esophagus. Complications of this surgery include leakage at the anastomosis site, gastrointestinal reflux, tracheomalacia due to compression of the proximal trachea by the distended esophagus during fetal development, and anastomotic stricture. Short bowel syndrome, intestinal dysfunction, and ileus are postoperative problems associated with complicated jejunal or ileal atresia repair. Renal dysfunction and urosepsis are not complications associated with primary repair of EA/TEF. Complications due to increased intraabdominal pressures are more often seen after repair of abdominal wall defects such as gastroschisis and omphalocele than after EA/TEF repair.

**References:** Bradshaw, W.: Gastrointestinal disorders. In Verklan, M., Walden, M. (Eds.): *Core Curriculum for Neonatal Intensive Care Nursing*, 4th ed. St. Louis, Saunders, 2010, p. 602.

Hansen, A.R., Lillehei, C.: Respiratory disorders. Part 1: Esophageal atresia and tracheoesophageal fistula. In Hansen, A.R., Puder, M. (Eds.): *Manual of Neonatal Surgical Intensive Care*, 2nd ed. Shelton, Conn., B.C. Decker/People's Medical Publishing House, 2009, pp. 159-167.

4. **(D)** The priority for this infant is to stabilize the abdomen by gastric decompression, to hold enteral feedings to allow the gastrointestinal system to rest, and to ensure that the infant is hydrated. An upper gastrointestinal tract contrast study is often obtained after initial assessment and stabilization in infants who do not require emergent surgical intervention. Obtaining further abdominal radiographs and measuring abdominal girth may be required; however, they are not the most immediate actions necessary for an infant with a bowel obstruction. Placement of a urinary catheter may be required; however, is not the most immediate action necessary for an infant with a bowel obstruction.

**References:** Pursley, D., Hansen, A.R., Puder, M.: Gastrointestinal disorders. Part 4: Obstructions. In Hansen, A.R., Puder, M. (Eds.): *Manual of Neonatal Surgical Intensive Care,* 2nd ed. Shelton, Conn., B.C. Decker/People's Medical Publishing House, 2009, pp. 159-167.

Silva, N.T., Young, J.A., Wales, P.W.: Understanding neonatal bowel obstructions: Building knowledge to advance practice. *Neonatal Network,* 25(5):303-318, 2006.

5. **(C)** Midgut volvulus is one of the more serious neonatal emergencies. A delay in diagnosis and treatment can result in significant bowel loss and septic shock. Malrotation is a congenital abnormality that results from abnormal intestinal rotation and fixation during the embryonic period. As a result, the mesentery is positioned incorrectly in the abdomen, which places it at risk of twisting and occlusion (volvulus). This can lead to a disruption of the blood supply and intestinal infarction. Pneumonia is a postoperative complication and is not the reason that midgut volvulus is a surgical emergency. Fluid and electrolyte imbalance is a common occurrence but does not precipitate a surgical emergency. Tissue injury from a necrotic gut or surgery can precipitate disseminated intravascular coagulation (DIC), but DIC is not the first priority in a patient with midgut volvulus.

**References:** Little, D.C., Smith, S.D.: Malrotation. In Holcomb, G.W., Murphy, J.P. (Eds.): *Ashcraft's Pediatric Surgery,* 5th ed. Philadelphia, Saunders, 2010, pp. 416-424.

Pursley, D., Hansen, A.R., Puder, M.: Gastrointestinal disorders. Part 4: Obstructions. In Hansen, A.R., Puder, M. (Eds.): *Manual of Neonatal Surgical Intensive Care,* 2nd ed. Shelton, Conn., B.C. Decker/People's Medical Publishing House, 2009, pp. 159-167.

6. **(A)** The infant is showing signs of significant bowel compromise resulting in shock and possible intestinal ischemia and infarction. Blood transfusion and dopamine therapy may be required for this infant; however, the priority is surgical repair and volume resuscitation. Because there are signs of significant bowel compromise, surgical repair is required emergently; delaying surgery could result in irreversible bowel injury and death.

**References:** Little, D.C., Smith, S.D.: Malrotation. In Holcomb, G.W., Murphy, J.P. (Eds.): *Ashcraft's Pediatric Surgery,* 5th ed. Philadelphia, Saunders, 2010, pp. 416-424.

Pursley, D., Hansen, A.R., Puder, M.: Gastrointestinal disorders. Part 4: Obstructions. In Hansen, A.R., Puder, M. (Eds.): *Manual of Neonatal Surgical Intensive Care,* 2nd ed. Shelton, Conn., B.C. Decker/People's Medical Publishing House, 2009, pp. 159-167.

7. **(B)** Opioids are the main treatment for postoperative pain in the neonate. Timing of pain reassessment after analgesic administration is based on the onset of action, peak effect, and duration of action of the analgesic. Fentanyl has an onset of action of 2 or 3 minutes, a peak effect at 3 or 4 minutes, and duration of action of 30 to 60 minutes. Pain reassessment should occur within 15 minutes, and not longer than 30 minutes, after administration of a bolus dose. Midazolam is a benzodiazepine with sedative, not analgesic, properties. Although sedation is often a goal after surgery, midazolam is not an effective treatment for pain. The frequency of acetaminophen administration in the

term infant is more than 4 hours, so it is too soon for an additional dose. Increasing the fentanyl infusion may be indicated; however, this large an increase may not be necessary, and reassessment of pain should occur much sooner than 2 hours after the dose increase.

**References:** American Academy of Pediatrics, Committee on Fetus and Newborn; American Academy of Pediatrics, Section on Surgery; Canadian Paediatric Society, Fetus and Newborn Committee: Prevention and management of pain in the neonate: An update. *Pediatrics,* 118(5):2231-2241, 2006.

Gardner, S.L, Enzman-Hines, M., Dickey, L.A.: Pain and pain relief. In Gardner, S.L., Carter, B.S., Enzman-Hines, M., et al. (Eds.): *Merenstein and Gardner's Handbook of Neonatal Intensive Care,* 7th ed. St. Louis, Mosby, 2011, pp. 223-269.

8. **(D)** Imperforate anus is classified as high or low depending on the level of the upper rectal pouch in relation to the puborectal muscle, which is the main muscle of continence. Infants with a low imperforate anus have a rectum that descends through the puborectalis and levator ani muscles and can be expected to have normal bowel continence after surgical repair. High defects may be associated with bowel incontinence due to impairment of the neurologic and muscular mechanisms of bowel control. Although it is impossible to fully predict bowel function in an individual patient, the nurse understands that typically bowel continence is related primarily to the level of the defect. The nurse shares with the family this knowledge of anticipated outcomes in children with similar conditions. The infant's sex is not the primary determinant of bowel incontinence. Eighty percent of females have low defects; males have an equal rate of high and low defects. Thus, bowel incontinence may occur more frequently in males, but this is due to the fact that more males have high defects. Bowel continence is not related to the presence or absence of a urogenital fistula.

**References:** Bradshaw, W.: Gastrointestinal disorders. In Verklan, M., Walden, M. (Eds.): *Core Curriculum for Neonatal Intensive Care Nursing,* 4th ed. St. Louis, Saunders, 2010, pp. 611-612.

Hartman, G.E., Boyajian, M.J., Choi, S.S., et al.: Surgical care of conditions presenting in the newborn. In MacDonald, M.G., Seshia, M.M.K., Mullett, M.D. (Eds.): *Avery's Neonatology: Pathophysiology and Management of the Newborn,* 6th ed. Philadelphia, Lippincott Williams & Wilkins, 2005, pp. 1122-1123.

9. **(D)** Hirschsprung disease is a congenital absence of the parasympathetic innervation to the distal intestine due to absence of ganglionic cells in the submucosal and myenteric plexuses of the intestine. This lack of intestinal innervation leads to a functional bowel obstruction. Hirschsprung disease affects the distal intestine and rectum. Acholic stools are associated with biliary atresia. Projectile vomiting is associated with pyloric stenosis. Oliguria is normal in the first 24 hours of life as the infant transitions to extrauterine life; beyond that, oliguria indicates renal dysfunction, which is not a common problem in Hirschsprung disease.

**References:** Bradshaw, W.: Gastrointestinal disorders. In Verklan, M., Walden, M. (Eds.): *Core Curriculum for Neonatal*

*Intensive Care Nursing,* 4th ed. St. Louis, Saunders, 2010, pp. 609-610.

Georgeson, K.E.: Hirschsprung's disease. In Holcomb, G.W., Murphy, J.P. (Eds.): *Ashcraft's Pediatric Surgery,* 5th ed. Philadelphia, Saunders, 2010, pp. 456-467.

10. **(D)** Gastroesophageal reflux (GER) is the retrograde movement of stomach contents into the esophagus and occurs frequently in both term and preterm neonates. When GER leads to pathologic symptoms, it is known as *gastroesophageal reflux disease* (GERD). Positioning the infant upright after feeding or with the head of the bed inclined to 30 degrees facilitates esophageal clearance and gastric emptying. In rare instances, postpyloric feeding may be necessary in severe cases of GERD; however, this is not the initial conservative management. Prokinetic agents are used to increase gastric emptying and thereby decrease reflux. Although medical management with prokinetic agents may be beneficial, such therapy typically is not initiated until conservative management has failed because of the potential adverse effects. Metoclopramide has been associated with irritability and the more serious side effects of dystonic reaction and tardive dyskinesia. Medical management with a histamine-2 receptor antagonist may be beneficial in the prevention and management of esophagitis or ulcers aggravated by gastric acid secretion and reflux, but they usually are not given unless conservative management of GERD has failed. These medications inhibit histamine receptors on the basolateral membrane of the parietal cells and thereby decrease gastric acid production.

**References:** Bradshaw, W.: Gastrointestinal disorders. In Verklan, M., Walden, M. (Eds.): *Core Curriculum for Neonatal Intensive Care Nursing,* 4th ed. St. Louis, Saunders, 2010, pp. 621-622.

Siddiqui, A., Hamilton, T., Nurko, S.: Gastrointestinal disorders. Part 10: Gastroesophageal reflux. In Hansen, A.R., Puder, M. (Eds.): *Manual of Neonatal Surgical Intensive Care,* 2nd ed. Shelton, Conn., B.C. Decker/People's Medical Publishing House, 2009, pp. 159-167.

11. **(C)** Pantoprazole use has been shown to increase the risk of gastroenteritis and pneumonia. Gastric acidity is a natural part of the body's immune response. Recent evidence has shown that interference with the body's gastric acidity, as occurs with the use of acid-blocker medications such as proton pump inhibitors and histamine-2 receptor blockers, may lead to increased bacterial colonization and subsequent gastroenteritis or community-acquired pneumonia. Pantoprazole is a proton pump inhibitor (PPI), not a histamine-2 receptor antagonist. PPIs suppress gastric acid secretion by inhibiting the proton pump, the parietal cell membrane enzyme $H^+,K^+$–adenosine triphosphatase. Pantoprazole should be administered 30 minutes before a meal when given orally. Pantoprazole is used in the treatment and prevention of esophagitis associated with gastroesophageal reflux disease.

**References:** Canani, R.B., Cirillo, P., Roggero, P., et al.: Therapy with gastric acidity inhibitors increases the risk of acute gastroenteritis and community-acquired pneumonia in children. *Pediatrics,* 117:e817-e820, 2006.

Siddiqui, A., Hamilton, T., Nurko, S.: Gastrointestinal disorders. Part 10: Gastroesophageal reflux. In Hansen, A.R., Puder, M. (Eds.): *Manual of Neonatal Surgical Intensive Care,* 2nd ed. Shelton, Conn., B.C. Decker/People's Medical Publishing House, 2009, pp. 159-167.

12. **(A)** The classic radiographic presentation of duodenal atresia is the "double bubble" appearance. Air is seen in the stomach and the upper duodenum, creating the double bubble, with no air below the site of atresia in the small or large intestine. Congenital diaphragmatic hernia would appear on radiographs as air-filled loops of bowel in the thoracic cavity and a mediastinal shift. In malrotation with midgut volvulus, radiographic studies classically show a distended stomach and proximal duodenum above the area where the bowel is twisted and scant gas distribution throughout the remaining bowel. An airless abdomen is an ominous sign and usually indicates intestinal infarction. Esophageal atresia and tracheoesophageal fistula is associated with varying radiographic findings, depending on the type of defect.

**References:** Aguayo, P., Ostlie, D.J.: Duodenal and intestinal atresia and stenosis. In Holcomb, G.W., Murphy, J.P. (Eds.): *Ashcraft's Pediatric Surgery,* 5th ed. Philadelphia, Saunders, 2010, pp. 400-415.

Bradshaw, W.: Gastrointestinal disorders. In Verklan, M., Walden, M. (Eds.): *Core Curriculum for Neonatal Intensive Care Nursing,* 4th ed. St. Louis, Saunders, 2010, p. 603.

13. **(A)** The intestines of an infant with a gastroschisis are often matted and edematous due to prolonged exposure to amniotic fluid. Malabsorption and delayed gastric motility or ileus are often postoperative complications in infants with a gastroschisis. Associated anomalies occur in 45% to 55% of infants with omphalocele and 10% to 15% of infants with gastroschisis. Although all abdominal wall defects potentially increase fluid losses, the anticipated fluid losses are greater in an infant with a gastroschisis because the bowel is exposed and therefore more at risk for insensible fluid loss. An omphalocele typically occurs at the umbilical ring and has a sac covering the defect, whereas a gastroschisis is typically to the right of the umbilicus and has no sac.

**References:** Fishman, S.J., Martin, C.R.: Gastrointestinal disorders. Part 1: Gastroschisis. In Hansen, A.R., Puder, M. (Eds.): *Manual of Neonatal Surgical Intensive Care,* 2nd ed. Shelton, Conn., B.C. Decker/People's Medical Publishing House, 2009, pp. 224-237.

Kelleher, C., Langer, J.C.: Congenital abdominal wall defects. In Holcomb, G.W., Murphy, J.P. (Eds.): *Ashcraft's Pediatric Surgery,* 5th ed. Philadelphia, Saunders, 2010, pp. 625-636.

14. **(C)** Infants with a gastroschisis or a ruptured omphalocele are at increased risk for loss of fluid, electrolytes, and heat through the exposed bowel. Excessive fluid loss can lead to hypovolemia, decreased perfusion, and metabolic acidosis. Although the risk of sepsis is a great concern in an infant with a gastroschisis, especially with delayed or staged repair, this is not the immediate preoperative concern. Neurologic compromise and seizure activity are not typically associated with gastroschisis. This infant has a gestational

age of 38 weeks, so respiratory distress syndrome is not likely.

**References:** Fishman, S.J., Martin, C.R.: Gastrointestinal disorders. Part 1: Gastroschisis. In Hansen, A.R., Puder, M. (Eds.): *Manual of Neonatal Surgical Intensive Care,* 2nd ed. Shelton, Conn., B.C. Decker/People's Medical Publishing House, 2009, pp. 224-237.

Kelleher, C., Langer, J.C.: Congenital abdominal wall defects. In Holcomb, G.W., Murphy, J.P. (Eds.): *Ashcraft's Pediatric Surgery,* 5th ed. Philadelphia, Saunders, 2010, pp. 625-636.

15. **(A)** Covering the bowel by placing the infant in a bowel bag that extends above the level of the defect maintains a sterile environment, prevents loss of fluid and heat, and allows for visualization of the bowel through the clear plastic. If a bowel bag is not available, the bowel may be covered with warm, saline-soaked gauze; however, caution should be used with this method to prevent bowel trauma resulting from adherence of the gauze to the bowel if the gauze is too dry, and bowel changes will not be visible. A bowel bag does not provide any protection to the bowel, so care should be used when handling the infant and the infant should be placed in a side-lying position to prevent kinking of the mesenteric vessel over the abdominal opening. Although use of a bowel bag does decrease the risk of infection, this is not its main function. The infant's privacy is maintained by other strategies, such as use of a private room, placement of screens around the bedside, and visitor surveillance.

**References:** Fishman, S.J., Martin, C.R.: Gastrointestinal disorders. Part 1: Gastroschisis. In Hansen, A.R., Puder, M. (Eds.): *Manual of Neonatal Surgical Intensive Care,* 2nd ed. Shelton, Conn., B.C. Decker/People's Medical Publishing House, 2009, pp. 224-237.

Kelleher, C., Langer, J.C.: Congenital abdominal wall defects. In Holcomb, G.W., Murphy, J.P. (Eds.): *Ashcraft's Pediatric Surgery,* 5th ed. Philadelphia, Saunders, 2010, pp. 625-636.

16. **(C)** Surgical repair is completed either by performing closure in a single procedure (primary repair) or by placing the bowel in a silo and performing several staged reductions. Ideally, a staged repair should be completed by 7 days to reduce the risk of infection. A staged repair is indicated with larger defects or in infants with respiratory or hemodynamic compromise who would not tolerate a primary repair and the resultant increase in intraabdominal pressure. There is no evidence to indicate that less pain is associated with a staged than with a primary repair. The risk of infection is greater with a staged repair than with a primary repair, because the abdomen remains open longer. Infants who require a staged repair typically have a longer postoperative course and later initiation of enteral feeds.

**References:** Fishman, S.J., Martin, C.R.: Gastrointestinal disorders. Part 1: Gastroschisis. In Hansen, A.R., Puder, M. (Eds.): *Manual of Neonatal Surgical Intensive Care,* 2nd ed. Shelton, Conn., B.C. Decker/People's Medical Publishing House, 2009, pp. 224-237.

Kelleher, C., Langer, J.C.: Congenital abdominal wall defects. In Holcomb, G.W., Murphy, J.P. (Eds.): *Ashcraft's Pediatric Surgery,* 5th ed. Philadelphia, Saunders, 2010, pp. 625-636.

17. **(D)** Because the exposed bowel is reduced into the abdominal cavity, intraabdominal pressure is increased. Complications of increasing intraabdominal pressure may include respiratory and hemodynamic compromise, and decreased perfusion of the lower extremities due to inferior vena cava compression, which can result in oliguria; cool, cyanotic lower extremities; and metabolic acidosis. Initial management includes volume resuscitation to improve cardiac output and lower extremity perfusion. Sepsis is a potential complication but not the most likely cause of deterioration in this situation. Decreased perfusion related to sepsis would be more generalized, not localized to the lower extremities. Postoperative pain is a potential complication but would not account for the decreased perfusion evident in this situation. Intracranial hemorrhage is not a likely complication in an infant of this gestational age.

**References:** Fishman, S.J., Martin, C.R.: Gastrointestinal disorders. Part 1: Gastroschisis. In Hansen, A.R., Puder, M. (Eds.): *Manual of Neonatal Surgical Intensive Care,* 2nd ed. Shelton, Conn., B.C. Decker/People's Medical Publishing House, 2009, pp. 224-237.

Kelleher, C., Langer, J.C.: Congenital abdominal wall defects. In Holcomb, G.W., Murphy, J.P. (Eds.): *Ashcraft's Pediatric Surgery,* 5th ed. Philadelphia, Saunders, 2010, pp. 625-636.

18. **(D)** If intraabdominal pressure continues to escalate, the infant is at risk for abdominal compartment syndrome. Measures should be taken to relieve the pressure and restore perfusion to the intraabdominal viscera. An epinephrine infusion may improve cardiac output by increasing heart rate and vasoconstriction, but it does not address the cause of the deterioration, which is compression of the abdominal organs and vessels. A furosemide bolus would likely worsen the hypotension as a result of diuresis and subsequent movement of fluid out of the vascular space. A sodium bicarbonate bolus may correct the metabolic acidosis but not the hypotension or anuria. Also, without further intervention, metabolic acidosis would likely reoccur.

**References:** Fishman, S.J., Martin, C.R.: Gastrointestinal disorders. Part 1: Gastroschisis. In Hansen, A.R., Puder, M. (Eds.): *Manual of Neonatal Surgical Intensive Care,* 2nd ed. Shelton, Conn., B.C. Decker/People's Medical Publishing House, 2009, pp. 224-237.

Kelleher, C., Langer, J.C.: Congenital abdominal wall defects. In Holcomb, G.W., Murphy, J.P. (Eds.): *Ashcraft's Pediatric Surgery,* 5th ed. Philadelphia, Saunders, 2010, pp. 625-636.

19. **(A)** Because duodenal atresia results from an early in utero event, there is a high incidence (30%) of associated anomalies. Common associated anomalies include trisomy 21 (30%), congenital heart disease (30%), intestinal malrotation (20%), tracheoesophageal abnormalities (10% to 20%), and anorectal defects (10% to 20%). Trisomy 18 is associated with cardiac, renal, and genital abnormalities, but not duodenal atresia. Turner syndrome is caused by complete or partial absence of one X chromosome and is associated with short stature and cardiac, renal, and musculoskeletal anomalies. Beckwith-Wiedemann syndrome is a triad consisting of omphalocele, macroglossia, and organomegaly.

**References:** Aguayo, P., Ostlie, D.J.: Duodenal and intestinal atresia and stenosis. In Holcomb, G.W., Murphy, J.P. (Eds.): *Ashcraft's Pediatric Surgery,* 5th ed. Philadelphia, Saunders, 2010, pp. 400-415.

Bradshaw, W.: Gastrointestinal disorders. In Verklan, M., Walden, M. (Eds.): *Core Curriculum for Neonatal Intensive Care Nursing,* 4th ed. St. Louis, Saunders, 2010, p. 603.

Lovvorn, H.N., Glenn, J.B., Pacetti, A.S., et al.: Neonatal surgery. In Gardner, S.L., Carter, B.S., Enzman-Hines, M., et al. (Eds.): *Merenstein and Gardner's Handbook of Neonatal Intensive Care,* 7th ed. St. Louis, Mosby, 2011, p. 824.

20. **(D)** The majority of infants with congenital diaphragmatic hernia (CDH) show respiratory distress and cyanosis immediately after birth. To avoid bowel distention, infants with CDH should be intubated and a large sump nasogastric tube should be inserted for gastric decompression. Timing of surgical repair varies based on the infant's condition and the size of the defect. Immediate surgical repair is associated with a higher mortality rate. The infant's condition should be first stabilized and the infant evaluated for associated conditions that may preclude extracorporeal membrane oxygenation or surgery. Airway anomalies are not commonly associated with CDH. Infants with CDH have been shown to have surfactant deficiency; however, surfactant replacement therapy is not always administered and would not be an immediate delivery room intervention.

**References:** Muratore, D.S., Wilson, J.M.: Congenital diaphragmatic hernia: Where are we and where do we go from here? *Seminars in Perinatology,* 24:418-428, 2000.

Ringer, S.A., Hansen, A.R.: Surgical emergencies in the newborn. In Cloherty, J.P., Eichenwald, E.C., Stark, A.R. (Eds.): *Manual of Neonatal Care,* 6th ed. Philadelphia, Lippincott Williams & Wilkins, 2008, pp. 621-622.

21. **(C)** The presence of abdominal viscera in the thoracic cavity prohibits intrauterine lung growth, which results in pulmonary hypoplasia. As a result of pulmonary hypoplasia, infants with congenital diaphragmatic hernia (CDH) have increased pulmonary vascular resistance, which places them at higher risk for pulmonary hypertension and right ventricular dysfunction. Bowel ischemia, hepatic dysfunction, and necrotizing enterocolitis are not typically associated with CDH.

**References:** Congenital Diaphragmatic Study Group: Defect size determines survival in infants with congenital diaphragmatic hernia. *Pediatrics,* 120:e651-e657, 2007.

Muratore, D.S., Wilson, J.M.: Congenital diaphragmatic hernia: Where are we and where do we go from here? *Seminars in Perinatology,* 24:418-428, 2000.

22. **(B)** Prematurity is the single greatest risk factor for necrotizing enterocolitis (NEC). Gestational age is inversely correlated with risk for necrotizing enterocolitis. Causes of NEC are not yet well defined and are often multifactorial. Infection may be a contributing factor. Intestinal ischemia, which may occur in sepsis, and the presence of bacteria in the intestinal tract have been shown to have some effect on the incidence of NEC. Enteral feeding may be a contributing factor in some instances. Although maternal cocaine use is a

risk factor for NEC due to the vasoconstrictive effects of the drug, it is not the single greatest risk factor.

**References:** Bradshaw, W.: Gastrointestinal disorders. In Verklan, M., Walden, M. (Eds.): *Core Curriculum for Neonatal Intensive Care Nursing,* 4th ed. St. Louis, Saunders, 2010, p. 613.

Eichenwald, E.: Necrotizing enterocolitis. In Cloherty, J.P., Eichenwald, E.C., Stark, A.R. (Eds.): *Manual of Neonatal Care,* 6th ed. Philadelphia, Lippincott Williams & Wilkins, 2008, pp. 608-615.

23. **(D)** In infants with necrotizing enterocolitis (NEC), an abnormal gas pattern, dilated loops of bowel, and pneumatosis intestinalis (intraluminal air) are often seen on abdominal radiographs. Pneumoperitoneum usually indicates intestinal perforation resulting in free air in the abdomen. Intestinal perforation is an absolute indication for surgical intervention, either by intestinal resection with enterostomy or peritoneal drainage. Relative indications for surgery include progressive clinical deterioration, portal venous gas, persistent fixed dilated bowel loops, abdominal wall edema or erythema, progressive pneumatosis, progressive acidosis, progressive thrombocytopenia, and leucopenia or leukocytosis. The presence of bacteria in the intestinal tract has been suggested as a contributing factor in the pathogenesis of NEC. Blood culture results may be positive or negative in infants with NEC. Positive blood culture findings indicate the presence of bacteria in the bloodstream but do not indicate a need for surgical intervention. Abdominal distention and lethargy are commonly seen in necrotizing enterocolitis; however, their presence alone does not indicate a need for surgery. Infants with NEC may develop respiratory failure and require intubation and mechanical ventilation. Although the need to reintubate this infant suggests disease progression, additional signs of clinical deterioration would be necessary to support the need for surgical intervention.

**References:** Bradshaw, W.: Gastrointestinal disorders. In Verklan, M., Walden, M. (Eds.): *Core Curriculum for Neonatal Intensive Care Nursing,* 4th ed. St. Louis, Saunders, 2010, p. 614.

Eichenwald, E.: Necrotizing enterocolitis. In Cloherty, J.P., Eichenwald, E.C., Stark, A.R. (Eds.): *Manual of Neonatal Care,* 6th ed. Philadelphia, Lippincott Williams & Wilkins, 2008, pp. 608-615.

24. **(B)** Infants in whom a large amount of bowel has been resected due to conditions such as necrotizing enterocolitis (NEC), bowel atresia, intestinal infarctions, and total colon aganglionosis often have short bowel syndrome because insufficient bowel is left for absorption of fluids and nutrients. Consequently, infants with a significant loss of small bowel, especially the ileum, are at risk for malabsorption. Infants with short bowel syndrome are often dependent on total parenteral nutrition and develop cholestasis and further hepatic dysfunction over time. Constipation is not typically a concern for infants with short bowel syndrome. More often these infants are at risk for loose stools caused by decreased transit time through the short bowel and limited water absorption if the colon is affected. Infections or changes in diet may increase the incidence of dumping or loose stools in this population. Infants who have lost the use of the ileum are

at risk for deficiencies of fat-soluble vitamins because fat-soluble vitamins are absorbed in the segment of the intestine. Although infants with short bowel syndrome may be at risk for recurrence of NEC or other abdominal complications such as gastrointestinal infections, dysmotility, or strictures, this is not the primary long-term nutritional concern for these infants.

**References:** Bradshaw, W.: Gastrointestinal disorders. In Verklan, M., Walden, M. (Eds.): *Core Curriculum for Neonatal Intensive Care Nursing,* 4th ed. St. Louis, Saunders, 2010, p. 616.

Eichenwald, E.: Necrotizing enterocolitis. In Cloherty, J.P., Eichenwald, E.C., Stark, A.R. (Eds.): *Manual of Neonatal Care,* 6th ed. Philadelphia, Lippincott Williams & Wilkins, 2008, pp. 608-615.

**25. (B)** Ninety percent of neonates with meconium ileus have cystic fibrosis, an autosomal recessive disorder. Because of this high incidence, all infants with meconium ileus should be evaluated for cystic fibrosis. Meconium ileus is not associated with trisomy 18. Cardiac, renal, and genital abnormalities may be associated with trisomy 18. Meconium ileus is not associated with DiGeorge syndrome. Cardiac defects, hypoplasia of the thymus, hypocalcemia, and microcephaly are seen in DiGeorge syndrome. Hirschsprung disease also results in bowel obstruction, but obstruction is caused by the absence of ganglionic cells in the colon, rather than by thick, inspissated meconium.

**References:** Bradshaw, W.: Gastrointestinal disorders. In Verklan, M., Walden, M. (Eds.): *Core Curriculum for Neonatal Intensive Care Nursing,* 4th ed. St. Louis, Saunders, 2010, p. 607.

Pursley, D., Hansen, A.R., Puder, M.: Gastrointestinal disorders. Part 4: Obstructions. In Hansen, A.R., Puder, M. (Eds.): *Manual of Neonatal Surgical Intensive Care,* 2nd ed. Shelton, Conn., B.C. Decker/People's Medical Publishing House, 2009, pp. 159-167.

## CHAPTER 17: METABOLIC AND ENDOCRINE DISORDERS

**1. (D)** Although postterm birth can pose some risk of hypoglycemia if the infant is not fed, the risk is low in an infant who is feeding. A 32-week, small-for-gestational-age infant has two major risk factors for hypoglycemia (prematurity and small for gestational age classification). Endogenous glucose stores are unlikely to be sufficient to overcome a prolonged period of fasting. A 34-week breast-feeding infant has one definite risk factor (prematurity) and one possible risk factor, if breast-feeding is not frequent and sufficient. Late hypoglycemia has been observed in such late preterm infants. A 36-week infant of a diabetic mother has two major risk factors for hypoglycemia (prematurity and a diabetic mother) and must be monitored closely.

**Reference:** Armentrout, D.: Glucose management. In Verklan, M., Walden, M. (Eds.): *Core Curriculum for Neonatal Intensive Care Nursing,* 4th ed. St. Louis, Saunders, 2010, pp. 172-181.

**2. (C)** Because a glucose bolus induces a surge of insulin secretion in the neonate, following the bolus with a continuous infusion of glucose or starting feedings will help eliminate the insulin surge and thereby eliminate rebound hypoglycemia. This neonate has no need of exogenous insulin; starting an insulin infusion

would make the problem worse. Repeating the glucose bolus will not solve the problem, because each new bolus will induce an insulin surge in the neonate. The pattern of peaks and valleys in blood glucose level will continue. Glucagon causes an endogenous release of glucose. If the glucagon bolus is not followed by a continuous infusion of either glucagon or glucose, rebound hypoglycemia can still occur.

**Reference:** Armentrout, D.: Glucose management. In Verklan, M., Walden, M. (Eds.): *Core Curriculum for Neonatal Intensive Care Nursing,* 4th ed. St. Louis, Saunders, 2010, pp. 172-181.

**3. (C)** As pregnancy progresses in the presence of diabetes, insulin resistance progressively worsens, and hyperglycemia and hyperaminoacidemia increase the rate of fetal growth. The fetal pancreas may respond to the excess glucose by producing more insulin, which causes beta cell hyperplasia, not hypoplasia. Although it is possible that a newborn's large size could be inherited from one or both parents, in the case of maternal diabetes, this is not the usual cause of macrosomia. The pregnancy of a woman with diabetes is more likely to be ended earlier, not later, and the neonate is more likely to be premature than postmature.

**Reference:** Armentrout, D.: Glucose management. In Verklan, M., Walden, M. (Eds.): *Core Curriculum for Neonatal Intensive Care Nursing,* 4th ed. St. Louis, Saunders, 2010, pp. 172-181.

**4. (A)** This infant is at high risk for hypoglycemia. The plasma glucose level must be confirmed by laboratory analysis as quickly as possible. Treatment should be started immediately to prevent sequelae of hypoglycemia such as brain damage. Although a blood sample should be sent, waiting for the results before taking action could be dangerous. If the infant does have hypoglycemia, brain damage could occur in the time taken to receive the results. Feeding the infant before drawing a specimen for plasma glucose measurement does not permit verification of the point-of-care test results. After this action, another 3 hours will be required before it is known if the infant is truly hypoglycemic and whether more intensive therapy is required.

**Reference:** Armentrout, D.: Glucose management. In Verklan, M., Walden, M. (Eds.): *Core Curriculum for Neonatal Intensive Care Nursing,* 4th ed. St. Louis, Saunders, 2010, pp. 172-181.

**5. (B)** This infant's history and laboratory findings suggest metabolic bone disease. The infant's bones are fragile and easily fractured (e.g., limbs, ribs). No contraindication to kangaroo care is suggested by this condition. A soy-based formula will not affect metabolic bone disease and may be nutritionally inferior to what the infant is receiving. Lack of mobility contributes to metabolic bone disease, so limiting mobility is incorrect.

**Reference:** Halbardier, B.H.: Fluid and electrolyte management. In Verklan, M., Walden, M. (Eds.): *Core Curriculum for Neonatal Intensive Care Nursing,* 4th ed. St. Louis, Saunders, 2010, pp. 156-171.

**6. (C)** A low thyroxine ($T_4$) level with an elevated level of thyroid-stimulating hormone (TSH) is pathognomonic for congenital hypothyroidism, because of the negative feedback control of the endocrine system. TSH level is not elevated in euthyroid sick syndrome (also called *nonthyroidal illness*). Neonatal Graves disease is associated with a high, rather than low, $T_4$ level. Thyroid-binding globulin deficiency does not manifest as an elevated TSH level.

**Reference:** Stokowski, L.: Endocrine disorders. In Verklan, M., Walden, M. (Eds.): *Core Curriculum for Neonatal Intensive Care Nursing,* 4th ed. St. Louis, Saunders, 2010, pp. 638-665.

7. **(C)** Transient hypothyroxinemia (low thyroxine and thyroid-stimulating hormone levels in the early weeks of life) occurs in up to 50% of low birth weight and extremely low birth weight infants. Thyroid dysgenesis, a common cause of congenital hypothyroidism, is a relatively rare condition. Neonatal thyrotoxicosis is a serious form of hyperthyroidism that is also relatively rare. Thyroid peroxidase deficiency is an inherited disorder of thyroid dyshormonogenesis and is not necessarily any more prevalent in preterm than in term infants. Thyroid peroxidase deficiency is the most common disorder of thyroid hormone synthesis.

**Reference:** Stokowski, L.: Endocrine disorders. In Verklan, M., Walden, M. (Eds.): *Core Curriculum for Neonatal Intensive Care Nursing,* 4th ed. St. Louis, Saunders, 2010, pp. 638-665.

8. **(D)** As blood glucose level rises, glucose begins spilling into the urine, followed by water, which results in osmotic diuresis. This can be dangerous for the very low birth weight infant. Weight gain is unlikely, because glucose utilization is poor. Ketonuria is not expected with neonatal hyperglycemia. Very low birth weight infants tend to have a deficiency, not an excess, of insulin.

**Reference:** Ogilvy-Stuart, A.L., Beardsall K.: Management of hyperglycemia in the preterm infant. *Archives of Disease in Childhood—Fetal and Neonatal Edition,* 95:126-131, 2010.

9. **(A)** Perinatal asphyxia is a significant risk factor for hypocalcemia in the neonate. Asphyxia stimulates a surge in calcitonin level, which inhibits the release of calcium from the bone. Hypophosphatemia is associated with hypercalcemia, not hypocalcemia. Hypocalcemia is not a feature of hypervitaminosis D. Subcutaneous fat necrosis is associated with hypercalcemia.

**Reference:** Hyman, S.J., Novoa, Y., Holzman, I.: Perinatal endocrinology: Common endocrine disorders in the sick and premature newborn. *Endocrinology Clinics of North America,* 38:509-524, 2009.

10. **(A)** Neonates have a limited repertoire of responses to illness, and the signs and symptoms of inborn errors of metabolism are often nonspecific and can mimic those of sepsis. Clinical evidence of a congenital heart defect is very different from the signs and symptoms of most inborn errors of metabolism. Clinical manifestations of necrotizing enterocolitis can include nonspecific findings, but also have a component specifically related to the abdomen and gastrointestinal tract, whereas most inborn errors of metabolism do not. The signs and symptoms of respiratory distress

syndrome are fairly specific and respond to specific treatments, unlike those of most inborn errors of metabolism.

**Reference:** Stokowski, L.: Metabolic disorders. In Kenner, C., Wright Lott, J. (Eds.): *Comprehensive Neonatal Care: An Interdisciplinary Approach,* 4th ed. St. Louis, Saunders, 2007. pp. 134-154.

11. **(C)** Infants who have fatty acid oxidation defects cannot break down fatty acids to supply energy, so energy needs must be met exogenously. Long periods of fasting (and other stressors) lead rapidly to hypoglycemia. Breast-feeding is allowable and encouraged for infants with medium-chain acyl–coenzyme A dehydrogenase deficiency (MCAD) because it is readily available. However, one must ensure that the infant is getting milk from the breast, or the infant may become hypoglycemic. Phenylalanine-free formula offers no benefit in MCAD. Phenylalanine-free formula is given to infants diagnosed with phenylketonuria. Protein is necessary to prevent tissue catabolism in infants with MCAD.

**Reference:** Stokowski, L.: Metabolic disorders. In Kenner, C., Wright Lott, J. (Eds.): *Comprehensive Neonatal Care: An Interdisciplinary Approach,* 4th ed. St. Louis, Saunders, 2007. pp. 134-154.

12. **(C)** A sizable goiter can compress and obstruct the trachea, leading to airway compromise. Positioning the infant with the head of bed elevated and head extended slightly will help maintain a patent airway. Otherwise, intubation might be necessary. If the goiter is caused by hyperthyroidism, cardiac effects are possible, but having a defibrillator on standby is not the most important intervention. The neonatal screen should be sent at the usual time to identify other potentially treatable metabolic problems. Not all goiters are corrected surgically. Many resolve spontaneously, and infants are fed as usual.

**Reference:** Stokowski, L.: Endocrine disorders. In Verklan, M., Walden, M. (Eds.): *Core Curriculum for Neonatal Intensive Care Nursing,* 4th ed. St. Louis, Saunders, 2010, pp. 638-665.

13. **(A)** An infant born to a mother who received magnesium sulfate is at risk of lethargy, hypotonia, and apnea. No treatment other than observation is usually necessary. Hypertension and fever, jitteriness and tachycardia, and tachypnea and hypoglycemia are not generally associated with a residual excess of magnesium.

**Reference:** Halbardier, B.H.: Fluid and electrolyte management. In Verklan, M., Walden, M. (Eds.): *Core Curriculum for Neonatal Intensive Care Nursing,* 4th ed. St. Louis, Saunders, 2010, pp. 156-171.

14. **(C)** Congenital adrenal hyperplasia caused by 21-hydroxylase deficiency is the most common cause of ambiguous genitalia in the newborn and is also the most common cause of virilization in a genetically female infant. Pure gonadal dysgenesis is less common than congenital adrenal hyperplasia, and genotype varies. Partial androgen insensitivity also occurs less frequently than congenital adrenal hyperplasia, and the genotype is 46,XY. Prenatal exposure to progestins is an uncommon cause of ambiguous genitalia.

Reference: Stokowski, L.: Endocrine disorders. In Verklan, M., Walden, M. (Eds.): *Core Curriculum for Neonatal Intensive Care Nursing,* 4th ed. St. Louis, Saunders, 2010, pp. 638-665.

15. **(C)** An apparent female with an inguinal hernia could be an XY child with complete or partial androgen insensitivity, and the "hernia" could be a testis. A workup is necessary to rule out these conditions. A hydrocele is a collection of fluid within the scrotum and is not associated with conditions that cause ambiguous genitalia. Physiologic phimosis is a common normal variant in male infants. Blood-tinged vaginal mucus is a common normal occurrence in female infants.

Reference: Stokowski, L.: Endocrine disorders. In Verklan, M., Walden, M. (Eds.): *Core Curriculum for Neonatal Intensive Care Nursing,* 4th ed. St. Louis, Saunders, 2010, pp. 638-665.

16. **(C)** The birth of a baby with ambiguous genitalia raises many distressing issues for parents (such as what to tell family and friends, how to deal with registering the birth and naming the baby, etc.), and a mental health professional can help the parents deal with these and other issues. Parents should never be told with certainty that their baby is a boy (or girl) in these cases; care professionals should not attempt to guess the gender in advance of test results and should keep their opinions to themselves. Suggesting that parents choose a name suitable for either a boy or a girl is not recommended. Once the gender is established, the name is a way of reinforcing the gender for the family. Keeping secrets reinforces feelings of guilt and shame. The parents can choose how, when, and how much information will be communicated, but trying to maintain strict secrecy about the baby's condition is not recommended and can isolate the parents from supportive family and friends.

Reference: Stokowski, L.: Endocrine disorders. In Verklan, M., Walden, M. (Eds.): *Core Curriculum for Neonatal Intensive Care Nursing,* 4th ed. St. Louis, Saunders, 2010, pp. 638-665.

## CHAPTER 18: HEMATOLOGIC DISORDERS

1. **(B)** Immunoglobulin M (IgM) is actively synthesized by the fetus in response to in utero infections. Although synthesis begins early in the pregnancy, increased levels are detectable beginning at 30 weeks' gestation. IgG is the major immunoglobulin present in the serum of the infant. It is transferred via the placenta and provides passive immunity against bacterial and viral infections. The majority of IgG is transferred in the third trimester. IgA is passed primarily in colostrum and breast milk and through the respiratory tract. Although its level can increase as a result of in utero infections, it is not detectable in the infant until 2 to 3 weeks after birth. IgE is synthesized in response to allergic reactions.

Reference: Lott, J.W.: Immunology and infectious disease. In Verklan, M., Walden, M. (Eds.): *Core Curriculum for Neonatal Intensive Care Nursing,* 4th ed. St. Louis, Saunders, 2010, pp. 696-697.

2. **(A)** Erythropoietin triggers erythropoiesis, or the production of erythrocytes. Although the primary reason for in utero synthesis of erythropoietin is hypoxia, infants born to women with pregnancy-induced hypertension also have a higher level of erythropoietin than normal. It can be anticipated that an excess amount of erythropoietin will result in polycythemia. Based on maternal history, there is no indication of maternal-fetal hemorrhage. Although neonates have a higher percentage of hemoglobin F than adults do, it does not result in polycythemia. It is not standard to strip blood from the umbilical cord into the baby at the time of delivery.

Reference: Diehl-Jones, W., Askin, D.F.: Hematologic disorders. In Verklan, M., Walden, M. (Eds.): *Core Curriculum for Neonatal Intensive Care Nursing,* 4th ed. St. Louis, Saunders, 2010, p. 667.

3. **(A)** The oxygen-hemoglobin dissociation curve determines the affinity of hemoglobin for oxygen. Factors shifting the curve to the left result in a higher affinity. These factors include the presence of fetal hemoglobin, decreased temperature, low $Paco_2$, higher pH, and low levels of 2,3-diphosphoglycerate (2,3-DPG). The level of 2,3-DPG is directly proportional to gestational age. Therefore, a 28-week-gestational-age infant with a low-normal temperature would show the greatest affinity for oxygen due to the high $Paco_2$. In a 30-week-gestational-age infant with a $Paco_2$ of 55, the oxygen-hemoglobin dissociation curve will be shifted to the right (decreased affinity for oxygen). In a 35-week-gestational-age infant with a temperature of 38.0° C (100.4° F), the curve will also be shifted to the right due to the high temperature. In a 38-week-gestational-age infant, a $Paco_2$ of 40 is normal, but the infant will have a higher level of 2,3-DPG based on gestational age. Thus the oxygen-hemoglobin dissociation curve will be shifted to the right.

Reference: Diehl-Jones, W., Askin, D.F.: Hematologic disorders. In Verklan, M., Walden, M. (Eds.): *Core Curriculum for Neonatal Intensive Care Nursing,* 4th ed. St. Louis, Saunders, 2010, p. 667.

4. **(D)** Because of the greater number of receptor sites for oxygen on fetal hemoglobin, newborn red blood cells carry a greater amount of oxygen on the hemoglobin than do adult red blood cells. Newborn RBCs are much more fragile than adult RBCs. RBCs have a life span of 60 to 70 days in term newborns and an even shorter life span in premature infants. The life span of an adult RBC is 100 to 120 days. The mean corpuscular volume is the relative size of the red blood cell. Newborn red blood cells are larger than adult red blood cells for the first 4 to 5 years of life.

Reference: Diehl-Jones, W., Askin, D.F.: Hematologic disorders. In Verklan, M., Walden, M. (Eds.): *Core Curriculum for Neonatal Intensive Care Nursing,* 4th ed. St. Louis, Saunders, 2010, pp. 668-669.

5. **(C)** Disseminated intravascular coagulation (DIC) is an acquired hemorrhagic disorder associated with underlying disease such as septic shock. Presenting signs of the DIC include sudden hemorrhage, prolonged oozing, petechiae, and purpura. In neonatal alloimmune thrombocytopenia, while fetal platelet counts are low, maternal platelet counts are usually normal. Thrombocytopenia results from maternal antibodies that cross the placenta and destroy fetal platelets. Babies present with petechiae and bleeding, but

not sudden hemorrhage. Babies of mothers with systemic lupus erythematosus and idiopathic (auto-immune) thrombocytopenic purpura have thrombocytopenia as a result of maternal autoantibodies. Mothers of these infants typically have low platelet counts. Babies show petechiae and bleeding, but not sudden hemorrhage.

**Reference:** Diehl-Jones, W., Askin, D.F.: Hematologic disorders. In Verklan, M., Walden, M. (Eds.): *Core Curriculum for Neonatal Intensive Care Nursing*, 4th ed. St. Louis, Saunders, 2010, pp. 679-683.

6. **(B)** Typical laboratory results for disseminated intravascular coagulation (DIC) are low platelet count, prolonged prothrombin time and prolonged partial thromboplastin time (although they may initially be normal), increased level of fibrin split products, low fibrinogen level, and increased level of D-dimer (the marker for DIC).

**Reference:** Diehl-Jones, W., Askin, D.F.: Hematologic disorders. In Verklan, M., Walden, M. (Eds.): *Core Curriculum for Neonatal Intensive Care Nursing*, 4th ed. St. Louis, Saunders, 2010, p. 681.

7. **(B)** One unit of cryoprecipitate supplies 100 to 150 mg of fibrinogen along with factors VIII and XIII. A transfusion of platelets results only in a higher platelet count. Fresh frozen plasma replaces all of the coagulation proteins. A transfusion of packed red blood cells results in a higher hematocrit.

**Reference:** Diehl-Jones, W., Askin, D.F.: Hematologic disorders. In Verklan, M., Walden, M. (Eds.): *Core Curriculum for Neonatal Intensive Care Nursing*, 4th ed. St. Louis, Saunders, 2010, pp. 689-690.

8. **(B)** Immediately after an acute blood loss, the hematocrit will be unchanged, because the body has not had a chance to equilibrate. Acute blood loss results in a decreased preload leading to decreased cardiac output as evidenced by low blood pressure, tachycardia, and poor perfusion (pallor, delayed capillary refill). Decreased hematocrit, unchanged blood pressure and heart rate, and hepatosplenomegaly are more typical of chronic blood loss. Respiratory distress can be expected.

**Reference:** Diehl-Jones, W., Askin, D.F.: Hematologic disorders. In Verklan, M., Walden, M. (Eds.): *Core Curriculum for Neonatal Intensive Care Nursing*, 4th ed. St. Louis, Saunders, 2010, p. 667.

9. **(D)** The preferred treatment for acute blood loss resulting in hypovolemia is transfusion of whole blood if available. In addition to increasing the volume returning to the heart, blood transfusion increases the oxygen-carrying capacity of the body. The use of group O, Rh-negative blood does not require that typing and crossmatching be performed before the transfusion. Placing preterm infants in Trendelenburg position is not recommended because it changes cerebral perfusion and increases potential for intraventricular hemorrhage. If immediate access to whole blood or packed red blood cells is not available, the next choice would be an isotonic volume expander. Although administering oxygen would increase the infant's $Po_2$, an increased $Po_2$ does not contribute significantly to

oxygen content. The most significant contributor to oxygen content is hemoglobin level.

**Reference:** Diehl-Jones, W., Askin, D.F.: Hematologic disorders. In Verklan, M., Walden, M. (Eds.): *Core Curriculum for Neonatal Intensive Care Nursing*, 4th ed. St. Louis, Saunders, 2010, p. 667.

10. **(C)** Because the infant is anemic and showing signs of hypoxemia, and has an underlying pulmonary condition, it would be appropriate to give a transfusion to increase oxygen-carrying capacity. Because the patient is symptomatic, it would not be beneficial to "wait and see" at this point. Although supplemental iron is important in the ongoing formation of red blood cells like Epogen, it is not for acute treatment. Because erythropoietin causes the production of the precursors of erythrocytes, it is not a treatment for a patient who is currently symptomatic with anemia. Epogen may prevent further transfusions in the course of therapy.

**Reference:** Manco-Johnson, M., Rodden, D., Hays, T.: Newborn hematology. In Gardner, S.L., Carter, B.S., Enzman-Hines, M., et al. (Eds.): *Merenstein and Gardner's Handbook of Neonatal Intensive Care*, 7th ed. St. Louis, Mosby, 2011, pp. 510-513.

11. **(C)** Angioedema, or subcutaneous hives, is a sign of an allergic reaction to blood. Bradycardia and restlessness are also signs of a transfusion reaction. Febrile reactions are very rare in newborns. Rather than tachycardia, bradycardia is a sign of a transfusion reaction. Irregular respirations and apnea can occur in a transfusion reaction. A histamine reaction to blood would probably result in hypotension rather than hypertension. Babies with transfusion reactions become pale rather than erythematic. Diaphoresis is a sign of a transfusion reaction, but an increasing level of jaundice is not. Irregular respirations would occur rather than tachypnea.

**References:** Diehl-Jones, W., Askin, D.F.: Hematologic disorders. In Verklan, M., Walden, M. (Eds.): *Core Curriculum for Neonatal Intensive Care Nursing*, 4th ed. St. Louis, Saunders, 2010, p. 687.

Manco-Johnson, M., Rodden, D., Hays, T.: Newborn hematology. In Gardner, S.L., Carter, B.S., Enzman-Hines, M., et al. (Eds.): *Merenstein and Gardner's Handbook of Neonatal Intensive Care*, 7th ed. St. Louis, Mosby, 2011, pp. 528, 532.

12. **(C)** In the case of maternal idiopathic thrombocytopenic purpura (autoimmune thrombocytopenia), maternal antibodies bind to platelet surface antigens, which makes the platelets susceptible to premature destruction. The immunoglobulin G molecules in intravenous immune globulin (IVIG) bind to the host antigens, form immune complexes, and block the antibodies that destroy the sensitized platelets. Modulation of complement activation is the mechanism of action of IVIG in the case of neutropenia. Decreasing the autoimmune hemolysis of erythrocytes is the mechanism of action of IVIG in pathologic autoimmune hyperbilirubinemia. Steroids have been found to increase production and mobilization of platelets from the platelet pool in idiopathic thrombocytopenic purpura.

**References:** Diehl-Jones, W., Askin, D.F.: Hematologic disorders. In Verklan, M., Walden, M. (Eds.): *Core Curriculum for Neonatal Intensive Care Nursing*, 4th ed. St. Louis, Saunders, 2010, p. 682.

Roberts, K., Brinker, D., Murante, B. Hematology and immunology. In Slota, M. (Ed.): *Core Curriculum for Pediatric Critical Care Nursing*, 2nd ed. St. Louis, Saunders, 2006, p. 623.

Scheinfeld, N., Godwin, J.: Intravenous Immunoglobulin. 2008. Available at: http://emedicine.medscape.com/article/210367. Accessed May 22, 2010.

13. **(B)** The physiologic signs of an adverse immune reaction to intravenous immune globulin include skin flushing, wheezing, tachycardia, nausea (emesis), and hypotension.

**Reference:** Scheinfeld, N., Godwin, J.: Intravenous Immunoglobulin. 2008. Available at: http://emedicine.medscape.com/article/210367. Accessed May 22, 2010.

14. **(D)** The Kleihauer-Betke test is used to confirm the presence of fetal blood cells in the maternal blood. In the case of a fetal-maternal hemorrhage, the results would be positive. A positive Apt test result distinguishes swallowed maternal blood from neonatal blood. A positive result on a direct Coombs test identifies newborn hemolytic disease by detecting serum antibodies (immunoglobulin G) attached to neonatal erythrocytes. A positive result on an indirect Coombs test identifies newborn hemolytic disease by detecting serum antibodies that are in the blood but are not attached to the maternal erythrocytes.

**References:** Manco-Johnson, M., Rodden, D., Hays, T.: Newborn hematology. In Gardner, S.L., Carter, B.S., Enzman-Hines, M., et al. (Eds.): *Merenstein and Gardner's Handbook of Neonatal Intensive Care*, 7th ed. St. Louis, Mosby, 2011, pp. 522-523.

Roberts, K., Brinker, D., Murante, B.: Hematology and immunology. In Slota, M. (Ed.): *Core Curriculum for Pediatric Critical Care Nursing*, 2nd ed. St. Louis, Saunders, 2006, p. 623.

15. **(A)** A 36-week-gestation infant with temperature instability is in a high risk category because there are two major risk factors for negative effects related to hyperbilirubinemia—gestational age of 36 weeks and temperature instability. A 38-week-gestation infant with sepsis has one major risk factor for negative effects related to hyperbilirubinemia—sepsis. A 39-week-gestation infant with visible jaundice in the first 24 hours has one major risk factor for significant hyperbilirubinemia—visible jaundice in the first 24 hours. A 40-week-gestation infant with ABO incompatibility and positive direct Coombs has one major risk factor for significant hyperbilirubinemia—ABO incompatibility with positive direct Coombs.

**Reference:** Kamath, B., Thilo, E. and Hernandez, J.: Jaundice. In Verklan, M. and Walden, M. (Eds.): *Core Curriculum for Neonatal Intensive Care Nursing*, 4th ed. St. Louis, Saunders Elsevier, 2011, p. 545.

16. **(A)** Many infants who are readmitted to the NICU from home with severe hyperbilirubinemia are already mildly dehydrated. This dehydration is then compounded by the increase in insensible water loss that occurs with phototherapy. Loose stools are actually helpful in clearing the bilirubin, although they may add to the level of dehydration if not monitored carefully. Naked term infants placed under fluorescent bulbs do not generally experience significant hyperthermia at room temperature. Bronze baby syndrome occurs as a side effect of phototherapy in infants with elevated conjugated or direct bilirubin levels. Hyperbilirubinemia related to breast-feeding is usually a result of elevated levels of indirect bilirubin.

**Reference:** Bradshaw, W.: Gastrointestinal disorders. In Verklan, M., Walden, M. (Eds.): *Core Curriculum for Neonatal Intensive Care Nursing*, 4th ed. St. Louis, Saunders, 2010, pp. 630-631.

17. **(B)** The metabolic acidosis must be corrected before the exchange. Acidosis increases the risk of bilirubin toxicity and causes the infant to be more susceptible to complications related to the exchange. It is no longer recommended to give a bolus of albumin prior to an exchange transfusion. Although the infant must be restrained before the exchange transfusion, this will occur after the correction of the metabolic acidosis. Emergency equipment (oxygen, suction, resuscitation equipment) should present during the exchange transfusion, but the acid-base status must be stabilized before the start of the procedure.

**Reference:** Bradshaw, W.: Gastrointestinal disorders. In Verklan, M., Walden, M. (Eds.): *Core Curriculum for Neonatal Intensive Care Nursing*, 4th ed. St. Louis, Saunders, 2010, pp. 630-632.

18. **(D)** Although this newborn does not strictly meet the criterion for polycythemia (venous hematocrit of 65%), the fact that she has some jitteriness and difficulty feeding may indicate that she is beginning to experience the effects of hyperviscosity. Because coexisting hypoglycemia is an important determinant of adverse neurologic outcomes and the baby's condition is stable at this point, the exchange could be delayed, provided the infant is watched carefully and her feeding and glucose level monitored. Immediately performing a partial exchange transfusion increases the risk of gastrointestinal complications. Because the infant is not experiencing any respiratory difficulties, the infant can continue to try to feed if possible.

**Reference:** Diehl-Jones, W., Askin, D.F.: Hematologic disorders. In Verklan, M., Walden, M. (Eds.): *Core Curriculum for Neonatal Intensive Care Nursing*, 4th ed. St. Louis, Saunders, 2010, p. 685.

19. **(D)** Breast-feeding infants of less than 38 weeks' gestation are at a high risk for developing hyperbilirubinemia and require closer surveillance. Early signs of acute bilirubin encephalopathy are lethargy, sleepiness, and poor suck. Four to six thoroughly wet diapers is the amount expected from a well-hydrated infant. Still passing meconium stools at 3 days of life is within normal limits. Beginning at this time, the breast-feeding infant will begin to have yellow seedy stools. Irritability and crying for a few hours each afternoon is a common sign of colic.

**Reference:** Management of hyperbilirubinemia in the newborn infant 35 or more weeks of gestation. American Academy of Pediatrics. Subcommittee on Hyperbilirubinemia. *Pediatrics*, 114(1):297-316, 2004.

20. **(A)** The maternal history and physical findings suggests fetal immune hydrops related to Rh/ABO sensitization. Because the fetus is already symptomatic and the mother has a history of stillbirths at around this gestational length, the prudent action would be to deliver the infant and provide neonatal intensive care.

Fetal thoracentesis would be appropriate if the fetus had a pleural effusion; however, this is not present according to the ultrasonography results. In addition, the fetus's condition is critical enough that delivery is warranted. Intrauterine transfusion would be an appropriate treatment to minimize fetal anemia, and amniocentesis would successfully reduce uterine volume, but the fetus's critical condition requires more than palliative care.

**Reference:** Bradshaw, W.: Gastrointestinal disorders. In Verklan, M., Walden, M. (Eds.): *Core Curriculum for Neonatal Intensive Care Nursing*, 4th ed. St. Louis, Saunders, 2010, pp. 633-635.

## CHAPTER 19: NEUROLOGIC DISORDERS

1. **(A)** A large, mobile scalp mass that crosses suture lines and extends into the neck is a sign of subgaleal hemorrhage. A primiparous mother and vacuum-assisted delivery are risk factors. The subgaleal space can hide large quantities of blood, and shock can occur from exsanguination. Seizures may occur after a difficult delivery but are not suggested by the information provided. Hydrocephalus may be present but is not caused by a difficult delivery and is not indicated by the description given. Craniosynostosis is the fusion of one or more sutures. It is not caused by a difficult delivery and the information provided does not suggest that it is present.

**References:** Blackburn, S.T., Ditzenberger, G.R.: Neurologic system. In Kenner, C.A., Lott, J.W. (Eds.): *Comprehensive Neonatal Care: An Interdisciplinary Approach*, 4th ed. St. Louis, Saunders, 2007, p. 289.

Furdon, S.A., Benjamin, K.: Physical assessment. In Verklan, M.T., Walden, M. (Eds.): *Core Curriculum for Neonatal Intensive Care Nursing*, 4th ed. St. Louis, Saunders, 2010, p. 138.

Lynam, L., Verklan, M.T.: Neurologic disorders. In Verklan, M.T., Walden, M. (Eds.): *Core Curriculum for Neonatal Intensive Care Nursing*, 4th ed. St. Louis, Saunders, 2010, p. 763.

2. **(C)** A common cause of neonatal seizures is metabolic encephalopathy. Signs and symptoms of neonatal seizures are usually subtle and nonspecific, but include lip smacking and bicycling and pedaling movements. Myoclonus is very rare in the neonatal period and manifests as jerking movements. Signs of hypercalcemia include bradycardia, hypotonia, and constipation. Behaviors indicating readiness to feed include rooting and nonnutritive sucking.

**References:** Blackburn, S.T., Ditzenberger, G.R.: Neurologic system. In Kenner, C.A., Lott, J.W. (Eds.): *Comprehensive Neonatal Care: An Interdisciplinary Approach*, 4th ed. St. Louis, Saunders, 2007, p. 279.

Lynam, L., Verklan, M.T.: Neurologic disorders. In Verklan, M.T., Walden, M. (Eds.): *Core Curriculum for Neonatal Intensive Care Nursing*, 4th ed. St. Louis, Saunders, 2010, p. 772.

3. **(D)** The underlying cause of up to 65% of neonatal seizures is hypoxic-ischemic encephalopathy. Hypocalcemia, not hypercalcemia is a common cause of neonatal seizures. Bacterial meningitis can lead to seizures, but together with viral central nervous system infections causes only 10% to 15% of all neonatal seizures. Subarachnoid hemorrhage is fairly common, especially in term infants delivered vaginally, but is a cause for seizures in fewer than 30% of cases.

**References:** Blackburn, S.T., Ditzenberger, G.R.: Neurologic system. In Kenner, C.A., Lott, J.W. (Eds.): *Comprehensive Neonatal Care: An Interdisciplinary Approach*, 4th ed. St. Louis, Saunders, 2007, p. 279.

Lynam, L., Verklan, M.T.: Neurologic Disorders. In Verklan, M.T., Walden, M. (Eds.): *Core Curriculum for Neonatal Intensive Care Nursing*, 4th ed. St. Louis, Saunders, 2010, p. 771.

4. **(D)** In the infant with posthemorrhagic hydrocephalus, the subgaleal shunt drains cerebrospinal fluid from the lateral ventricles to the space between the periosteum of the skull and the aponeurotic membrane, where it is eventually reabsorbed. A Blalock-Taussig shunt surgically connects the pulmonary artery to the subclavian artery. The ductus venosus in the fetus connects the umbilical vein to the inferior vena cava. Cerebral spinal fluid drains from the lateral ventricles to the third ventricle via the foramina of Monro.

**Reference:** Lam, H.P., Heilman, C.B.: Ventricular access device versus ventriculosubgaleal shunt in post hemorrhagic hydrocephalus associated with prematurity. *Journal of Maternal-Fetal and Neonatal Medicine*, 22(11):1097-1101, 2009.

5. **(D)** Periventricular leukomalacia (PVL) is the necrosis and then thinning or liquefaction of cerebral white matter secondary to ischemia and occurs primarily in the preterm infant. Increased neutrophil count in the cerebrospinal fluid indicates meningitis. Postterm infants are at no increased risk for PVL. The finding of PVL on head ultrasonography is significant, because PVL is associated with motor deficits, visual impairment, and possibly intellectual deficits.

**References:** Blackburn, S.T., Ditzenberger, G.R.: Neurologic system. In Kenner, C.A., Lott, J.W. (Eds.): *Comprehensive Neonatal Care: An Interdisciplinary Approach*, 4th ed. St. Louis, Saunders, 2007, p. 287.

Lynam, L., Verklan, M.T.: Neurologic disorders. In Verklan, M.T., Walden, M. (Eds.): *Core Curriculum for Neonatal Intensive Care Nursing*, 4th ed. St. Louis, Saunders, 2010, p. 778.

6. **(D)** Sarnat staging is helpful in differentiating between mild and more severe hypoxic-ischemic encephalopathy to determine prognosis and possible treatment with hypothermia. Moderate to severely affected infants display stupor, hypotonia, and depressed deep tendon reflexes. Mildly affected infants demonstrate autonomic excitation, normal deep tendon reflexes, and hyperalertness.

**References:** Blackburn, S.T., Ditzenberger, G.R.: Neurologic system. In Kenner, C.A., Lott, J.W. (Eds.): *Comprehensive Neonatal Care: An Interdisciplinary Approach*, 4th ed. St. Louis, Saunders, 2007, p. 282.

Lynam, L., Verklan, M.T.: Neurologic disorders. In Verklan, M.T., Walden, M. (Eds.): *Core Curriculum for Neonatal Intensive Care Nursing*, 4th ed. St. Louis, Saunders, 2010, p. 775.

7. **(D)** Abnormal movements that do not cease with gentle passive flexion of the extremity are characteristic of neonatal seizures, and this maneuver aids in differentiating between seizures and jitteriness. Changes in vital signs are not specific to seizures and may not always occur with seizure activity. On a bedside electroencephalogram, seizure activity is characterized by a sudden sustained increase in baseline voltage. Postictal states are extremely rare in the neonate.

Reference: Lynam, L., Verklan, M.T.: Neurologic disorders. In Verklan, M.T., Walden, M. (Eds.): *Core Curriculum for Neonatal Intensive Care Nursing,* 4th ed. St. Louis, Saunders, 2010, p. 773.

8. **(C)** Hydrocephalus is very common in infants with myelomeningocele, as is Arnold-Chiari malformation, which causes hydrocephalus in 70% of affected infants. Seizures are not associated with a diagnosis of myelomeningocele. Although postoperative wound infection and skin breakdown may occur, use of aseptic technique and good nursing care minimize the risk of these complications.

Reference: Lynam, L., Verklan, M.T.: Neurologic disorders. In Verklan, M.T., Walden, M. (Eds.): *Core Curriculum for Neonatal Intensive Care Nursing,* 4th ed. St. Louis, Saunders, 2010, p. 759.

9. **(B)** Ninety percent of intraventricular/periventricular hemorrhages (IVHs/PVHs) occur in the first 72 hours after birth. Only about half of IVHs/PVHs occur in the first day of life. It is beneficial to have information about an intraventricular bleed and any ventriculomegaly early in life to guide treatment, allow early intervention, and determine prognosis. Waiting until after 30 weeks may miss a window of opportunity.

References: Blackburn, S.T., Ditzenberger, G.R.: Neurologic system. In Kenner, C.A., Lott, J.W. (Eds.): *Comprehensive Neonatal Care: An Interdisciplinary Approach,* 4th ed. St. Louis, Saunders, 2007, p. 285.

Lynam, L., Verklan, M.T.: Neurologic disorders. In Verklan, M.T., Walden, M. (Eds.): *Core Curriculum for Neonatal Intensive Care Nursing,* 4th ed. St. Louis, Saunders, 2010, p. 770.

10. **(B)** Clinical presentation of major intraventricular hemorrhage includes a sudden drop in hematocrit or failure to respond to transfusions, full anterior fontanelle, change in activity level, and decreased tone. Anemia of prematurity would result in a more gradual drop in hematocrit. Upper gastrointestinal bleeding is uncommon in the neonate. Iatrogenic anemia from laboratory blood draws would result in a more gradual drop in hematocrit and could be anticipated from careful recording of intake and output.

Reference: Blackburn, S.T., Ditzenberger, G.R.: Neurologic system. In Kenner, C., Lott, J.W. (Eds.): *Comprehensive Neonatal Care: An Interdisciplinary Approach,* 4th ed. St. Louis, Saunders, 2007, p. 286.

11. **(D)** Outcomes of intraventricular/periventricular hemorrhage vary, and hemorrhage alone does not account for all neurologic deficits, so early intervention is necessary. Infants with lower-grade bleeds may have no sequelae or neurodevelopmental disability similar to that of premature infants without bleeds. Even mildly affected infants may have subtle learning disabilities not detected until school age. Infants with grade IV bleeds have hydrocephalus, but not all require shunt placement. Fewer than 20% of infants with lesser-grade bleeds have hydrocephalus. Spontaneous regression can occur.

Reference: Lynam, L., Verklan, M.T.: Neurologic disorders. In Verklan, M.T., Walden, M. (Eds.): *Core Curriculum for Neonatal Intensive Care Nursing,* 4th ed. St. Louis, Saunders, 2010, p. 769.

12. **(B)** In the absence of pathology (e.g., hydrocephalus, craniosynostosis), head circumference is a measure of brain growth. Daily weight is a measure of overall growth and is not specific to the brain. Head ultrasonography details anatomic structures and measures ventricular size but is not used to measure brain growth or size. The Dubowitz examination assesses gestational age at birth.

Reference: Furdon, S.A., Benjamin, K.: Physical assessment. In Verklan, M.T., Walden, M. (Eds.): *Core Curriculum for Neonatal Intensive Care Nursing,* 4th ed. St. Louis, Saunders, 2010, p. 136.

13. **(D)** Intracranial pressure (ICP) is lowest with the head in the midline and the head of the bed elevated 30 degrees. Turning the head to the side compresses the jugular vein, which impedes venous drainage and increases ICP. An infant with a large head who is placed upright in a swing or infant seat may tip the head forward with the chin down and obstruct venous drainage or compromise the airway. An infant lying prone would have the head turned sharply to one side or the other, which impedes venous drainage.

Reference: Blackburn, S.T., Ditzenberger, G.R.: Neurologic system. In Kenner, C., Lott, J.W. (Eds.): *Comprehensive Neonatal Care: An Interdisciplinary Approach,* 4th ed. St. Louis, Saunders, 2007, p. 283, 286.

14. **(C)** Since most myelomeningoceles are in the lumbar region, meticulous care is needed to shield the incision and dressings from urine and stool contamination. Depending on the size of the defect, the incision can be under some tension, and careful positioning is required to prevent dehiscence. Infants with myelomeningocele frequently also have hydrocephalus, which cannot be prevented even by good nursing care. Initially, infants need to be positioned prone or side lying to prevent pressure on the incision until healing occurs. Holding the infant for feeding would put pressure on the back. Surgery does not restore normal function of the legs; it only preserves the function that is present.

Reference: Blackburn, S.T., Ditzenberger, G.R.: Neurologic system. In Kenner, C., Lott, J.W. (Eds.): *Comprehensive Neonatal Care: An Interdisciplinary Approach,* 4th ed. St. Louis, Saunders, 2007, p. 270.

15. **(D)** Only a grade IV intraventricular/periventricular hemorrhage (IVH/PVH) involves bleeding into the parenchyma. Decerebrate posturing is a sign of neurologic dysfunction; it is not specific to grade IV hemorrhage and is not seen in premature infants. Periventricular echogenicity may be insignificant or may indicate periventricular leukomalacia, and may be present with or without hemorrhage. Both grade III and grade IV IVH/PVH is associated with ventricular dilation.

Reference: Lynam, L., Verklan, M.T.: Neurologic disorders. In Verklan, M.T., Walden, M. (Eds.): *Core Curriculum for Neonatal Intensive Care Nursing,* 4th ed. St. Louis, Saunders, 2010, p. 769.

16. **(A)** Infants who have fever and seizures would undergo a workup for herpes infection, which is treated with acyclovir. Morphine may be indicated if the infant is experiencing withdrawal symptoms. Neonatal abstinence can cause fever and seizures, but not

usually by 3 hours of age and not without other signs and symptoms. There is no specific immunoglobulin for herpesvirus infection. Hypothermia is used in the management of hypoxic-ischemic encephalopathy (HIE). This infant does not have a history or signs and symptoms of HIE.

**References:** Lott, J.W.: Immunology and infectious disease. In Verklan, M.T., Walden, M. (Eds.): *Core Curriculum for Neonatal Intensive Care Nursing,* 4th ed. St. Louis, Saunders, 2010, pp. 715-716.

Lynam, L., Verklan, M.T.: Neurologic disorders. In Verklan, M.T., Walden, M. (Eds.): *Core Curriculum for Neonatal Intensive Care Nursing,* 4th ed. St. Louis, Saunders, 2010, p. 779.

17. **(D)** A large base deficit and low Apgar score at 5 minutes are indicative of severe perinatal depression and meet the criteria for treatment with hypothermia. Infants with more severe hypoxic-ischemic encephalopathy (HIE) have hypotonia. $Po_2$ is not considered in the criteria for hypothermia. More severe HIE is characterized by stupor or coma, not irritability. A $Pco_2$ of 55 would not affect the decision to treat with hypothermia. A base deficit of −9 and hyperalertness would be considered mild HIE, which does not require hypothermia treatment.

**References:** Blackburn, S.T., Ditzenberger, G.R.: Neurologic system. In Kenner, C.A., Lott, J.W. (Eds.): *Comprehensive Neonatal Care: An Interdisciplinary Approach,* 4th ed. St. Louis, Saunders, 2007, p. 282.

Lynam, L., Verklan, M.T.: Neurologic disorders. In Verklan, M.T., Walden, M. (Eds.): *Core Curriculum for Neonatal Intensive Care Nursing,* 4th ed. St. Louis, Saunders, 2010, p. 775.

18. **(C)** Rapid volume expansion may cause rupture of germinal matrix vessels resulting in intraventricular hemorrhage (IVH). A large patent ductus arteriosus is a risk factor for IVH. Closure would be beneficial. Central nervous system malformation may carry a slightly higher risk of seizure activity but not of IVH. The risk of IVH decreases with advancing gestational age.

**Reference:** Lynam, L., Verklan, M.T.: Neurologic disorders. In Verklan, M.T., Walden, M. (Eds.): *Core Curriculum for Neonatal Intensive Care Nursing,* 4th ed. St. Louis, Saunders, 2010, p. 769.

19. **(C)** Rapid volume expansion may cause rupture of germinal matrix vessels. Fluid overload may cause pulmonary edema regardless of the rate of infusion. The kidneys of a newborn are less effective at excreting excess fluid than those of an older infant. Fluid administration in the neonate is controlled by volumetric infusion pumps. Vascular access catheters rarely are a limiting factor in the rate of fluid administration in neonates.

**Reference:** Lynam, L., Verklan, M.T.: Neurologic disorders. In Verklan, M.T., Walden, M. (Eds.): *Core Curriculum for Neonatal Intensive Care Nursing,* 4th ed. St. Louis, Saunders, 2010, p. 769.

20. **(D)** Erb palsy is the injury of cranial nerves V and VI in the brachial plexus due to excessive stretching, rotation, or lateral flexion of the neck during a difficult delivery. These nerves innervate the upper arm, affecting movement. Respiratory distress is a sign of phrenic nerve paralysis. Facial drooping is a sign of facial

nerve palsy. A hand held in a claw posture is a sign of Klumpke paralysis, which involves injury to spinal nerves in the region of C6 to T1.

**Reference:** Lynam, L., Verklan, M.T.: Neurologic Disorders. In Verklan, M.T., Walden, M. (Eds.): *Core Curriculum for Neonatal Intensive Care Nursing,* 4th ed. St. Louis, Saunders, 2010, p. 764.

21. **(D)** Initial management of Erb palsy is aimed at resting the involved extremity until swelling and inflammation subside. Surgical repair is undertaken much later only if there is no spontaneous recovery. Erb palsy is not caused by viral infection, so antiviral medication would not be helpful. Passive range-of-motion exercise and physical therapy are usually initiated after 5 to 10 days.

**Reference:** Lynam, L., Verklan, M.T.: Neurologic disorders. In Verklan, M.T., Walden, M. (Eds.): *Core Curriculum for Neonatal Intensive Care Nursing,* 4th ed. St. Louis, Saunders, 2010, p. 765.

22. **(A)** Cranial nerve IX is responsible for taste, swallowing, and gagging. Cranial nerve XII is responsible for tongue movement and symmetric movements allowing sucking. The cerebral cortex is the seat of the intellect. Peripheral nerves support movement and sensation of the extremities. The autonomic nervous system regulates automatic functions such as heart rate, breathing, secretions, and gastrointestinal motility.

**References:** Blackburn, S.T., Ditzenberger, G.R.: Neurologic system. In Kenner, C.A., Lott, J.W. (Eds.): *Comprehensive Neonatal Care: An Interdisciplinary Approach,* 4th ed. St. Louis, Saunders, 2007, pp. 275-276.

Lynam, L., Verklan, M.T.: Neurologic disorders. In Verklan, M.T., Walden, M. (Eds.): *Core Curriculum for Neonatal Intensive Care Nursing,* 4th ed. St. Louis, Saunders, 2010, p. 754.

23. **(B)** Early-onset meningitis is noted for rapid progression to shock. Infants who show signs of early shock should undergo a lumbar puncture as soon as possible when in stable condition and able to tolerate the procedure. Blueberry muffin rash is indicative of viral infection. Pulmonary hypertension may accompany critical illness in the newborn period but is not indicative of meningitis. Later-onset meningitis presents with subtle and nonspecific symptoms.

**Reference:** Lynam, L., Verklan, M.T.: Neurologic disorders. In Verklan, M.T., Walden, M. (Eds.): *Core Curriculum for Neonatal Intensive Care Nursing,* 4th ed. St. Louis, Saunders, 2010, p. 779.

24. **(C)** Although treatment for seizures is controversial, benzodiazepines have been used successfully in neonates to treat seizures refractory to phenobarbital. Vitamin $B_6$ is useful in the treatment of a very rare type of seizure caused by a congenital abnormality of pyridoxine dependency but would not be effective for seizures of any other cause and is not used unless other causes have been ruled out. Excess absorption of medications such as lidocaine may cause seizure activity. Neuromuscular blockers would mask seizures by stopping any movements but would not treat the abnormal electrical discharges in the brain.

**Reference:** Blackburn, S.T., Ditzenberger, G.R.: Neurologic system. In Kenner, C., Lott, J.W. (Eds.): *Comprehensive Neonatal Care: An Interdisciplinary Approach,* 4th ed. St. Louis, Saunders, 2007, p. 280.

25. **(A)** Hypothermia therapy for hypoxic-ischemic encephalopathy is aimed at preventing secondary damage from the reperfusion phase, which begins by 6 to 12 hours after the insult. Unchecked, this phase is characterized by hyperexcitability and cytotoxic edema, damage from the release of free radicals and nitric oxide, inflammatory changes, and imbalances in inhibitory and excitatory neurotransmitters with secondary neuronal death due to necrosis or apoptosis. Studies have shown that 6 hours is the therapeutic window before further cell death occurs. Starting cooling as soon as possible also decreases cerebral metabolism and edema. Waiting until 12 hours would not be effective. Head and body cooling program criteria require initiation of therapy by 6 hours after birth. Upon admission, stabilization and assessment of the infant for inclusion criteria are priorities.

**References:** Blackburn, S.T., Ditzenberger, G.R.: Neurologic system. In Kenner, C.A., Lott, J.W. (Eds.): *Comprehensive Neonatal Care: An Interdisciplinary Approach,* 4th ed. St. Louis, Saunders, 2007, pp. 281-282.

Lynam, L., Verklan, M.T.: Neurologic disorders. In Verklan, M.T., Walden, M. (Eds.): *Core Curriculum for Neonatal Intensive Care Nursing,* 4th ed. St. Louis, Saunders, 2010, p. 777.

26. **(B)** The neonatal brain is dependent on glucose and cannot use alternative substrate. The neonatal central nervous system is quickly and significantly affected by hypoglycemia. Glycogen stores are minimal or nonexistent in the premature infant, and the brain requires oxygen and glucose for the energy for growth and metabolism. Blood glucose levels of less than 30 mg/dl are associated with increased cerebral blood flow in an attempt to maintain glucose levels. Hyperglycemia does not have this effect.

**Reference:** Lynam, L., Verklan, M.T.: Neurologic disorders. In Verklan, M.T., Walden, M. (Eds.): *Core Curriculum for Neonatal Intensive Care Nursing,* 4th ed. St. Louis, Saunders, 2010, p. 751.

27. **(B)** The criteria for brain death in the pediatric population are generally agreed upon as electroencephalographic silence, absence of cerebral blood flow, and absence of brainstem function. Anencephalic infants generally have brainstem function and can breathe unassisted; therefore, they do not meet brain death criteria. Anencephalic infants lack cerebral tissue and thus would not have cerebral blood flow. Parents are advocates for their infants and, with the help of staff, decide if and when to withdraw support, but they do not have to make the determination of brain death, which requires the expertise of a neurologist. Ethics committees make recommendations that aid staff and family in resolving difficult dilemmas but do not mandate care or determine brain death.

**References:** Driscoll, K.M., Sudia-Robinson, T.: Legal and ethical issues of neonatal care. In Kenner, C.A., Lott, J.W. (Eds.): *Comprehensive Neonatal Care: An Interdisciplinary Approach,* 3rd ed. St. Louis, Saunders, 2003, pp. 56-57.

Lynam, L., Verklan, M.T.: Neurologic disorders. In Verklan, M.T., Walden, M. (Eds.): *Core Curriculum for Neonatal Intensive Care Nursing,* 4th ed. St. Louis, Saunders, 2010, pp. 753-754.

28. **(A)** Neuromuscular blockade masks signs of agitation and pain. Since sensation remains intact, analgesics should be used before and during administration of paralytics. Neuromuscular blockers prevent acetylcholine from binding to the receptors on the muscle end plate, thus blocking depolarization, but do nothing to block sensory or pain receptors. Neostigmine is used to reverse the effects of a nondepolarizing agent and would cancel out the effects if given concurrently. Atropine, an anticholinergic, is frequently given with neuromuscular blockers before intubation to block vagal tone, but neuromuscular blockers do not have anticholinergic effects.

**References:** Heiss-Harris, G.M., Bailey, T.: Common invasive procedures. In Verklan, M.T., Walden, M. (Eds.): *Core Curriculum for Neonatal Intensive Care Nursing,* 4th ed. St. Louis, Saunders, 2010, p. 304.

Walden, M.: Pain assessment and management. In Verklan, M.T., Walden, M. (Eds.): *Core Curriculum for Neonatal Intensive Care Nursing,* 4th ed. St. Louis, Saunders, 2010, p. 344.

Young, T.E., Mangum, B.: *NeoFax,* 22nd ed. Montvale, N.J., Thomson Reuters, 2009, pp. 211-213.

## CHAPTER 20: RENAL AND GENITOURINARY DISORDERS

1. **(A)** Circumcision is avoided until the time of surgical repair. The foreskin may be needed for urethroplasty and/or penile shaft skin coverage. An abnormal amount of urine output is not a complication associated with isolated hypospadias. Surgical correction is anticipated to occur at 6 to 12 months of age. Urinary tract infections are not increased as a result of hypospadias, and antibiotic prophylaxis is not warranted.

**Reference:** Botwinski, C.: Renal and genitourinary disorders. In Verklan, M.T., Walden, M. (Eds.): *Core Curriculum for Neonatal Intensive Care Nursing,* 4th ed. St. Louis, Saunders, 2010, pp. 741-742.

2. **(B)** A voiding cystourethrogram is performed as soon as the infection has been controlled to assess for vesicoureteral reflux, which occurs in a substantial percentage of neonates with urinary tract infections and is associated with renal scarring. Hypospadias is a visual diagnosis. Ultrasonography and renal flow studies are tests for the diagnosis of renal vein thrombosis. Renal ultrasonography and renal scans are used for the diagnosis of polycystic kidney disease.

**Reference:** Botwinski, C.: Renal and genitourinary disorders. In Verklan, M.T., Walden, M. (Eds.): *Core Curriculum for Neonatal Intensive Care Nursing,* 4th ed. St. Louis, Saunders, 2010, pp. 741-742.

3. **(C)** Renal function is dependent on local prostaglandin production, which is inhibited by indomethacin administration. Indomethacin use is almost always associated with decreased urine output, elevated serum creatinine level, and hyponatremia. Low-dose dopamine leads to selective renal vasodilation and an increase in urine output in the preterm infant. Furosemide leads to prostaglandin production, which results in increased renal blood flow. It acts primarily at the ascending limb of Henle, leading to urinary losses of sodium, potassium, chloride, calcium, and magnesium. Renal effects of aminophylline include diuresis and increased urinary calcium excretion.

**References:** Frost, M.S., Fashaw, L., Hernandez, J.A., et al.: Neonatal nephrology. In Gardner, S.L., Carter, B.S., Enzman-Hines, M., et al. (Eds.): *Merenstein and Gardner's Handbook of Neonatal Intensive Care,* 7th ed. St. Louis, Mosby, 2011, p. 723.

Young, T.E., Mangum, B.: *NeoFax,* 22nd ed. Montvale, N.J., Thomson Reuters, 2009, pp. 164-165.

4. **(D)** Normal kidney mass is replaced by cysts, with the amount of cystic tissue determining the severity of the disease. The prognosis for this disease depends on the degree of damage to the kidney. Elevation in blood pressure is thought to be related to a decrease in arterial renal perfusion and an increase in renin levels. Complete or partial nephrectomy of the affected kidney can halt this problem. A voiding cystourethrogram is a diagnostic test to identify obstruction to urine flow; it is not intended to serve as a routine measure of urinary function. Glucosuria may be attributed to alterations in renal function, but not specifically to multicystic dysplastic kidney disease. Infants are at risk for failure to thrive and need aggressive enteral nutrition, but weight is not a critical parameter to measure.

**References:** Frost, M.S., Fashaw, L., Hernandez, J.A., et al.: Neonatal nephrology. In Gardner, S.L., Carter, B.S., Enzman-Hines, M., et al. (Eds.): *Merenstein and Gardner's Handbook of Neonatal Intensive Care,* 7th ed. St. Louis, Mosby, 2011, pp. 739-740.

Parker, L.: Genitourinary dysfunction. In Kenner, C.A., Wright Lott, J.W. (Eds.): *Comprehensive Neonatal Care: An Interdisciplinary Approach,* 4th ed. Philadelphia, Saunders, 2007, pp. 191-192.

5. **(C)** Postrenal causes are those leading to obstruction of urine flow distal to the kidney. Posterior urethral valves obstruct the flow of urine from the kidney and bladder. Abnormalities of the bladder wall may develop, along with vesicoureteral reflux, leading to parenchymal renal damage. Hypotension is classified as a prerenal cause of acute renal failure. Perinatal asphyxia is considered a prerenal cause because it leads to a decrease in renal blood flow resulting in compromise in renal function. Indomethacin administration leads to prerenal and intrinsic renal failure because local prostaglandin production is inhibited by indomethacin.

**References:** Botwinski, C.: Renal and genitourinary disorders. In Verklan, M.T., Walden, M. (Eds.): *Core Curriculum for Neonatal Intensive Care Nursing,* 4th ed. St. Louis, Mosby, 2010, pp. 728-731.

Parker, L.: Genitourinary dysfunction. In Kenner, C.A., Wright Lott, J.W. (Eds.): *Comprehensive Neonatal Care: An Interdisciplinary Approach,* 4th ed. Philadelphia, Saunders, 2007, p. 187.

6. **(D)** Ureteropelvic junction obstruction prevents the flow of urine from the kidney into the bladder. This results in a backup of urine and subsequent dilation of the structures of the kidney and can lead to intrinsic renal failure. Hypospadias is not associated with blockage of urine from the kidney leading to hydronephrosis. A patent urachus creates a connection between the bladder and the umbilicus and does not cause an obstruction to kidney outflow. A urinary tract infection can result from urinary stasis and anomalies associated with hydronephrosis, but is not a cause of hydronephrosis.

**Reference:** Botwinski, C.: Renal and genitourinary disorders. In Verklan, M.T., Walden, M. (Eds.): *Core Curriculum for Neonatal Intensive Care Nursing,* 4th ed. St. Louis, Saunders, 2010, p. 736.

7. **(A)** Furosemide (Lasix) inhibits active chloride transport in the ascending limb of the loop of Henle and results in increased excretion of several substances, particularly sodium, potassium, chloride, and calcium. Glucose homeostasis is not influenced by the use of furosemide. Hyponatremia, not hypernatremia, is a side effect of furosemide due to increased excretion. Chloride is lost as an effect of furosemide therapy.

**Reference:** Young, T.E., Mangum, B.: *NeoFax,* 22nd ed. Montvale, N.J., Thomson Reuters, 2009, p. 232.

8. **(D)** If the blood pressure cuff is too small for the extremity, the measurement will be higher than the true reading, and if the cuff is too large, the measurement will be artificially low. Measuring with an appropriately sized cuff is critical to obtaining an accurate measurement, which will guide treatment. Urine output and the concentrating ability of the kidney are important but are not primary indices in hypertension, and monitoring them is not as critical as measuring blood pressure. Restricting fluid intake is not part of the treatment for hypertension. Targeting weight gain is unrelated to the monitoring of hypertension.

**Reference:** Botwinski, C.: Renal and genitourinary disorders. In Verklan, M.T., Walden, M. (Eds.): *Core Curriculum for Neonatal Intensive Care Nursing,* 4th ed. St. Louis, Saunders, 2010, pp. 731-733.

9. **(B)** Vomiting is a symptom of incarceration due to obstruction of the normal passage of abdominal contents. An incarcerated inguinal hernia does not directly affect urinary output. Apnea and bradycardia are not associated with incarceration of the involved intestine. Transillumination of the scrotum cannot detect incarcerated inguinal hernia, but is helpful distinguishing a hydrocele from a hernia.

**Reference:** Tappero, E., Witt, C.: Neonatal gastrointestinal surgical conditions. In Longobucco, D.B., Ruth, V.A. (Eds.): *Neonatal Surgical Procedures: A Guide for Care and Management.* Santa Rosa, Calif., NICU Ink, 2007, pp. 181-186.

10. **(C)** Congenital adrenal hyperplasia, or adrenogenital syndrome, usually presents with early signs such as lethargy, diarrhea, poor feeding, and vomiting. If salt-wasting disease is present, profound hyponatremia may occur, typically after 7 days of age. Later symptoms may include further electrolyte abnormalities, hypoglycemia, metabolic acidosis, and shock. Hyperthyroidism presents with irritability, tremors, hyperactivity, sweating, hyperthermia, vomiting, diarrhea, and tachycardia. Intraventricular hemorrhage is unusual in a term infant, and the majority of these occur within the first 2 days of age. Low breast milk supply may lead to jaundice, poor feeding, dehydration, and elevated serum sodium levels.

**Reference:** Stokowski, L.: Endocrine disorders. In Verklan, M.T., Walden, M. (Eds.): *Core Curriculum for Neonatal Intensive Care Nursing,* 4th ed. St. Louis, Saunders, 2010, pp. 650-654.

11. **(C)** Perinatal asphyxia is the most common cause of intrinsic acute renal failure. Cellular damage occurs in the glomerular, tubular, and collecting systems and results in dysfunction of these components of the renal system. Acute renal failure leads to an increase in creatinine level, hyponatremia, and a decrease in osmolality. The hyponatremia is due to the decreased excretion of free water, most likely caused by an increase in the secretion of antidiuretic hormone. This also results in the decrease in plasma osmolality.

**References:** Botwinski, C.: Renal and genitourinary disorders. In Verklan, M.T., Walden, M. (Eds.): *Core Curriculum for Neonatal Intensive Care Nursing,* 4th ed. St. Louis, Saunders, 2010, pp. 729-730.

Parker, L.: Genitourinary dysfunction. In Kenner, C.A., Wright Lott, J.W. (Eds.): *Comprehensive Neonatal Care: An Interdisciplinary Approach,* 4th ed. Philadelphia, Saunders, 2007, p. 188.

12. **(A)** Enalapril is known to lead to hypotension primarily in infants who are volume depleted. Electrolyte imbalance is not associated with enalapril use and would not lead to hypotension. Undiagnosed congenital heart disease has no bearing on the effect of enalapril on the vascular system. The speed of administration of the medication is not related to the effects seen.

**Reference:** Young, T.E., Mangum, B.: *NeoFax,* 22nd ed. Montvale, N.J., Thomson Reuters, 2009, p. 145.

13. **(D)** Correction of electrolyte abnormalities and hypervolemia is much faster when hemodialysis is used. Peritoneal dialysis can be conducted in the home. Hemodialysis requires administration of heparin to the infant, whereas peritoneal dialysis does not. Peritoneal dialysis is an appropriate treatment for multicystic dysplastic kidneys.

**Reference:** Frost, M.S., Fashaw, L., Hernandez, J.A., et al.: Neonatal nephrology. In Gardner, S.L., Carter, B.S., Enzman-Hines, M., et al. (Eds.): *Merenstein and Gardner's Handbook of Neonatal Intensive Care,* 7th ed. St. Louis, Mosby, 2011, pp. 730-731.

14. **(A)** Hyperkalemia may be caused by a metabolic acidosis, which pulls potassium out of the cells into the serum and leads to hyperkalemia. Giving sodium bicarbonate is a temporary measure to reduce the effects of the hyperkalemia by enhancing cellular uptake of potassium and thus lowering the serum potassium level. Myocardial excitability is lessened by administration of calcium, not sodium bicarbonate. Sodium bicarbonate does not directly influence renal excretion of potassium. Sodium bicarbonate administration raises serum pH. Metabolic acidosis, not alkalosis, facilitates potassium release from the cell and increases the serum potassium level.

**Reference:** Halbardier, B.H.: Fluid and electrolyte management. In Verklan, M.T., Walden, M. (Eds.): *Core Curriculum for Neonatal Intensive Care Nursing,* 4th ed. St. Louis, Saunders, 2010, pp. 163-165.

15. **(D)** Cystic renal disease is the most common cause of abdominal masses in newborns. Ascites is a generalized fluid collection that may lead to firmness over the entire abdomen, but it does not present as a mass. An ovarian tumor would be an extremely unusual problem

in a newborn. Testicular torsion manifests as a firm, discolored (red to blue) scrotum that may be painful.

**References:** Frost, M.S., Fashaw, L., Hernandez, J.A., et al.: Neonatal nephrology. In Gardner, S.L., Carter, B.S., Enzman-Hines, M., et al. (Eds.): *Merenstein and Gardner's Handbook of Neonatal Intensive Care,* 7th ed. St. Louis, Mosby, 2011, pp. 737-739.

Goodwin, M.: Abdomen assessment. In Tappero, E.P., Honeyfield, M.E (Eds.): *Physical Assessment of the Newborn,* 4th ed. Santa Rosa, Calif., NICU Ink, 2009, pp. 105-114.

## CHAPTER 21: GENETICS AND CONGENITAL ANOMALIES

1. **(C)** A dominant gene is expressed even if only one copy of the gene is present. In an autosomal dominant disorder, there is a 50% chance that the offspring of a given pregnancy will have the disorder. Although an autosomal dominant disorder has a 50% chance of inheritance with each pregnancy, it is not possible to predict whether or not future babies will or will not have the disorder. Both sexes are affected by autosomal dominant disorders.

**Reference:** Schiefelbien, J.: Genetics: From bench to bedside. In Verklan, M., Walden, M. (Eds.): *Core Curriculum for Neonatal Intensive Care Nursing,* 4th ed. St. Louis, Saunders, 2010, pp. 400-401.

2. **(A)** The genetic term *deletion* is defined as a loss of a chromosomal segment. Mosaicism is the nondisjunction of an anaphase lag that occurs during mitosis. This results in different compositions of genetic material within one individual. Translocation is the shifting of one segment of a chromosome to another site at which it is not normally located. Nondisjunction occurs when chromosomes are not successful in disjoining during meiosis or mitosis.

**Reference:** Schiefelbien, J.: Genetics: From bench to bedside. In Verklan, M., Walden, M. (Eds.): *Core Curriculum for Neonatal Intensive Care Nursing,* 4th ed. St. Louis, Saunders, 2010, p. 402.

3. **(C)** *VATER* is an acronym for *v*ertebral anomalies, *a*nal atresia, *t*racheoesophageal fistula, and *r*adial and *r*enal dysplasia. Three or more of the defects must be present for the diagnosis of VATER association. Abdominal mass, myelodysplasia, cardiac anomalies, ventricular septal defect, and a single umbilical artery are not features of VATER association. VACTERL association occurs when cardiac anomalies and limb defects accompany anomalies of the VATER association.

**Reference:** Schiefelbien, J.: Genetics: From bench to bedside. In Verklan, M., Walden, M. (Eds.): *Core Curriculum for Neonatal Intensive Care Nursing,* 4th ed. St. Louis, Saunders, 2010, p. 411.

4. **(B)** A disruption is an abnormality of morphogenesis caused by disruptive forces acting on the developing structures. Defects that result from amniotic bands are an example of disruption. A sequence is a group of anomalies resulting from a cascade of events initiated by a single malformation. Pierre Robin is an example of a sequence. A deformation is an alteration of morphogenesis caused by unusual forces on previously normal tissue. Clubfoot and plagiocephaly are examples of deformation. A malformation is an abnormality of morphogenesis caused by an intrinsic abnormal

developmental process. Examples are neural tube defects, cleft lip, and cleft palate.

**References:** Schiefelbien, J.: Genetics: From bench to bedside. In Verklan, M., Walden, M. (Eds.): *Core Curriculum for Neonatal Intensive Care Nursing,* 4th ed. St. Louis, Saunders, 2010, p. 409.

Sterk, L.: Congenital anomalies. In Verklan, M., Walden, M. (Eds.): *Core Curriculum for Neonatal Intensive Care Nursing,* 4th ed. St. Louis, Saunders, 2010, p. 783.

5. **(A)** An X-linked disorder is caused by an abnormal gene on the X chromosome. In X-linked recessive disorders, male offspring are affected and carrier females transmit the disorder. In almost all cases, only male offspring have the disorder. The mother will require genetic counseling with subsequent pregnancies. A dominant inheritance pattern requires that only one copy of a defective gene be present for its effect to be expressed. An individual with the faulty gene will always express the effect of the gene. An X-linked dominant disorder affects both sexes, but females have twice the risk of manifesting the disorder because their chances of receiving a mutant X chromosome are doubled. Because this mother is a carrier but does not have the disorder, the disorder cannot have a dominant inheritance pattern. An autosomal recessive inheritance pattern requires that the corresponding genes on both chromosomes of a pair be defective for the gene's effect to be expressed. The faulty gene is on an autosome (non–sex determining chromosome) and therefore either sex can be affected. The maternal history in this case suggests that the disorder is X-linked. An autosomal dominant inheritance pattern requires that only one copy of a defective gene be present for its effect to be expressed. An individual with the defective gene will always express the effect of the gene. Either parent can pass the gene on to sons or daughters. Because this mother is a carrier but does not have the disorder, the disorder cannot have a dominant inheritance pattern.

**Reference:** Schiefelbien, J.: Genetics: From bench to bedside. In Verklan, M., Walden, M. (Eds.): *Core Curriculum for Neonatal Intensive Care Nursing,* 4th ed. St. Louis, Saunders, 2010, pp. 400-401.

6. **(D)** Osteogenesis imperfecta is caused by mutations of *COL1A1* and *COL1A2* genes on chromosome bands 17q21 and 17q22. Patau syndrome, also known as trisomy 13, occurs as a result of an extra chromosome 13. Down syndrome, also known as trisomy 21, occurs as a result of an extra chromosome 21. Edwards syndrome, also known as trisomy 18, occurs as a result of an extra chromosome 18.

**Reference:** Sterk, L.: Congenital anomalies. In Verklan, M., Walden, M. (Eds.): *Core Curriculum for Neonatal Intensive Care Nursing,* 4th ed. St. Louis, Saunders, 2010, p. 794.

7. **(D)** Klinefelter syndrome is a genetic disorder related to several factors, including advanced maternal age, parental nondisruption errors, maternal meiosis errors, and production of XY sperm by older fathers. All of these factors increase the risk of the disease. Monosomy is the presence of only one chromosome of a normal pair, such as in Turner syndrome. Monosomy

is not a cause of Klinefelter syndrome. Paternal meiosis errors occur in germ cells during the formation of sperm and are not implicated in Klinefelter syndrome. In partial trisomy, some of a chromosome is missing due to nondisjunction, chromosome lag, or mosaicism. Partial trisomy is not a cause of Klinefelter syndrome.

**References:** Schiefelbien, J.: Genetics: From bench to bedside. In Verklan, M., Walden, M. (Eds.): *Core Curriculum for Neonatal Intensive Care Nursing,* 4th ed. St. Louis, Saunders, 2010, p. 402.

Sterk, L.: Congenital anomalies. In Verklan, M., Walden, M. (Eds.): *Core Curriculum for Neonatal Intensive Care Nursing,* 4th ed. St. Louis, Saunders, 2010, p. 793.

8. **(C)** Additional clinical features of trisomy 21 include brachycephaly with flattened occiput, low-set and malformed ears, generalized hypotonia, hyperflexibility of the joints, clinodactyly of the fifth fingers, wide spacing between the first and second toes, and loose skinfolds in the posterior neck. Clinical features of trisomy 13 include microphthalmos, malformed ears, umbilical hernia, omphalocele, cutaneous hemangiomas, and hand deformities. Clinical features of trisomy 18 include low birth weight in a term infant, ears that are low set and/or of abnormal shape, micrognathia and microstomia, rocker-bottom feet, clenched hand with flexed fingers, and flexion contraction of the middle two fingers. Clinical features of Turner syndrome include low posterior hairline with the appearance of a short neck, small stature, low-set ears, broad chest with widely spaced nipples, limb abnormalities, and ptosis of the eyelids.

**Reference:** Sterk, L.: Congenital anomalies. In Verklan, M., Walden, M. (Eds.): *Core Curriculum for Neonatal Intensive Care Nursing,* 4th ed. St. Louis, Saunders, 2010, pp. 786-787.

9. **(D)** DiGeorge syndrome is one of several velocardiofacial syndromes caused by a deletion in chromosome band 22q11. Fluorescence in situ hybridization is a genetic testing method used to detect microdeletions on chromosomes. A rectal biopsy is indicated in patients with Hirschsprung disease. Although congenital heart defects are common in infants with DiGeorge syndrome, there is no urgent need to obtain an electrocardiogram, nor would its findings be diagnostic of DiGeorge syndrome. The oxygen challenge test uses 100% oxygen to differentiate persistent pulmonary hypertension of the newborn from a congenital heart defect.

**References:** Matthews, A., Robin, N.H.: Genetic disorders, malformation, and inborn errors of metabolism. In Gardner, S.L., Carter, B.S., Enzman-Hines, M., et al. (Eds.): *Merenstein and Gardner's Handbook of Neonatal Intensive Care,* 7th ed. St. Louis, Mosby, 2011, pp. 792-793.

Sadowski, S.: Cardiovascular disorders. In Verklan, M., Walden, M. (Eds.): *Core Curriculum for Neonatal Intensive Care Nursing,* 4th ed. St. Louis, Saunders, 2010, p. 542.

Schiefelbien, J.: Genetics: From bench to bedside. In Verklan, M., Walden, M. (Eds.): *Core Curriculum for Neonatal Intensive Care Nursing,* 4th ed. St. Louis, Saunders, 2010, p. 406.

Sterk, L.: Congenital anomalies. In Verklan, M., Walden, M. (Eds.): *Core Curriculum for Neonatal Intensive Care Nursing,* 4th ed. St. Louis, Saunders, 2010, p. 791.

10. **(B)** A sequence is a group of anomalies resulting from a cascade of events initiated by a single malformation. Pierre Robin is an example of a sequence. The initial event in Pierre Robin sequence is mandibular hypoplasia, which occurs between the seventh and eleventh weeks of gestation. The tongue is held high in the oral cavity, which causes a cleft in the palate by preventing closure of the palatal shelves. A nonrandom occurrence of multiple anomalies is classified as an association. VATER association (*v*ertebral anomalies, *a*nal atresia, *t*racheoesophageal fistula, *r*adial and *r*enal dysplasia) and CHARGE association (*c*oloboma of the eye, *h*eart anomaly, choanal *a*tresia, *r*etardation, and *g*enital and *e*ar anomalies) are examples. An alteration of morphogenesis caused by unusual forces on previously normal tissue is classified as a deformation. Clubfoot and plagiocephaly are examples of deformations. An abnormality of morphogenesis caused by disruptive forces acting on the developing structure is a malformation. Examples of malformations are neural tube defects, cleft lip, and cleft palate. A single malformation may lead to a cascade of events, resulting in a sequence.

**Reference:** Schiefelbien, J.: Genetics: From bench to bedside. In Verklan, M., Walden, M. (Eds.): *Core Curriculum for Neonatal Intensive Care Nursing*, 4th ed. St. Louis, Saunders, 2010, p. 409.

## CHAPTER 22: IMMUNOLOGIC DISORDERS AND INFECTIONS

1. **(C)** A CSF glucose less than 25 mg/dl is abnormal and could indicate meningitis. Normal mean glucose values are 79-83 mg/dl (range 64-106 mg/dl) for preterm infants, and 51-55 mg/dl (range 32-78 mg/dl) for term infants. Normal mean CSF protein values are 75-150 mg/dl (range 31-292 mg/dl) for preterm infants, and 47-67 mg/dl (range 17-240 mg/dl) for term infants. An abnormal CSF leukocyte count is $\geq 22/mm^3$ for preterm infants, and $\geq 25/mm^3$ for term infants with 70% polymorphonucleocytes.

**References:** Lott, J. W. Infectious disease. In Verklan, M. T. and Walden, M. (Eds.): *Core Curriculum for Neonatal Intensive Care Nursing*. St. Louis, Saunders Elsevier, 2010, p.704.

Venkatesh, M. P., Adams, K. M. and Weisman, L. E. In Gardner, W. L., Carter, B. S., Enzman-Hines, M., and Hernandez, J. A. (Eds.): *Neonatal Intensive Care*. St. Louis, Mosby Elsevier, 2011, p. 568.

2. **(B)** Infants born to mothers who received antimicrobial therapy for suspected chorioamnionitis should undergo a full diagnostic evaluation, consisting of a complete blood count with differential and blood culture, and should receive empiric therapy for at least 48 hours depending on clinical course and laboratory results. Infants may undergo a limited evaluation if neither chorioamnionitis nor neonatal sepsis is suspected. Infants may be observed for 48 hours or longer without further evaluation or therapy if maternal chorioamnionitis is not suspected, there are no signs of neonatal sepsis, the infant's gestational age is 35 weeks or longer, and maternal intrapartum antimicrobial prophylaxis was given 4 hours or more before delivery to prevent group B streptococcal disease. If the foregoing conditions are met and the infant's gestational age is

38 weeks or longer, the infant may be discharged home after 24 hours if other discharge criteria are met and a caregiver able to comply fully with instruction for home observation will be present.

**Reference:** American Academy of Pediatrics Committee on Infectious Diseases: *Red Book*, 28th ed. Elk Grove Village, Ill., The Academy, 2009, p. 633.

3. **(C)** Serial CRP measurements at 24 and 48 hours improve sensitivity to 82%-84% and improve positive predictive value to 83%-100%. Serial measurements may be helpful in monitoring resolution of infection and guiding antibiotic therapy. CRP values are not affected by gestational age. CRP response is better in gram-negative infection than in CoNS. CRP sensitivity is only 60% during the early stages of the infectious process.

**Reference:** Venkatesh, M. P., Adams, K. M. and Weisman, L. E. In Gardner, W. L., Carter, B. S., Enzman-Hines, M., and Hernandez, J. A. (Eds.): *Neonatal Intensive Care*. St. Louis, Mosby Elsevier, 2011, p. 568-569.

4. **(D)** The lower limit of the total neutrophil count is $1750/mm^3$ at birth and rises to $7200/mm^3$ by 12 hours of age. It then declines to approximately $1720/mm^3$ by 72 hours of age. Values suggestive of infection include the following:

> Neutropenia: neutrophil count of $<1750/mm^3$
> Ratio of immature to total neutrophils (I:T) of >0.2
> Absolute band count of $>2000/mm^3$
> Total white blood cell (WBC) count of $<5000/mm^3$

From the WBC count ($4.7 \times 10^3/mm^3$) and differential (27% segmented neutrophils, 8% bands), the absolute neutrophil count (ANC) is calculated as follows:

> ANC = (% segmented cells + % immature cells) × WBCs
> ANC = (0.27+ 0.08) × 4700
> ANC = (0.35) × 4700 = $1645/mm^3$

I:T ratio is calculated as follows:

> Mature cells = segmented cells
> Immature cells = bands, metamyelocytes, myelocytes, promyelocytes
> I:T = (% immature cells) ÷ (% mature cells + % immature cells)
> I:T = (0.08) ÷ (0.27 + 0.08)
> I:T = 0.08 ÷ 0.35
> I:T = 0.23

For a WBC count of $8.25 \times 10^3/mm^3$; segs 52%; bands 12%, the ANC and I:T ratio are 5280 cells/mm³ and 0.18 respectively. An ANC of 5280 is within the expected range for age. An I:T ratio of 0.18 is slightly elevated, but still below the value suggestive of infection. Some perinatal factors (e.g., prolonged oxytocin induction, stressful labor, prolonged crying) may increase the ratio. For a WBC count of $6.1 \times 10^3/mm^3$; segs 32%; bands 4%, the ANC is 2196 and I:T ratio is 0.11; both values are within the expected range for age.

For a WBC count of $15 \times 10^3/\text{mm}^3$, with 17% segmented neutrophils and 3% bands, the calculated ANC and I:T ratio are $3000/\text{mm}^3$ and 0.15, respectively. Both values are within the expected range for age.

**Reference:** Polin, R.A., Parravicini, E., Regan, J.A., et al.: Bacterial sepsis and meningitis. In Taeusch, H.W., Ballard, R.A., Gleason, C.A. (Eds.): *Avery's Diseases of the Newborn*, 8th ed. Philadelphia, Saunders, 2005, p. 560.

5. **(C)** Maternal hypertension is associated with decreased total neutrophil counts. The cause is uncertain. Stressful labor and neonatal seizures are associated with an increased neutrophil count. Uncomplicated respiratory distress syndrome has no effect on the total neutrophil count in newborns.

**Reference:** Kapur, R., Yoder, M.C., Polin, R.A.: The immune system: Developmental immunology. In Martin, R.J., Fanaroff, A.A., Walsh, M.C. (Eds.): *Fanaroff and Martin's Neonatal-Perinatal Medicine: Diseases of the Fetus and Infant*, 8th ed. Philadelphia, Mosby, 2006, p. 797.

6. **(B)** Infectious pustulosis is usually caused by *Staphylococcus aureus*. Lesions are commonly found in the axillae, groin, and periumbilical area. Benign rashes, such as erythema toxicum and transient pustular melanosis, typically have a generalized distribution. Cultures of benign rashes produce negative results or grow contaminating organisms, such as *Staphylococcus epidermidis*. Eosinophils are seen on a Wright stain preparation of erythema toxicum. Neutrophils, but no organisms, are seen on a Gram stain preparation of neonatal pustular melanosis. The characteristic rash of *Candida* diaper dermatitis is confluent and intensely erythematous with satellite lesions. Laboratory analysis reveals fungal elements rather than bacteria. *S. epidermidis* infection does not present as described in the scenario, although it may be isolated as a contaminant in a benign rash culture.

**Reference:** Puopolo, K.M.: Bacterial and fungal infections. In Cloherty, J.P., Eichenwald, E.C., Stark, A.R. (Eds.): *Manual of Neonatal Care*, 6th ed. Philadelphia, Lippincott Williams & Wilkins, 2008, p. 297.

7. **(C)** Hydrocephalus with generalized calcifications and chorioretinitis are clinical findings suggestive of congenital toxoplasmosis. Herpes infection is associated with keratoconjunctivitis, skin vesicles, and acute central nervous system findings. Clinical findings in rubella include cataracts, cloudy cornea, pigmented retina, blueberry muffin syndrome, and certain cardiac abnormalities. Cytomegalovirus infection is associated with microcephaly, periventricular calcifications, thrombocytopenia, jaundice, and hearing loss.

**Reference:** Pan, E.S., Cole, F.S., Weintrub, P.S.: Viral infections of the fetus and newborn. In Taeusch, H.W., Ballard, R.A., Gleason, C.A. (Eds.): *Avery's Diseases of the Newborn*, 8th ed. Philadelphia, Saunders, 2005, p. 496.

8. **(D)** The use of sulfonamides, such as sulfamethoxazole/trimethoprim (Bactrim), is contraindicated in newborns because these agents displace bilirubin from albumin-binding sites. Ticarcillin has expanded gram-negative activity and can be used to treat susceptible *Pseudomonas* infections in newborns. Amikacin is indicated for treatment of infections with aerobic gram-negative organisms. Ceftazidime is used to treat sepsis and meningitis caused by susceptible gram-negative organisms.

**Reference:** Kapur, R., Yoder, M.C., Polin, R.A.: The immune system: Developmental immunology. In Martin, R.J., Fanaroff, A.A., Walsh, M.C. (Eds.): *Fanaroff and Martin's Neonatal-Perinatal Medicine: Diseases of the Fetus and Infant*, 8th ed. Philadelphia, Mosby, 2006, p. 802.

9. **(A)** Hand washing has been shown to be the most effective means of preventing nosocomial infections. Studies have demonstrated that administration of intravenous immune globulin (IVIG) does not decrease the incidence of nosocomial infection in newborns, possibly because pooled IVIG does not contain adequate amounts of antibodies specific against the pathogens that commonly cause nosocomial infection. Antibiotic prophylaxis in the newborn does not prevent nosocomial infection and may result in colonization or infection with fungi or drug-resistant strains of bacteria. The use of gowns by nursery personnel does not significantly alter infection rates in infants.

**Reference:** Adams-Chapman, I., Stoll, B.J.: Nosocomial infections in the nursery. In Taeusch, H.W., Ballard, R.A., Gleason, C.A. (Eds.): *Avery's Diseases of the Newborn*, 8th ed. Philadelphia, Saunders, 2005, p. 585.

10. **(D)** A preterm infant weighing less than 2000 g whose mother's hepatitis B surface antigen (HBsAg) status is unknown should receive hepatitis B immune globulin (HBIG, 0.5 ml) within 12 hours of birth if the mother's status cannot be determined, because the vaccine has potentially decreased immunogenicity in these infants. Term infants born to mothers not tested during pregnancy for HBsAg can receive HBIG up to 7 days after birth while maternal HBsAg results are awaited. The recommendations for term infants should be followed for preterm infants with birth weights of more than 2000 g.

**Reference:** American Academy of Pediatrics Committee on Infectious Diseases: *Red Book*, 28th ed. Elk Grove Village, Ill., The Academy, 2009, p. 354.

11. **(A)** Human immunodeficiency virus (HIV) has been isolated from breast milk and can be transmitted through breast-feeding. In the United States, HIV-infected women should be counseled not to breast-feed even if neonatal prophylaxis is given. If the infant has been given hepatitis B vaccine and hepatitis B immune globulin, breast-feeding by a mother positive for hepatitis B surface antigen poses no additional risk of hepatitis B infection for the infant.

**Reference:** American Academy of Pediatrics Committee on Infectious Diseases: *Red Book*, 28th ed. Elk Grove Village, Ill., The Academy, 2009, pp. 121, 354.

12. **(C)** Immunoglobulin G (IgG) placental transport begins at about 20 weeks' gestation, and the term infant has a complete store of maternal IgG antibodies, which protects the newborn from many viral and bacterial infections during the first months of life. IgA is not transferred transplacentally in significant amounts. IgE normally is produced only with induction of inflammation. Maternal-fetal transfer of IgM does not occur due to the large size of the IgM molecule. An

elevated concentration of IgM is indicative of infection in the fetus or newborn.

**Reference:** Williams, C.B., Cole, F.S.: Immunology of the fetus and newborn. In Taeusch, H.W., Ballard, R.A., Gleason, C.A. (Eds.): *Avery's Diseases of the Newborn,* 8th ed. Philadelphia, Saunders, 2005, p. 454.

13. **(D)** The rate of transmission is 60% to 100% during primary and secondary syphilis and decreases to 40% with early latent infection and 8% with late latent infection.

**Reference:** American Academy of Pediatrics Committee on Infectious Diseases: *Red Book,* 28th ed. Elk Grove Village, Ill., The Academy, 2009, p. 639.

14. **(B)** *Staphylococcus aureus* is a gram-positive coccus-shaped organism that is coagulase positive. *Escherichia coli* is a gram-negative rod. *Listeria monocytogenes* is typically a gram-positive rod. *Staphylococcus epidermidis* is a gram-positive, coagulase-negative cocci.

**Reference:** Puopolo, K.M.: Bacterial and fungal infections. In Cloherty, J.P., Eichenwald, E.C., Stark, A.R. (Eds.): *Manual of Neonatal Care,* 6th ed. Philadelphia, Lippincott Williams & Wilkins, 2008, p. 289.

15. **(D)** Coagulase-negative staphylococci are the organisms that most commonly cause nosocomial infections in the NICU, accounting for approximately 50% of bloodstream infections. *Enterococcus,* group B streptococci, and *Staphylococcus aureus* organisms each are responsible for fewer than 10% of nosocomial bloodstream infections.

**Reference:** Heath, J.A., Zerr, D.M.: Infections acquired in the nursery: Epidemiology and control. In Remington, J.S., Klein, J.O., Wilson, C.B., et al. (Eds.): *Infectious Disease of the Fetus and Newborn Infant,* 6th ed. Philadelphia, Saunders, 2006, p. 1183.

16. **(A)** Anemia occurs in 22% of infants receiving zidovudine. Zidovudine may cause granulocytopenia; therefore, neutropenia rather than neutrophilia is an adverse effect of its use. There are no common cardiovascular side effects related to zidovudine use. Electrolyte disturbances are not commonly reported with this drug.

**Reference:** Young, T. E., Mangum, B., and Thomson Reuters clinical editorial staff: *Neofax 2010,* 23rd ed. Montvale, NJ, 2010, p. 98.

17. **(A)** A gestational age of less than 26 weeks, hyperglycemia, and postnatal steroid therapy are risk factors for invasive fungal dermatitis, caused by microorganisms such as *Aspergillus* or *Candida* species, in the first 2 weeks of life. The characteristic lesions typically appear on dependent surfaces such as the back or abdomen. Parvovirus B19 infections may be associated with an erythematous facial rash and a symmetric maculopapular, lacelike, and often pruritic rash on the trunk, arms, buttocks, and thighs. Clinical manifestations of infection with *Escherichia coli* and *Staphylococcus epidermidis* do not typically include erosive skin lesions.

**Reference:** Bendel, C.M.: Candidiasis. In Remington, J.S., Klein, J.O., Wilson, C.B., et al. (Eds.): *Infectious Disease of the Fetus and Newborn Infant,* 6th ed. Philadelphia, Saunders, 2006, p. 1114.

## CHAPTER 23: DERMATOLOGIC DISORDERS

1. **(B)** Providing environmental humidity for preterm infants reduces insensible water loss. Routine bathing of a 24-week-gestational-age infant should be done with plain water only. Daily bathing may result in excessive drying and is not recommended. The safety of chemical solvents has not been established for preterm infants. Tape and other adhesives may be loosened from the skin with warm water. Skin disinfectants used for invasive procedures, such as povidone-iodine or chlorhexidine, should be completely removed from the skin to prevent absorption.

**References:** Houska-Lund, C., Durand, D.J.: Skin and skin care. In Gardner, S.L., Carter, B.S., Enzman-Hines, M., et al. (Eds.): *Merenstein and Gardner's Handbook of Neonatal Intensive Care,* 7th ed. St. Louis, Mosby, 2011, pp. 482-501.

Witt, C.: Neonatal dermatology. In Verklan, M., Walden, M. (Eds.): *Core Curriculum for Neonatal Intensive Care Nursing,* 4th ed. St. Louis, Saunders, 2010, pp. 813-831.

2. **(D)** Fewer fibrils connect the dermis and epidermis, which causes stripping of the epidermis when adhesives are removed. Because preterm infants have immature sweat glands, they have poor tolerance of excessive heat. The presence of fewer layers in the stratum corneum is a risk factor for insensible water loss in preterm infants. Lack of subcutaneous fat is a cause of heat loss in preterm infants.

**Reference:** Witt, C.: Neonatal dermatology. In Verklan, M., Walden, M. (Eds.): *Core Curriculum for Neonatal Intensive Care Nursing,* 4th ed. St. Louis, Saunders, 2010, pp. 813-831.

3. **(B)** Epidermolysis bullosa is characterized by vesicles and fragile skin. Interventions are needed to prevent secondary infections, which may result in death. Epidermolysis bullosa is not a cause of jaundice in infants. Neurologic dysfunction is not a characteristic of epidermolysis bullosa. Extremely dry and scaly skin is associated with congenital ichthyosis.

**Reference:** Witt, C.: Neonatal dermatology. In Verklan, M., Walden, M. (Eds.): *Core Curriculum for Neonatal Intensive Care Nursing,* 4th ed. St. Louis, Saunders, 2010, pp. 813-831.

4. **(C)** Strawberry hemangiomas increase in size for 6 months before spontaneously regressing. Treatment options for hemangiomas include corticosteroid therapy, laser surgery, or cryosurgery. Infants with intact hemangiomas do not have an increased risk of infection. Strawberry hemangiomas are not associated with genetic or chromosomal abnormalities.

**Reference:** Witt, C.: Neonatal dermatology. In Verklan, M., Walden, M. (Eds.): *Core Curriculum for Neonatal Intensive Care Nursing,* 4th ed. St. Louis, Saunders, 2010, pp. 813-831.

5. **(D)** Scalded skin syndrome is caused by a staphylococcal infection. Isolation and antibiotic therapy are needed to prevent the spread of the bacteria. Cutis aplasia is the congenital absence of an area of skin. It is not infectious. Erythema toxicum is a benign skin variation and pustular melanosis is a transient, benign condition. Neither requires treatment.

**Reference:** Witt, C.: Neonatal dermatology. In Verklan, M., Walden, M. (Eds.): *Core Curriculum for Neonatal Intensive Care Nursing,* 4th ed. St. Louis, Saunders, 2010, pp. 813-831.

6. **(B)** The four types of congenital ichthyosis all are hereditary: ichthyosis vulgaris (autosomal dominant), X-linked ichthyosis, lamellar ichthyosis (autosomal recessive), and bullous ichthyosis (autosomal dominant). Although adequate zinc is necessary for skin health, zinc deficiency is not a cause of ichthyosis. Congenital ichthyosis is not caused by an infectious agent. Maternal ingestion of mercury may cause central nervous system damage in the fetus but does not cause ichthyosis.

**Reference:** Witt, C.: Neonatal dermatology. In Verklan, M., Walden, M. (Eds.): *Core Curriculum for Neonatal Intensive Care Nursing,* 4th ed. St. Louis, Saunders, 2010, pp. 813-831.

### CHAPTER 24: AUDITORY AND OPHTHALMOLOGIC DISORDERS

1. **(A)** The incidence of retinopathy of prematurity is significantly higher in preterm infants with a birth weight of less than 1 kg and gestational age of less than 28 weeks.

**Reference:** Askin, D.F., Diehl-Jones, W.: Ophthalmologic and auditory disorders. In Verklan, M., Walden, M. (Eds.): *Core Curriculum for Neonatal Intensive Care Nursing,* 4th ed. St. Louis, Saunders, 2010, pp. 832-849.

2. **(B)** During and after an eye examination, infants should be evaluated for bradycardia and apnea. Infants may be restless after receiving mydriatic eye drops and undergoing an eye examination. Hypertension may result from mydriatic eye drops and eye examinations. Subconjunctival hemorrhage may be the result of birth trauma.

**Reference:** Askin, D.F., Diehl-Jones, W.: Ophthalmologic and auditory disorders. In Verklan, M., Walden, M. (Eds.): *Core Curriculum for Neonatal Intensive Care Nursing,* 4th ed. St. Louis, Saunders, 2010, pp. 832-849.

3. **(A)** Hearing screening is recommended for all newborns. Failure on the hearing screening is an indication for referral for further evaluation.

**Reference:** Askin, D.F., Diehl-Jones, W.: Ophthalmologic and auditory disorders. In Verklan, M., Walden, M. (Eds.): *Core Curriculum for Neonatal Intensive Care Nursing,* 4th ed. St. Louis, Saunders, 2010, pp. 832-849.

4. **(A)** Hearing screening aids in identifying infants at high risk for hearing loss. Infants who fail the screening should be referred for further evaluation. Failure on the hearing screening is not diagnostic of hearing loss. Gentamicin is a potentially ototoxic medication and can lead to permanent hearing loss. Repetition of the same screening test is not indicated. Infants who fail a hearing screening require further evaluation.

**Reference:** Askin, D.F., Diehl-Jones, W.: Ophthalmologic and auditory disorders. In Verklan, M., Walden, M. (Eds.): *Core Curriculum for Neonatal Intensive Care Nursing,* 4th ed. St. Louis, Saunders, 2010, pp. 832-849.

5. **(A)** Symptoms of a chlamydial eye infection include severe eyelid edema and purulent discharge. Silver nitrate is ineffective in preventing chlamydial conjunctivitis, and it is no longer the standard agent for eye prophylaxis. Eye prophylaxis should be administered as soon as possible after birth. Assessment of the eyes should be ongoing. If initial treatment with erythromycin ointment was ineffective, the infant will develop symptoms of conjunctivitis.

**Reference:** Askin, D.F., Diehl-Jones, W.: Ophthalmologic and auditory disorders. In Verklan, M., Walden, M. (Eds.): *Core Curriculum for Neonatal Intensive Care Nursing,* 4th ed. St. Louis, Saunders, 2010, pp. 832-849.

## Multisystem Considerations

### CHAPTER 25: MATERNAL-FETAL COMPLICATIONS

1. **(C)** Maternal use of sulfonylureas increases the incidence of neonatal hyperbilirubinemia and hypoglycemia. Apnea is not commonly seen in a 37-week-gestational-age infant. Infants of diabetic mothers are at risk for polycythemia and hyperviscosity. They are at greater risk of developing hypoglycemia than hyperglycemia.

**References:** Jacobson, G.F., Ramos, G.A., Ching, J.Y., et al.: Comparison of glyburide and insulin for the management of gestational diabetes in a large managed care organization. *American Journal of Obstetrics and Gynecology,* 93:118-124, 2005.

Moore, T.: Glyburide for the treatment of gestational diabetes. *Diabetes Care,* 30(suppl 2):S209-S213, 2007.

2. **(D)** Offspring of women treated with phenobarbital, phenytoin, and primidone have been reported to have abnormal clotting and hemorrhage, which appears to be caused by a decrease in vitamin K–dependent clotting factors. The exact mechanism of the defect is unknown but may involve phenobarbital induction of fetal liver microsomal enzymes that deplete the already low reserves of fetal vitamin K. Listlessness is a vague symptom of many concerns in the newborn. Hyperreflexia in the newborn may be seen in withdrawal from illicit drugs or from serotonin reuptake inhibitors and with cerebral palsy. Hypoventilation may be caused by pulmonary or cardiac disorders and should be investigated. It also may occur if the mother received opiates during the 4 hours immediately before delivery.

**Reference:** Meader, K.J., Pennel, P.B., Harden, C.L., et al.; Hope Work Group: Pregnancy registries in epilepsy: A consensus statement on health outcomes. *Neurology,* 71:1109-1117, 2008.

3. **(D)** Maternal thyroid hormones (triiodothyronine [$T_3$] and thyroxine [$T_4$]) cross the placenta in small amounts. The fetus depends on maternal $T_4$ in the first trimester of pregnancy until the fetal thyroid begins to concentrate iodine and produce $T_4$. During the second and third trimesters, the fetus is independent of maternal stores. Maternal thyroid hormones are believed to be important for fetal neurologic development in the first trimester. Tachycardia is associated with hyperthyroidism. A neonatal goiter is associated with maternal ingestion of thyroid medications. Hyperthyroidism is unlikely in the situation described.

**Reference:** Endocrine Society: Management of thyroid dysfunction during pregnancy and postpartum: An endocrine society clinical practice guideline. *Journal of Clinical Endocrinology and Metabolism,* 92(8 suppl):S1-S45, 2007.

4. **(D)** Alterations in placental perfusion and gas exchange occur when the mother's condition involves

a significant decrease in cardiac output. Reduced cardiac output leads to decreased uterine blood flow and diminished placental perfusion with a resulting impairment in the exchange of nutrients, oxygen, and metabolic wastes. Congestive heart failure in the newborn is associated with fetal-neonatal cardiac defects rather than a decrease in maternal cardiac output. Decreased placental flow from a decrease in maternal cardiac output may cause lower birth weight, intrauterine growth restriction, diminished brain growth, or pregnancy loss, but unless the infant is born very prematurely, intracranial hemorrhage is not an issue. Respiratory distress syndrome (RDS) is associated with prematurity. If the infant is born before term, RDS can be a complication.

**Reference:** Khairy, P., Ouyang, D.W., Fernandes, S.M., et al.: Pregnancy outcomes in women with congenital heart disease. *Circulation,* 113:517-524, 2006.

5. **(D)** Anticoagulants are often used to decrease the risk of thrombophlebitis, especially in women with artificial valves. Oral anticoagulants (e.g., warfarin sodium) cross the placenta and have been associated with fetal malformations when administered during the first trimester. Malformations associated with maternal warfarin use include nasal hypoplasia, stippled epiphyses, limb deformities, absent or nonfunctioning kidneys, anal dysplasia, deafness, seizures, Dandy-Walker syndrome, and focal cerebellar atrophy. Hypotension can develop if there is excessive bleeding in the fetus. Warfarin inhibits the synthesis of vitamin K–dependent clotting factors. Fetal hemorrhage is more likely to occur than microcytic anemia when there are low concentrations of these factors. Although warfarin sodium is a teratogenic medication, it is not associated with ambiguous genitalia.

**Reference:** Cotrufo, M., De Feo, M., De Santo, L.S., et al.: Risk of warfarin during pregnancy with mechanical valve prostheses. *Obstetrics and Gynecology,* 100(5 pt 1):1040, 2002.

6. **(D)** There is a genetic component to the development of asthma. However, if the asthma is well controlled during pregnancy, neonatal risks are low. Low birth weight is more common when maternal asthma has been poorly controlled. Respiratory distress is unlikely. Pulmonary hypoplasia is associated with conditions that compress the lung or limit lung growth as well as conditions that result in oligohydramnios.

**Reference:** National Asthma Education Prevention Program Working Group: *Managing Asthma During Pregnancy: Recommendations for Pharmacologic Treatment—Update 2004.* NIH Publication No. 05-3279. Bethesda, Md., U.S. Department of Health and Human Services, National Institutes of Health, National Heart, Lung and Blood Institute, 2004.

7. **(C)** Phenylketonuria (PKU) is an inherited disorder in which an enzymatic defect precludes conversion of the essential amino acid phenylalanine to tyrosine. The result of this defect is an accumulation of excessive amounts of phenylalanine in the blood. Dietary treatment needs to be maintained throughout life, and once dietary restriction is instituted, phenylalanine levels drop quickly. If reproductive-age women with PKU have high blood phenylalanine levels when they become pregnant, offspring will often have microcephaly and/or mental retardation. The incidence of low birth weight, cardiac defects, and characteristic facial features in these infants is also increased. Infants born to mothers with PKU usually do not have PKU themselves. Unilateral renal agenesis typically occurs sporadically. Bilateral renal agenesis can occur as an isolated defect or as part of a syndrome. Blindness is not a common finding in infants born to mothers with PKU. Microcephaly, rather than macrosomia, is commonly associated with PKU. Hypocalcemia is not a common finding. Although maternal PKU often results in low infant birth weight, intrauterine growth restriction is not a common finding. Hearing impairment also is not a common finding.

**Reference:** Maillot, F., Lilburn, M., Baudin, J., et al.: Factors influencing outcomes in the offspring of mothers with phenylketonuria during pregnancy: The importance of variation in maternal blood phenylalanine. *American Journal of Clinical Nutrition,* 88(5):700-705, 2008.

8. **(D)** Cigarette smoke contains some 4000 compounds, including carbon monoxide and nicotine, which cross the placenta and may affect the fetus. Research findings suggest neurotoxic effects of prenatal tobacco exposure on the newborn, including neonatal withdrawal symptoms. Prenatal nicotine exposure produces a dose-related response in the neonate. Although hypertonicity is common in withdrawal syndromes, seizures are generally not seen with nicotine withdrawal. Loose stools are associated with heroine and methadone withdrawal. Symptoms of withdrawal seen in the neonate include hypertonicity and irritability, but not respiratory depression.

**Reference:** Stroud, L.R., Paster, R.L., Goodwin, M.S., et al.: Maternal smoking during pregnancy and neonatal behavior. *Pediatrics,* 123(5):842-848, 2009.

9. **(B)** Screening newborns for the presence of drugs or drug metabolites in the hair and meconium is a more reliable method of detecting drug and alcohol exposure during pregnancy than are other methods (testing of urine and blood). Hair and meconium testing gives information about substance exposure over time, not just the presence or absence of a given substance at the time of the testing. Regardless, the level of substance exposure does not always correlate with the degree of clinical impact. Cocaine metabolites can be found in adult urine for up to 72 hours after ingestion. This will lead to a positive urine drug screen result in the mother, but not necessarily in the newborn. Although cocaine may be found in breast milk, the toxicology testing is performed using maternal urine.

**References:** Araojo, R., McCure, S., Feibus, K.: Substance abuse in pregnant women: Making improved detection and good clinical outcome. *Clinical Pharmacology and Therapeutics,* 83:521-524, 2008.

Fike, D.: Substance-exposed newborn. In Kenner, C.A., Wright Lott, J.W. (Eds.): *Comprehensive Neonatal Care: An Interdisciplinary Approach,* 4th ed. St. Louis, Saunders, 2007, pp. 404-436.

Koren, G., Hutson, J., Garen, J. Methods for detection of drug and alcohol exposure during pregnancy. *Clinical Pharmacology and Therapeutics* 83: 631-634, 2008.

10. **(B)** Obese pregnant women are more likely to have infants with macrosomia, which is associated with a higher frequency of shoulder dystocia. Infants of obese women are not at increased risk for spontaneous prematurity. However, obese women may have the comorbidities of hypertension and diabetes, which are medical indications for induction, and infants of these women may be at increased risk for prematurity. Microcephaly is not found at increased rates in the offspring of obese pregnant women. There is no evidence suggesting a causal relationship between maternal obesity and congenital heart defects.

**References:** Cedergren, M.: Maternal obesity and the risk of adverse pregnancy outcome. *Obstetrics and Gynecology*, 103:219-224, 2004.

Dietl, J.: Maternal obesity and complications during pregnancy. *Journal of Perinatal Medicine*, 33:100, 2005.

James, D. and Maher, M.: Caring for the extremely obese woman during pregnancy and birth. *The American Journal of Maternal Child Nursing* 34(1):24-30, 2009.

Morin, K., Reilly, L.: Caring for obese pregnant women. *Journal of Gynecologic, Obstetric, and Neonatal Nursing*, 36(5):482-489, 2007.

11. **(C)** In placenta previa, the placenta lies abnormally low in the uterus and may partially or completely cover the internal cervical os. The amount of fetal compromise relates to the extent of the placenta previa, the severity of maternal hemorrhage, the degree of the resulting fetal hypoxia, and gestational age at delivery. Placenta accreta is abnormal placental implantation in which anchoring placental villi attach to the myometrium. This can cause hemorrhage, disseminated intravascular coagulation, and need for hysterectomy in the mother. Unless it is associated with a placenta previa, placenta accreta poses more risk for the mother than for the fetus or newborn. In circumvallate placenta, the area from the chorionic plate to the extraplacental membranes is a raised ring due to folding or rolling of the membranes. Circumvallate placenta can be associated with recent or old hemorrhage. It is noted on examination after delivery. A succenturiate lobe, or accessory lobe, is one that is joined to the main placenta by a bridge or is entirely separated by a membrane. It is seen in 3% to 6% of placentas and increases the risk of postpartum hemorrhage and infection if it is retained.

**References:** Eller, A.G., Porter, T.F., Soisson, P., et al.: Optimal management strategies for placenta accreta. *British Journal of Obstetrics and Gynecology*, 116(5):648-654, 2009.

Maloney-Schuler, D., Lee, S.: *The Placenta: To Know Me Is to Love Me: A Reference Guide for Gross Placental Examination.* St. Mary's, Iowa, DSM PathWorks, 1998.

Oyelese, Y., Smulian, J.C.: Placenta previa, placenta accreta, and vasa previa. *Obstetrics and Gynecology*, 107(4):927-941, 2006.

12. **(A)** Magnesium sulfate is the most commonly used agent in the United States for the prevention of maternal seizures. Hypotonia and central nervous system depression have been reported as side effects in the neonate. Neonatal hypotension and hypertension are not common side effects of maternal magnesium sulfate therapy. Magnesium sulfate has no effect on the newborn's blood glucose level.

**Reference:** Creasy, R.K., Iams, J.D.: Preterm labor and delivery. In Creasy, R.K., Resnik, R. Iams, J.D., et al. (Eds.): *Creasy and Resnik's Maternal-Fetal Medicine: Principles and Practice*, 6th ed. Philadelphia, Saunders, 2009.

13. **(D)** The 2000 National Institutes of Health Consensus Statement supports giving a single course of corticosteroids to pregnant women at risk for preterm birth because it reduces the risk of death, respiratory distress syndrome, and intraventricular hemorrhage in preterm infants. Repeated antenatal corticosteroid therapy should not be routinely used because it carries risks to the fetus of impaired somatic and brain growth, adrenal suppression, neonatal sepsis, chronic lung disease, and death. Steroids are used to accelerate fetal lung maturity but have no affect on birth weight. Adrenal gland activity is not suppressed by steroid therapy. Risk of intraventricular hemorrhage is not increased by the use of prenatal steroids.

**Reference:** American College of Obstetricians and Gynecologists Committee Opinion No. 402: Antenatal corticosteroid therapy for fetal maturation. *Obstetrics and Gynecology*, 111:805, 2008.

14. **(D)** Measurement of umbilical artery velocity is used as a method of fetal surveillance for intrauterine growth restriction. Reversal of diastolic flow is highly predictive of in utero fetal demise within 24 hours and warrants immediate evaluation and/or delivery. A nonreactive result on the nonstress test indicates a lack of fetal heart rate acceleration in response to fetal movement. Many factors contribute to a nonreactive nonstress test result, including medications, maternal smoking, fetal structural or chromosomal anomaly, and fetal sleep cycles. The biophysical profile (BPP) includes the nonstress test and four parameters measured with ultrasonography. These parameters are amniotic fluid volume, fetal activity, fetal breathing movements, and fetal tone. The BPP is felt to assess indicators of both acute and chronic hypoxia. A score of 0 or 2 is given for each parameter. When the total score is 6 or less, intervention is warranted. Results of the contraction stress test (CST) are negative when there are no late fetal heart rate decelerations after uterine contractions. A negative CST result indicates adequate uteroplacental reserve.

**References:** Harman, C.R.: Assessment of fetal health. In Creasy, R.K., Resnik, R., Iams, J.D., et al. (Eds.): *Creasy and Resnik's Maternal-Fetal Medicine: Principles and Practice*, 6th ed. Philadelphia, Saunders, 2009, pp. 361-396.

Signore, C., Freeman, R., Spong, C.: Antenatal testing—a reevaluation. *Obstetrics and Gynecology*, 113(3):687-701, 2009.

15. **(A)** Effects of maternal narcotics administration on the neonate are related to dose, route, and timing. The effects of narcotics may be reversed by administration of the narcotic antagonist naloxone. The indications for naloxone administration in newborns are continued respiratory depression after positive pressure ventilation (PPV) has restored a normal heart rate and color, and a history of maternal narcotic

administration within the previous 4 hours. Dextrose is given to correct hypoglycemia. Epinephrine is given when the heart rate is lower than 60 beats/minute after 30 seconds of PPV and another 30 seconds of PPV combined with chest compressions. It is best administered via an umbilical artery catheter but may also be given via an endotracheal tube.

**Reference:** Kattwinkel, J., Bloom, R.S., American Heart Association, American Academy of Pediatrics: *Textbook of Neonatal Resuscitation*, 5th ed. Dallas, American Heart Association, 2006, pp. 7-10.

## CHAPTER 26: PAIN ASSESSMENT AND MANAGEMENT

1. **(D)** *Clinical utility* refers to the usefulness of a measure in supporting decision making about health-related practice for an individual infant in a particular setting and circumstance. *Feasibility* refers to how easily a given measure can be used in practice.

**Reference:** Stevens, B., Gibbins, S.: Clinical utility and clinical significance in the assessment and management of pain in vulnerable infants. *Clinics in Perinatology*, 29(3):459-468, 2002.

2. **(C)** Infants' responses to pain are affected by gestational age, frequency of prior painful procedures, time since last painful procedure, duration of hospitalization, and use of analgesics during the neonatal period. There is no evidence that opioid use, neurologic integrity, or intraventricular hemorrhage contributes to an inconsistent, less robust pattern of pain response in infants.

**References:** Craig, K., Whitfield, M., Grunau, R., et al.: Pain in the preterm neonate: Behavioral and physiological indices. *Pain*, 52:287-299, 1993.

Grunau, R., Holsti, L., Whitfield, M., et al.: Are twitches, startles, and body movements pain indicators in extremely low birth weight infants? *Clinical Journal of Pain*, 16(1):37-45, 2000.

Johnston, C., Stevens, B.: Experience in a neonatal intensive care unit affects pain response. *Pediatrics*, 98:925-930, 1996.

3. **(C)** Procedures should not be performed at the same time as other, nonemergency caregiving. Evidence suggests that after exposure to a painful stimulus, a preterm infant's pain sensitivity is accentuated due to increased excitability of nociceptive neurons in the dorsal horn of the spinal cord. There is not enough information to draw the conclusion that the infant is experiencing withdrawal. A more thorough assessment is required before changing opioid therapy. There are no data to indicate that a different pain tool is required.

**References:** Fitzgerald, M., Millard, C., McIntosh, N.: Cutaneous hypersensitivity following peripheral tissue damage in newborn infants and its reversal with topical anaesthesia. *Pain*, 39:31-36, 1989.

Fitzgerald, M., Shaw, A., McIntosh, N.: The postnatal development of the cutaneous flexor reflex: A comparative study in premature infants and newborn rat pups. *Developmental Medicine and Child Neurology*, 30:520-526, 1988.

4. **(C)** Parents have many concerns and fears about their infants' pain and about the drugs used in the treatment of pain. Suggesting sucrose as an alternative intervention and telling the parent that addiction is a psychologic dependence on a drug do not address or explore the parent's concerns. If the nurse does not provide analgesia, then the nurse is not advocating for the infant.

**References:** Franck, L.S., Allen, A., Cox, S., et al.: Parent's views about infant pain in neonatal intensive care. *Clinical Journal of Pain*, 21(2):133-139, 2005.

Gale, G., Franck, L.S., Kools, S., et al.: Parents' perceptions of their infant's pain experience in the NICU. *International Journal of Nursing Studies*, 41(1):51-58, 2004.

5. **(C)** Preterm infants have the neural anatomy and physiologic development to perceive and respond to painful stimuli at approximately midgestation. However, the brain's ability to modulate pain is much more limited due to immaturity of the pain descending pathways and limited cognitive capabilities. Adequate preemptive analgesia does not eliminate the need for postoperative pain management. Neuroanatomy, neurophysiology, and neurochemical systems are sufficiently developed in the bowel. Neurotransmitter response is not exaggerated after bowel surgery.

**References:** Anand, K., Carr, D.B.: The neuroanatomy, neurophysiology, and neurochemistry of pain, stress and analgesia in newborns and children. *Pediatric Clinics of North America*, 36:795-822, 1989.

Andrews, K., Fitzgerald, M.: The cutaneous withdrawal reflex in human neonates: Sensitization, receptive fields, and the effects of contralateral stimulation. *Pain*, 56:95-102, 1994,

Mitchell, A., Boss, B.: Adverse effects of pain on the nervous systems of newborns and young children: A review of the literature. *Journal of Neuroscience Nursing*, 34(5):228.e-236.e, 2002.

6. **(D)** A key principle of family-centered neonatal care is that parents and health care professionals must talk openly and honestly about acute and chronic pain associated with medical diseases, as well as about pain associated with operative, diagnostic, and therapeutic procedures. Providing 24% sucrose 2 minutes before the examination and asking the mother to watch her daughter's response to the examination while the nurse assists the ophthalmologist do not explore the mother's concerns nor facilitate family-centered care. Although it will be helpful to have the mother perform comfort measures, in the spirit of family-centered care, the nurse must first explore the mother's concerns and explain the benefits of the comfort measures.

**Reference:** Agency for Health Care Policy and Research: Acute Pain Management in Infants, Children, and Adolescents: Operative and Medical Procedures: Quick Reference Guide for Clinicians. Rockville, Md., U.S. Department of Health and Human Services, 1992.

7. **(B)** The safety and efficacy of sucrose for preterm and term infants has been reported in many studies. A systematic review of 21 randomized controlled trials found that administration of sucrose decreased crying time, heart rate, facial action, and composite pain scores during heel lance and venipuncture. There are no data concerning the maximum number of doses per day. Sucrose is indicated for procedural pain, not irritability. Sucrose modifies pain through opioid pathways. Some studies indicate that infants exposed to

methadone before birth are not comforted in the same fashion as infants not exposed to methadone.

**References:** Stevens, B., Yamada J., Ohlsson A.: Sucrose for analgesia in newborn infants undergoing painful procedures. *Cochrane Database of Systematic Reviews*, Issue 3:CD001069, 2004.

Stevens, B., Yamada, J., Beyene, J., et al.: Consistent management of repeated procedural pain with sucrose in preterm neonates: Is it effective and safe for repeated use over time? *Clinical Journal of Pain*, 21(6):543-548, 2005.

8. **(D)** Facial expression, crying, and body movement are the most widely studied behavioral responses to pain in infants. Responses are influenced by many factors, such as gestational age or maturation and frequency of undergoing painful procedures. Behavioral indicators are more specific than physiologic indicators. Infants do communicate pain and do so in nonverbal ways, such as facial action, cry response, body movements, and physiologic responses. Multiple tools assist in distinguishing between pain and stress.

**References:** Grunau, R., Craig, K.D.: Pain expression in neonates: Facial action and cry. *Pain*, 28:395-410, 1987.

Grunau, R., Johnston, C.C., Craig, K.D.: Neonatal facial and cry responses to invasive procedures and non-invasive procedures. *Pain*, 4:295-305, 1990.

Stevens, B., Johnston, C.: Physiological responses of preterm infants to a painful stimulus. *Nursing Research*, 43:226-231, 1994.

9. **(C)** Comfort measures may be sufficient for an infant undergoing ventricular tapping. EMLA cream (eutectic mixture of local anesthetics) reduces pain during circumcision, venipuncture, arterial puncture, and percutaneous venous catheter placement. There is no evidence to support the use of EMLA during ventricular taps. Opioids are used in clinical situations in which severe pain is assessed or anticipated. Continuous opioid infusions should not be given until there is assessment of continuous pain. Although the infant's pain responses should be documented, some comfort management needs to be provided for this infant.

**References:** Simons, S.H., Anand, K.J.S.: Pain control: Opioid dosing, population kinetics and side-effects. *Seminars in Fetal and Neonatal Medicine*, 11:260-267, 2006.

Taddio, A., Ohlsson, A., Einarson, T., et al.: A systematic review of lidocaine-prilocaine cream (EMLA) in the treatment of acute pain in infants. *Pediatrics*, 101:e1, 1998.

10. **(B)** The mechanism of action of nonnutritive sucking is thought to be related to its effect on nonopioid pathways, which are activated as long as the infant sucks on the pacifier. The pain-relieving properties of sucking are related to the number of sucks per minute, not gestational age. Once the pacifier is removed from the infant's mouth, the pain-relieving effects of nonnutritive sucking cease.

**References:** Boyle, E.M., Freer, Y., Khan-Orakzai, Z., et al.: Sucrose and non-nutritive sucking for the relief of pain in screening for retinopathy of prematurity: A randomised controlled trial. *Archives of Disease in Childhood—Fetal and Neonatal Edition*, 91(3):F166-F168, 2006. Epub January 20, 2006.

Campos, R.: Soothing pain-elicited distress in infants with swaddling and pacifiers. *Child Development*, 60:781-792, 1989.

Carbajal, R., Chauvet, X., Couderc, S., et al.: Randomised trial of analgesic effects of sucrose, glucose, and pacifiers in term neonates. *British Medical Journal*, 319(7222):1393-1397, 1999.

11. **(A)** The time of peak effect for fentanyl is 3 to 4 minutes, and it is the preferred analgesic when immediate pain relief is the goal. The time of peak effect for morphine is 45 minutes and the time of peak effect for meperidine is 20 minutes. Thus, neither would be the analgesic of choice in an emergency situation. Midazolam is a barbiturate without analgesic properties and should not be used for pain relief.

**Reference:** Anand K.J.S., International Evidence-Based Group for Neonatal Pain: Consensus statement for the prevention and management of pain in the newborn. *Archives of Pediatric and Adolescent Medicine*, 155:173-180, 2001.

## CHAPTER 27: PERINATAL SUBSTANCE ABUSE

1. **(B)** Alcohol is a known teratogen causing growth restriction, facial anomalies, and severe central nervous system dysfunction. Perinatal exposure to heroin may cause neonatal abstinence syndrome and low birth weight, but is not a cause of facial anomalies. Perinatal exposure to cocaine or amphetamines is associated with low birth weight and central nervous system dysfunction or irritability, but not with facial anomalies.

**Reference:** Pitts, K.: Perinatal substance abuse. In Verklan, M., Walden, M. (Eds.): *Core Curriculum for Neonatal Intensive Care Nursing*, 4th ed. St. Louis, Saunders, 2010, pp. 41-71.

2. **(D)** Cocaine-exposed infants are restless, irritable, tremulous, and hypertonic. Perinatal exposure to cocaine is associated with low birth weight. The startle reflex is easily elicited in infants exposed to cocaine. Infants do not experience withdrawal from cocaine.

**References:** Pitts, K.: Perinatal substance abuse. In Verklan, M., Walden, M. (Eds.): *Core Curriculum for Neonatal Intensive Care Nursing*, 4th ed. St. Louis, Saunders, 2010, pp. 41-71.

Weiner, S.M., Finnegan, L.P. Drug withdrawal in the neonate. In Gardner, S.L., Carter, B.S., Enzman-Hines, M., et al. (Eds.): *Merenstein and Gardner's Handbook of Neonatal Intensive Care*, 7th ed. St. Louis, Mosby, 2011, pp. 201-222.

3. **(D)** The Neonatal Abstinence Scoring System should be used every 4 hours for 96 hours to detect the onset and progression of withdrawal symptoms and to evaluate the effectiveness of therapeutic interventions. Assessment should begin at 2 hours of age. The initial score determines the need for additional assessment. If the infant's score is 8 or higher, scoring should be done every 2 hours for at least 24 hours. Pharmacologic treatment should be considered if three successive scores are 8 or higher.

**Reference:** Pitts, K.: Perinatal substance abuse. In Verklan, M., Walden, M. (Eds.): *Core Curriculum for Neonatal Intensive Care Nursing*, 4th ed. St. Louis, Saunders, 2010, pp. 41-71.

4. **(D)** Neonatal abstinence scores of 8 or less are indicative of control of withdrawal symptoms. Tremors may decrease with swaddling, but this factor alone is not useful in evaluating treatment efficacy. Although respiratory rate is part of the Neonatal Abstinence Scoring System, this rate alone is not used to evaluate

the effectiveness of treatment. The infant should develop a rhythmic sleep-wake cycle.

**Reference:** Pitts, K.: Perinatal substance abuse. In Verklan, M., Walden, M. (Eds.): *Core Curriculum for Neonatal Intensive Care Nursing,* 4th ed. St. Louis, Saunders, 2010, pp. 41-71.

5. **(B)** Clonidine, chlorpromazine, diazepam, methadone, morphine, paregoric, phenobarbital, and tincture of opium are used to treat opioid withdrawal in infants. Fentanyl is a narcotic analgesic, and midazolam is a benzodiazepine. Neither drug is used in the treatment of opioid withdrawal in infants. The administration of naloxone, a narcotic antagonist, may result in rapid withdrawal and seizures in the infant.

**Reference:** Pitts, K.: Perinatal substance abuse. In Verklan, M., Walden, M. (Eds.): *Core Curriculum for Neonatal Intensive Care Nursing,* 4th ed. St. Louis, Saunders, 2010, pp. 41-71.

6. **(D)** Infants with perinatal cocaine exposure are irritable and restless. Swaddling and decreasing environmental stimulation are effective strategies. Supine positioning for sleep is recommended for full-term infants to reduce the risk of sudden infant death syndrome. Pharmacologic therapy is not used in managing the symptoms of perinatal cocaine exposure. Cocaine-exposed infants are at risk for poor nutritional intake. These infants need small, frequent feedings.

**Reference:** Pitts, K.: Perinatal substance abuse. In Verklan, M., Walden, M. (Eds.): *Core Curriculum for Neonatal Intensive Care Nursing,* 4th ed. St. Louis, Saunders, 2010, pp. 41-71.

7. **(A)** Meconium analysis is a noninvasive method that can be used to detect perinatal drug exposure as early as the second trimester. Signs associated with neonatal abstinence syndrome, such as tremors or irritability, may also be caused by glucose or electrolyte imbalances. Maternal history may be used to determine whether neonatal drug screening is needed. Urine toxicologic testing detects only recent maternal drug use, within 5 days or less.

**Reference:** Pitts, K.: Perinatal substance abuse. In Verklan, M., Walden, M. (Eds.): *Core Curriculum for Neonatal Intensive Care Nursing,* 4th ed. St. Louis, Saunders, 2010, pp. 41-71.

# Section III: Professional Caring and Ethical Practice

## CHAPTER 28: FAMILY INTEGRATION

1. **(C)** Several psychologic tasks have been identified that the mother and family must accomplish to cope with the crisis of a premature birth or the birth of a sick infant. These include preparation for the possible loss of the infant, acknowledgment of failure to deliver a term infant, adaptation to the intensive care environment, resumption of interaction with the infant after the threat of loss has passed, and preparation for taking the infant home. Refusing to participate in the infant's care will not establish a healthy parent-child relationship. Discussing the infant with family members may help a mother express her feelings, but it is not one of the psychologic tasks she must

accomplish. Allowing friends and family to touch and hold the infant is not a psychologic task related to coping with the crisis.

**Reference:** Kenner, C.: Families in crisis. In Verklan, M.T., Walden, M. (Eds.): *Core Curriculum for Neonatal Intensive Care Nursing,* 4th ed. St. Louis, Saunders, 2010, p. 348.

2. **(B)** Chronic grief is frequently seen in parents of a disabled child, who is a constant reminder of loss. Denied grief is not a recognized form of grief. Unresolved grief may occur in families who are not dealing with their loss, regardless of the amount of time that has passed since the loss. Anticipatory grief occurs before an actual loss.

**Reference:** Kenner, C.: Families in crisis. In Verklan, M.T., Walden, M. (Eds.): *Core Curriculum for Neonatal Intensive Care Nursing,* 4th ed. St. Louis, Saunders, 2010, p. 355.

3. **(C)** Predictors of good maternal parenting outcomes include moderate to high anxiety levels, seeking information about the infant, demonstrating warmth toward the infant, making positive eye contact, and exhibiting effective caregiving. Visits that last for a short period of time, limited verbal interaction with the staff, and not seeking out information related to the infant's condition may be predictors of poor parenting outcomes.

**Reference:** Kenner, C.: Families in crisis. In Verklan, M.T., Walden, M. (Eds.): *Core Curriculum for Neonatal Intensive Care Nursing,* 4th ed. St. Louis, Saunders, 2010, p. 354.

4. **(A)** Interventions to encourage family-infant bonding include showing the infant to the family in the delivery room, encouraging the parents to participate in caretaking activities, modeling nurturing parenting behavior, and encouraging sibling visitation. All members of the family should be addressed to encourage family-infant bonding. The nurse should encourage family participation in caregiving because it promotes bonding. Quickly explaining all of the medical conditions and equipment in great detail may cause fear and decrease family-infant bonding.

**Reference:** Kenner, C.: Families in crisis. In Verklan, M.T., Walden, M. (Eds.): *Core Curriculum for Neonatal Intensive Care Nursing,* 4th ed. St. Louis, Saunders, 2010, p. 357.

5. **(C)** Mothers and fathers often have "incongruent grieving" in which they do not grieve at the same pace. This incongruence frequently leads to marital discord because of misconceptions about feelings and inability to communicate. Delayed grief occurs at a later time. Abnormal grief is delayed or complicated grief. Anticipatory grief occurs before an actual loss.

**Reference:** Kenner, C.: Families in crisis. In Verklan, M.T., Walden, M. (Eds.): *Core Curriculum for Neonatal Intensive Care Nursing,* 4th ed. St. Louis, Saunders, 2010, p. 355.

6. **(B)** Interventions for parents experiencing loss include physically bringing the family together and providing privacy; providing the family with mementos such as photographs, identification bracelet, footprints, and so on; and talking with the family about possible end-of-life care and arrangements. Assisting the parents in understanding the importance

of including siblings is an appropriate nursing intervention.

**Reference:** Kenner, C.: Families in crisis. In Verklan, M.T., Walden, M. (Eds.): *Core Curriculum for Neonatal Intensive Care Nursing,* 4th ed. St. Louis, Saunders, 2010, p. 355.

7. **(D)** Adolescents are at a turning point; they are moving from childhood into adulthood and often have conflict with the family. Adolescent parents may be trying to take on adult responsibilities while feeling that they are being treated like children. Teenagers have difficulty anticipating the long-term implications of their decisions. Teenage parents often have unrealistic expectations of their role as parents and lack parenting skills.

**Reference:** Kenner, C.: Families in crisis. In Verklan, M.T., Walden, M. (Eds.): *Core Curriculum for Neonatal Intensive Care Nursing,* 4th ed. St. Louis, Saunders, 2010, p. 351.

8. **(C)** An abnormal visiting pattern may be a sign of inadequate bonding. Behavior showing adaptation would be the mother's changing her schedule to accommodate the care schedule of the infant. Normal parenting would be characterized by a more consistent visitation pattern and longer visits. Positive attachment behavior is characterized by frequent parental visits, demonstration of parenting skills such as holding the infant and changing the infant's diapers, and positive comments when talking to or about the infant.

**Reference:** Kenner, C.: Families in crisis. In Verklan, M.T., Walden, M. (Eds.): *Core Curriculum for Neonatal Intensive Care Nursing,* 4th ed. St. Louis, Saunders, 2010, pp. 356-359.

9. **(D)** Parents are given a lot of information in a short period of time, and many medical conditions are foreign to parents. The nurse should periodically assess the parents' understanding of their infant's condition and their interpretation of the information that has been given to them. Information must be reinforced throughout the hospital stay. When a person is anxious, little information is actually heard or retained. Parents are an integral part of the infant's care and should be encouraged to see, hold, and participate in care as the infant's condition allows. Closing the curtain will isolate the family from the infant and increase stress and anxiety. To reduce anxiety, families should be informed of the infant's condition and the plan of care.

**Reference:** Kenner, C.: Families in crisis. In Verklan, M.T., Walden, M. (Eds.): *Core Curriculum for Neonatal Intensive Care Nursing,* 4th ed. St. Louis, Saunders, 2010, p. 352.

10. **(C)** The stages of grief include shock, denial or panic, anger, and acceptance. The statement "This is all your fault!" is consistent with anger. In the shock stage of grief, comments such as "Why me?" or "It's not fair" are expected. Denial behavior would include not accepting or not even acknowledging the loss. Acceptance behavior would not include statements of anger.

**Reference:** Kenner, C.: Families in crisis. In Verklan, M.T., Walden, M. (Eds.): *Core Curriculum for Neonatal Intensive Care Nursing,* 4th ed. St. Louis, Saunders, 2010, p. 355.

## CHAPTER 29: DISCHARGE PLANNING AND TRANSITION TO HOME

1. **(B)** Neonates and families undergo many transitions during hospitalization. The most anticipated and significant transition is the discharge to home. Successful transition of the high-risk neonate from hospital to home requires a thorough understanding of the identified criteria for discharge, as well as coordination and progression of activities that ready the neonate and parent for home care. Coordinated, comprehensive discharge planning with a safe transition to home is critical for the health and well-being of high-risk infants and their families. Discharge planning begins on admission to the intensive care nursery and continues throughout hospitalization. Each plan must be individualized to patient and family. Discharge planning is the responsibility of the discharging facility.

**References:** Charsha, D.A.: Care of the extremely low birth weight infant. In Verklan, M.T., Walden, M. (Eds.): *Core Curriculum for Neonatal Intensive Care Nursing,* 4th ed. Philadelphia, Saunders, 2010, p. 444.

Hummel, P.: Discharge planning and transition to home care. In Verklan, M.T., Walden, M. (Eds.): *Core Curriculum for Neonatal Intensive Care Nursing,* 4th ed. Philadelphia, Saunders, 2010, p. 383.

2. **(D)** Preterm infants in medically stable condition who remain in the hospital at 2 months of chronologic age should be given all inactivated vaccines recommended for that age. Full doses of vaccine are recommended by the American Academy of Pediatrics.

**Reference:** American Academy of Pediatrics: Immunization in special clinical circumstances. In Pickering, L.K. (Ed.): *2009 Red Book: Report of the Committee on Infectious Diseases,* 28th ed. Elk Grove Village, Ill., The Academy, 2009, p. 68.

3. **(C)** The increased frequency of oxygen desaturation and episodes of apnea or bradycardia while sitting in car safety seats suggests that preterm infants (<37 weeks' gestation) should undergo a period of observation in a car safety seat, preferably their own, before hospital discharge. An observation period of 90 to 120 minutes or the duration of travel, whichever is longer, is suggested. Some hospitals require a car seat observation period for infants with respiratory compromise in addition to infants born at less than 37 weeks' gestation. The group for which a car seat observation period is recommended by the American Academy of Pediatrics is premature infants born at less than 37 weeks' gestation.

**Reference:** American Academy of Pediatrics, Committee on Injury, Violence, and Poison Prevention and Committee on Fetus and Newborn: Safe transportation of preterm and low birth weight infants at hospital discharge. *Pediatrics,* 123:1425-1429, 2009.

4. **(B)** Preterm infants in medically stable condition who remain in the hospital at 2 months of chronologic age should be given all vaccines recommended for that age: DTaP, Hib, IPV, pneumococcal conjugate (PCV), and HepB. Rotavirus vaccine is also recommended at two months of age, however current formulations of the vaccine contain live virus. To prevent horizontal transmission in the NICU, immunization for rotavirus

is often performed on the day of discharge. Hepatitis A vaccine is recommended at 12 months of age. Oral poliovirus vaccine is a live vaccine and is not recommended. Influenza vaccine is not recommended until a chronologic age of 6 months.

**References:** American Academy of Pediatrics: Immunization in special clinical circumstances. In Pickering, L.K. (Ed.): *2009 Red Book: Report of the Committee on Infectious Diseases,* 28th ed. Elk Grove Village, Ill., The Academy, 2009, p. 68.

Department of Health and Human Services, Centers for Disease Control and Prevention: Recommended Immunization Schedules for Persons Aged 0-18 Years, 2010. Available at http://www.aap.org. Accessed 12/12/10.

5. **(C)** Rickets in infants attributable to inadequate vitamin D intake and decreased exposure to sunlight continues to be reported in the United States. It is now recommended that all infants, including those who are exclusively breast-fed, have a minimum intake of 400 IU of vitamin D per day beginning soon after birth. Supplemental folic acid, supplemental vitamin E, and human milk fortifier are not recommended for this population.

**Reference:** American Academy of Pediatrics: Prevention of rickets and vitamin D deficiency in infants, children, and adolescents. *Pediatrics,* 122:1142-1152, 2008.

6. **(C)** The National Institutes of Health Consensus Development Conference on Infantile Apnea and Home Monitoring defines an *apparent life-threatening event* (ALTE) as "an episode that is frightening to the observer and is characterized by some combination of apnea, color change, change in muscle tone, choking, or gagging." The terms *near-miss sudden infant death syndrome* and *aborted crib death* should be abandoned, because they may be misleading. Obstructive apnea is defined as absence of airflow with continued respiratory effort, associated with blockage of the airway. Obstructive apnea accounts for almost a third of apnea episodes in premature infants.

**Reference:** Farrell, P.A., Weiner, G.M., Lemons, J.A.: SIDS, ALTE, apnea, and the use of home monitors. *Pediatrics in Review,* 23:3-9, 2002.

7. **(C)** For family members who have watched their infant progress from total technologic dependency to a state of normalcy, the prospect of having the infant at home removed from the intensive care environment can be terrifying. Some families begin to find many excuses to delay discharge. Lack of a parent-infant bond is unlikely since the parent has been visiting regularly. Parents are an integral part of the discharge planning process. Conflict is unlikely to have developed with this highly cooperative parent.

**Reference:** Spitzer, A.R.: Care of the family in the neonatal intensive care unit. In Spitzer, A. (Ed.): *Intensive Care of the Fetus and Neonate,* 2nd ed. Philadelphia, Mosby, 2005, p. 1403.

8. **(A)** Routine health promotion and screening is an important part of the care of extremely low birth weight infants. The primary goal of health screening is early recognition and diagnosis of potential significant health conditions and neurodevelopmental disabilities. Preparing the infant for transition to primary care begins early in the hospitalization. Blood typing and screening is not a test done to prepare an infant for discharge. Each birthing hospital should establish a universal newborn hearing screening program. Significant hearing loss is one of the most significant abnormalities present at birth. In 2005, the American Academy of Pediatrics endorsed a report from the American College of Medical Genetics which recommended that all states screen newborn infants for 29 treatable genetic conditions and an additional 25 conditions that may be detected by screening. Routine screening for germinal matrix hemorrhage and intraventricular hemorrhage should be performed in infants of less than 30 weeks' gestation or less than 1250 g. A "discharge" head ultrasonography should be performed at term.

**References:** American Academy of Pediatrics, Committee on Fetus and Newborn: Hospital discharge of the high-risk neonate. *Pediatrics,* 122:1119-1126, 2008.

Charsha, D.A.: Care of the extremely low Birth weight infant. In Verklan, M.T., Walden, M. (Eds.): *Core Curriculum for Neonatal Intensive Care Nursing,* 4th ed. Philadelphia, Saunders, 2010, p. 444.

9. **(C)** The most common cause of cardiac arrest in infants and children is respiratory problems. Although heart disease may be a factor, it is not the leading cause of cardiac arrest in infants and children. Abnormal heart rhythms are an infrequent cause of cardiac arrest in infants.

**Reference:** American Heart Association: *BLS for Healthcare Providers.* Dallas, The American Heart Association, 2006, p. 47.

10. **(A)** Preterm infants should be placed supine for sleeping just as term infants should, and the parents of preterm infants should be counseled about the importance of supine sleeping in preventing sudden infant death syndrome. The American Academy of Pediatrics recommends that hospitalized preterm infants should be kept predominantly in the supine position, at least from the postmenstrual age of 32 weeks onward, so that they become acclimated to supine sleeping before discharge. Infant monitoring need not have been discontinued for the sleeping guidelines to be followed. The American Academy of Pediatrics has recommended that infant home monitoring not be used as a strategy to prevent sudden infant death syndrome.

**Reference:** American Academy of Pediatrics, Committee on Fetus and Newborn: Hospital discharge of the high-risk neonate. *Pediatrics,* 122: 1119-1126, 2008.

## CHAPTER 30: PATIENT SAFETY

1. **(D)** For multiple reasons, medication errors are more common in the NICU than in other units in the hospital. Also, these errors result in more harm to the patient compared with similar errors involving adult patients. Although multiple studies have been published examining the most common errors in the NICU, no one specific type of error (such as wrong dose) has been shown to be more common than other types of errors. Voluntary error reporting frequently results in underreporting of all errors in the hospital, not just in the NICU.

**References:** Fortescue, E., Kaushal, R., Landrigan, C., et al.: Prioritizing strategies for preventing medication errors and adverse drug events in pediatric inpatients. *Pediatrics,* 111:722-729, 2003.

Kaushal, R., Bates, D., Landrigan, C., et al.: Medication errors and adverse drug events in pediatric inpatients. *Journal of the American Medical Association,* 285:2114-2120, 2001.

2. **(D)** Independent double-checks have been shown to prevent 95% of medication errors when performed correctly. *Independent* means that each RN compares the medication with the order and the medication label, checking the important components (minimally, the "Five Rights") separately. Although pharmacy personnel serve as another check before dispensing, errors still occur at this stage.

**References:** Mills, P.D., Neily, J., Kinney, L.M., et al.: Effective interventions and implementation strategies to reduce adverse drug events in the Veterans Affairs (VA) system. *Qual Saf Health Care* 2008; 17: 37-46.

Institute for Safe Medication Practices: ISMP Medication Safety Alert! The Virtues of Independent Double Checks—They Really Are Worth Your Time! Available at: http://www.ismp.org/Newsletters/acutecare/articles/20030306.asp. Retrieved February 2, 2008.

3. **(C)** A safety culture is one that is focused on reducing safety problems by using a nonpunitive approach to errors, sharing error reports as a method for learning and improving, and focusing on systems issues. An atmosphere of mutual trust is established in which all staff members can talk freely about safety problems and how to solve them without fear of retribution. Often, when a safety culture is present, error reporting increases because staff feel confident about reporting issues. A no-blame approach reduces the accountability of health care professionals for following established safety procedures.

**Reference:** Edwards, W.: Patient safety in the neonatal intensive care unit. *Clinics in Perinatology,* 32:97-106, 2005.

4. **(C)** A nonpunitive approach to patient safety errors includes achieving a balance between understanding human error and holding health care professionals accountable for following established safety procedures. A no-blame approach reduces the accountability of health care professional for adhering to established safety procedures. When a nonpunitive approach is followed, the focus of patient safety efforts is on systems issues. A nonpunitive approach does not disregard reckless behavior of an employee who knowingly violates a rule.

**Reference:** Clifton-Koeppel, R.: What nurses can do right now to reduce medication errors in the NICU. *Newborn and Infant Nursing Reviews,* 8(2):72-82, 2008.

5. **(C)** Distractions are a major contributing factor to medication errors in health care. Reducing distractions in the health care environment is a challenge and requires a combination of interventions, including behavioral changes in health care providers, work flow modifications, and use of new technology. Although there are multiple sources of distractions, one study demonstrated that other staff members are the most common source.

**References:** Pape, T.: Applying airline safety practice to medication administration. *MedSurg Nursing,* 12:77-93, 2003.

Relihan, E., O'Brien, V., O'Hara, S., et al.: The impact of a set of interventions to reduce interruptions and distractions to nurses during medication administration. *Qual Saf Health Care,* 19: 1-6, 2010.

6. **(D)** Because NICU patients are nonverbal and unable to respond to patient identification prompts, there is an increased risk of misidentification errors compared to adult patients. Other reasons for increased risk include identification bands that are small and hard to keep in place and the possible presence of twins or higher sibling multiples. Current available research does not indicate an increased risk for wrong-drug errors in NICU patients. Due to the use of weight-based dosing, infants in the NICU are at an increased risk of wrong-dose errors. However, increased risk of patient misidentification has been specifically identified for NICU patients.

**Reference:** Gray, J.E., Suresh, G., Ursprung, R., et al.: Patient misidentification in the neonatal intensive care unit. *Pediatrics,* 117:43-47, 2006.

7. **(B)** Most of the safety events in the NICU are not reported via a voluntary reporting system but rather are identified via a "trigger" tool that is used concurrently or retrospectively. Most patient safety events in the NICU are preventable. The majority of patient safety events identified using a trigger tool result in harm to the patient. Trigger methods have been shown to be superior to other identification strategies such as voluntary reporting, nontriggered chart review, and administrative databases in the identification of adverse events in the NICU. System issues and communication problems are the most common causes of errors.

**Reference:** Sharek, P., Horbar, J., Mason, W., et al.: Adverse events in the neonatal intensive care unit: Development, testing and findings of an NICU-focused trigger tool to identify harm in North American NICUs. *Pediatrics,* 118:1332-1340, 2006.

## CHAPTER 31: RESEARCH

1. **(A)** A dependent variable represents the outcome variable or result of interest in a study. An extraneous variable is one that may obscure the relationship between the dependent and independent variables. An antecedent variable occurs before the study and has the potential to affect the dependent variable. An independent variable is the phenomenon that has a presumed effect on the dependent variable.

**References:** Sullivan-Bolyai, S. and Grey, M. In Lo-Biondo-Wood, G., Haber, J.: *Nursing Research: Methods and Critical Appraisal for Evidence-Based Practice,* 5th ed. St. Louis, Mosby, 2002, p. 206.

Norwood, S.L.: *Research Essentials: Foundations for Evidence Based Practice.* Boston, Pearson, 2010, p. 101.

2. **(D)** Generalizability is the characteristic that allows study results to be applied to a similar phenomenon in a different population. Validity refers to the ability of an instrument to measure the attribute that it is intended to measure. Validity is an essential element of generalizability. Reliability refers to the ability of an instrument to consistently measure the attribute of interest. Testability refers to the degree to which a

variable lends itself to being measured, observed, and analyzed.

**Reference:** Norwood, S.L.: *Research Essentials: Foundations for Evidence-Based Practice.* Boston, Pearson, 2010, p 223.

3. **(D)** Randomization refers to the random assignment of study subjects to either control or treatment groups for the purposes of an experimental study. Blinding refers to the withholding of information from the study subjects, the persons implementing the study, or both. Control refers to a number of strategies used in research to hold study conditions constant so that true relationships between variables can be understood. Anonymity refers to a study participant's right to privacy and the expectation that the data a participant provides cannot be linked to that study participant. Anonymity is an essential element of ethically conducted research.

**Reference:** Norwood, S.L.: *Research Essentials: Foundations for Evidence-Based Practice.* Boston, Pearson, 2010, p. 75.

4. **(C)** Evidence-based practice is the result of integrating research, clinical expertise, and patient-family values and expectations into patient care. Although corporate directives should include the implementation of evidence-based practice, they are not an essential component of evidence-based practice. Clinician preferences are not considered a component of evidence-based practice and should be incorporated only when they are in line with current research and patient-family values and expectations. Quality improvement is a core competency that all health care professionals should possess and is an essential component of an optimal health care system. However, it is not an essential component of evidence-based practice. Efficiency and waste reduction are also important processes for an optimal practice environment, but cost-cutting measures are not an essential component of evidence-based practice.

**Reference:** Norwood, S.L.: *Research Essentials: Foundations for Evidence-Based Practice.* Boston, Pearson, 2010, p. 13.

5. **(D)** Reliability refers to the ability of an instrument to consistently measure the attribute of interest. Validity refers to the ability of an instrument to measure the attribute that it is intended to measure. Accuracy indicates the degree to which the value obtained for an attribute is congruent with its true value. Precision denotes the exactness with which an attribute is measured.

**Reference:** Norwood, S.L.: *Research Essentials: Foundations for Evidence-Based Practice.* Boston, Pearson, 2010, p. 257.

6. **(D)** Systematic reviews or meta-analyses, especially of randomized controlled trials, provide the highest level of evidence on which to base nursing practice. Descriptive studies are observational studies that give an overview of a particular phenomenon. Case-control studies are retrospective investigations of risk factors that compare a group which has a particular outcome of interest with a group which does not. Reports from expert committees can provide useful information to guide practice. None of these three types of data source represents the highest level of evidence.

**Reference:** DiCenso, A, Ciliska, D., and Guyatt, G. In DiCenso, A., Guyatt, G., and Ciliska, D: *Evidence-Based Nursing: A Guide to Clinical Practice.* St. Louis, Elsevier Mosby, 2005, p. 13.

## CHAPTER 32: LEGAL ISSUES

1. **(C)** The plaintiff must prove the following four things in a malpractice case: that the nurse had a duty to the patient, that there was a breach of that duty, that harm or damage did occur to the patient, and that breech of the nurse's duty resulted in harm (proximal cause). Intent is a purposeful action or plan. Malpractice can be unintentional. Accountability is being responsible and accounting for actions and not a specific element that must be proven by the plaintiff.

**Reference:** Verklan, M.T.: Legal Issues. In Verklan, M.T., Walden, M. (Eds.): *Core Curriculum for Neonatal Intensive Care Nursing,* 4th ed. St. Louis, Saunders, 2010, pp. 865-881.

2. **(C)** State nurse practice acts define the boundaries of nursing practice. Standards of care are what the average prudent nurse would do under similar circumstances. Practice guidelines are developed by professional associations to guide nursing practice. The American Nurses Association developed a Code of Ethics for nurses. Scope of practice may vary from state to state.

**References:** Williams, P.H., Sudia-Robinson, T.: Legal and ethical issues of neonatal care. In Kenner, C.A., Wright Lott, J.W. (Eds.): *Comprehensive Neonatal Care: An Interdisciplinary Approach,* 4th ed. St. Louis, Saunders, 2007, pp. 606-614.

Verklan, M.T.: Legal Issues. In Verklan, M.T., Walden, M. (Eds.): *Core Curriculum for Neonatal Intensive Care Nursing,* 4th ed. St. Louis, Saunders, 2010, pp. 865-881.

3. **(D)** Inappropriate comments that are admissions of legal liability regarding medical or nursing events should be avoided. Critical thinking was not demonstrated by the nurse in this situation. The nurse still has responsibility in this case. The nursing process is not being followed in this situation. The nurse does not document any nursing interventions done to further assess or correct blood pressure changes.

**Reference:** Verklan, M.T.: Legal Issues. In Verklan, M.T., Walden, M. (Eds.): *Core Curriculum for Neonatal Intensive Care Nursing,* 4th ed. St. Louis, Saunders, 2010, pp. 865-881.

4. **(D)** The nursing process forms the foundation for nursing education, practice, and documentation. Failure to follow the five steps of the nursing process is the number one cause of all patient injuries. Unfamiliarity with institutional protocol, lack of sufficient orientation and training, and lack of comprehensive standards of care all can lead to errors and injury; however, none of these is not reported as the leading cause.

**Reference:** Verklan, M.T.: Legal Issues. In Verklan, M.T., Walden, M. (Eds.): *Core Curriculum for Neonatal Intensive Care Nursing,* 4th ed. St. Louis, Saunders, 2010, pp. 865-881.

5. **(A)** Standard of care is what the average, reasonable, and prudent nurse would do under similar circumstances. The nursing process forms the foundation for nursing education, practice, and documentation. Scope of practice is developed by each state and

defines the boundaries of nursing. Policy and procedure are developed by the specific institution. Policy establishes the purpose of an activity, whereas procedure establishes how an activity will be carried out (the steps in performing the activity).

**Reference:** Verklan, M.T.: Legal Issues. In Verklan, M.T., Walden, M. (Eds.): *Core Curriculum for Neonatal Intensive Care Nursing,* 4th ed. St. Louis, Saunders, 2010, pp. 865-881.

6. **(A)** The nurse's legal responsibility in witnessing by signature an informed consent is to ensure that the parent voluntarily signed the consent form. The nurse's signature does not imply agreement with the diagnosis or procedure. The nurse does not witness that the physician's explanation was complete. The responsibility for obtaining informed consent remains with the person performing the procedure. The nurse's signature does not indicate that the nurse assessed and confirmed the parent's understanding of the risks, benefits, and alternatives.

**Reference:** Guido, G.W.: Legal and ethical issues. In Yoder-Wise, P.S. (Ed.): *Leading and Managing in Nursing,* 4th ed. St. Louis, Mosby, 2007, pp. 59-89.

7. **(B)** Autonomy addresses personal freedom and the right to choose what will happen to one's own person. Justice is treating all persons equally and fairly. Beneficence means that the actions one takes should promote good. Nonmaleficence means to do no harm.

**References:** Guido, G.W.: Legal and ethical issues. In Yoder-Wise, P.S. (Ed.): *Leading and Managing in Nursing,* 4th ed. St. Louis, Mosby, 2007, pp. 59-89.

Swaney, J., English, N., Carter, B.S.: Ethics, values, and palliative care in neonatal intensive care. In Gardner, S.L., Carter, B.S., Enzman-Hines, M., et al. (Eds.): *Merenstein and Gardner's Handbook of Neonatal Intensive Care,* 7th ed. St. Louis, Mosby, 2011, pp. 962-985.

## CHAPTER 33: ETHICAL ISSUES

1. **(B)** Bioethics seeks to determine the most morally desirable course of action in the context of conflicting values and multiple treatment variables. Ethics is the study of rational processes. Narrative ethics is ethical reasoning based in a story. Principle-based ethics consists of fundamental principles that form the foundation of ethical deliberation.

**Reference:** Swaney, J.R., English, N., Carter, B.S.: Ethics, values, and palliative care in neonatal intensive care. In Gardner, S.L., Carter, B.S., Enzman-Hines, M., et al. (Eds.): *Merenstein and Gardner's Handbook of Neonatal Intensive Care,* 7th ed. St. Louis, Mosby, 2011, pp. 962-985.

2. **(D)** *Autonomy* means that individuals have the right to make decisions for themselves. *Beneficence* means acting to benefit others. *Nonmaleficence* means doing no harm. *Justice* means fairness. Veracity, confidentiality, privacy, fidelity, and truth telling are rules for the professional-patient relationship. "Do no harm," "do good," "be truthful," and "be respectful" are phrases that define beneficence and nonmaleficence, but do not define justice and autonomy.

**Reference:** Beauchamp, T., Childress, J.: *Principles of Biomedical Ethics,* 6th ed. New York, Oxford University Press, 2008, pp. 99, 149, 197, 240.

3. **(A)** The rule of double effect is invoked to justify claims that a single act having two foreseen effects, one good and one harmful, is not always morally problematic. The agent's intention must be for the good effect, not the bad, and the bad effect must not be a means to the good effect. The good and bad effects must be weighed in proportion to one another. Fentanyl has the good effect of relieving pain and the foreseeable harmful effect of slowing respirations. The rule of double effect can be relied upon to distinguish between pain management during end of life and hastening death due to slowed respirations. Anaphylaxis is a serious adverse effect of antibiotic administration and would not outweigh the benefit of the antibiotic. Sedation is the intended good effect of midazolam. Stooling is the intended good effect of suppositories.

**Reference:** Beauchamp, T., Childress, J.: *Principles of Biomedical Ethics,* 6th ed. New York, Oxford University Press, 2008, pp. 162-166.

4. **(D)** The parents are the legal decision makers and bear the consequences of their decisions. The neonatologist has the obligation to provide the parents with information about the risks, benefits, and outcomes for the infant related to a specific medical condition or course of care. The primary nurse is part of the medical team, and the nurse's role is to provide support and relay information. The ethics committee can only provide guidance and help improve communication between the medical team and the parents.

**References:** Beauchamp, T., Childress, J.: *Principles of Biomedical Ethics,* 6th ed. New York, Oxford University Press, 2008, p. 171.

Griswold, K., Fanaroff, J.: An evidenced-based overview of prenatal consultation with a focus on infants born at the limits of viability. *Pediatrics,* 125(4):e931-e937, 2010.

5. **(A)** Nonmaleficence is the obligation not to inflict harm on others. "Do good" is the principle of beneficence. Fairness is the principle of justice. Autonomy is self-rule or self-governance.

**Reference:** Beauchamp, T., Childress, J.: *Principles of Biomedical Ethics,* 6th ed. New York, Oxford University Press, 2008, p. 149.

6. **(D)** Ethics committees are multidisciplinary in composition and are designed to ensure emotional stability, objectivity, and consistency. They help facilitate better communication among the medical team and families. The ethics committee is a consultative group only and cannot mandate an action or write orders. The ethics committee facilitates the understanding of information about a case. It does not change the plan of care.

**Reference:** Swaney, J.R., English, N., Carter, B.S.: Ethics, values, and palliative care in neonatal intensive care. In Gardner, S.L., Carter, B.S., Enzman-Hines, M., et al. (Eds.): *Merenstein and Gardner's Handbook of Neonatal Intensive Care,* 7th ed. St. Louis, Mosby, 2011, pp. 962-985.

7. **(D)** Open communication allows for all facts to be presented sensitively and thoroughly to create a relationship of trust. Charting accurately is critical to information sharing among the medical team; however, accurate documentation does not prevent ethical conflicts. Withholding information from the family erodes

the professional-parent relationship. Issues should be discussed openly between the medical team and the family to provide clear and open communication.

**References:** Beauchamp, T., Childress, J.: *Principles of Biomedical Ethics,* 6th ed. New York, Oxford University Press, 2008, p. 189.

Swaney, J.R., English, N., Carter, B.S.: Ethics, values, and palliative care in neonatal intensive care. In Gardner, S.L., Carter, B.S., Enzman-Hines, M., et al. (Eds.): *Merenstein and Gardner's Handbook of Neonatal Intensive Care,* 7th ed. St. Louis, Mosby, 2011, pp. 962-985.

8. **(B)** Informed consent is the individual's autonomous authorization to perform medical interventions or participate in research. Justice is the distribution of benefits, risks, and costs among members of society in relation to health care needs in a manner that is fair. Beneficence is doing good or benefiting others. Nonmaleficence is an obligation to cause no harm.

**Reference:** Beauchamp, T., Childress, J.: *Principles of Biomedical Ethics,* 6th ed. New York, Oxford University Press, 2008, p. 119.

9. **(C)** A treatment dilemma occurs when the outcome of a course of action is uncertain and there is a risk that a treatment decision, such as to resuscitate or not to resuscitate, will result in an undesirable outcome. Compassion is an attitude of active regard for another's welfare accompanied by an emotional response of sympathy, tenderness, and discomfort at another's misfortune and suffering. The description of the infant may indicate that this infant is not viable and that resuscitation would cause suffering for the infant. An ethical dilemma is the need to choose between alternatives that can be justified by moral rules or principles. Benevolence is the character trait of doing things to benefit others.

**References:** Beauchamp, T., Childress, J.: *Principles of Biomedical Ethics,* 6th ed. New York, Oxford University Press, 2008, p. 162.

Griswold, K., Fanaroff, J.: An evidenced-based overview of prenatal consultation with a focus on infants born at the limits of viability. *Pediatrics,* 125(4):e931-e937, 2010.

10. **(A)** Veracity is truthfulness or honesty. Fidelity is being loyal to a promise. Autonomy is the right of individuals to make decisions for themselves. Confidentiality is entrusting someone with information with the expectation that it will be kept private.

**Reference:** Beauchamp, T., Childress, J.: *Principles of Biomedical Ethics,* 6th ed. New York, Oxford University Press, 2008, p. 288.

## CHAPTER 34: AACN SYNERGY MODEL FOR PATIENT CARE

1. **(A)** A request for a social work consultation would be most effective to address the parents' transportation problem during this crisis period. Allowing the parents to verbalize their frustrations is acceptable but is not the best option to solve the immediate transportation concern. Speaking with the surgeon and reviewing clinical aspects of the disease process will not lead to a resolution of the parents' transportation problem.

This question illustrates the nurse characteristic of collaboration.

**Reference:** Kenner, C.: Families in crisis. In Verklan, M.T., Walden, M. (Eds.): *Core Curriculum for Neonatal Intensive Care Nursing,* 4th ed. St. Louis, Saunders, 2010, pp. 349-350.

2. **(A)** Given the disruption of work flow caused by having all of the work stations installed in one day, which could potentially compromise patient safety, the nurse should address this matter with the NICU nurse manager as an initial intervention. The nurse serving on the team may not have the authority to request a staged installation. Involvement of the director of neonatology or the hospital administrator may be necessary, but not as an initial intervention.

This question illustrates the nurse characteristic of systems thinking.

**Reference:** Smith, J.: Patient safety. In Verklan, M.T., Walden, M. (Eds.): *Core Curriculum for Neonatal Intensive Care Nursing,* 4th ed. St. Louis, Saunders, 2010, pp. 368-370.

3. **(C)** It is important for the mother to realize that omphalocele development is not the result of recreational drug use. A drug treatment program may be appropriate as a future intervention but does not address the mother's initial bedside concerns. Although the mother will likely meet with the social worker for counseling, the social worker may not be available at the time of the first bedside visit. The pediatric surgeon is most helpful in explaining the operative process and postsurgical course.

This question illustrates the nurse characteristic of facilitator of learning.

**Reference:** Bradshaw, W.: Gastrointestinal disorders. In Verklan, M.T., Walden, M. (Eds.): *Core Curriculum for Neonatal Intensive Care Nursing,* 4th ed. St. Louis, Saunders, 2010, pp. 595-596.

4. **(C)** Given that the mother has expressed concerns about both the surgical and nursing staff, a team meeting would be the best course of action. Speaking only to the surgeon would not resolve the issues related to the quality of nursing care. A quality issue may be identified as a result of an internal review process, but contacting the quality care coordinator would not be appropriate as an initial intervention. Provision of website resources should be accompanied by a discussion of the care needs of the individual infant and the infant's particular surgical repair.

This question illustrates the nurse characteristic of caring practices.

**Reference:** Kenner, C.: Families in crisis. In Verklan, M.T., Walden, M. (Eds.): *Core Curriculum for Neonatal Intensive Care Nursing,* 4th ed. St. Louis, Saunders, 2010, pp. 352-353.

5. **(C)** Ongoing, unit-based meetings will provide staff with the essential information about the initiative. Because this is not a formal research study but rather an evaluation of different skin care products available in the marketplace, recruitment is not necessary. Notification of the nurse manager of noncompliant staff would lend a punitive aspect to the initiative and would be counterproductive. Posting patient names in a public place would be a violation of the Health Insurance Portability and Accountability Act.

This question illustrates the nurse characteristic of clinical inquiry.

**Reference:** Smith, J.: Patient safety. In Verklan, M.T., Walden, M. (Eds.): *Core Curriculum for Neonatal Intensive Care Nursing,* 4th ed. St. Louis, Saunders, 2010, pp. 370-371.

6. **(C)** The best initial action is to allow the parents to verbalize their emotions, with the recognition that men and women may express their grief in different ways. Meeting with the chaplain may be helpful after the acute phase, but not initially. The neonatologist is unable to provide any more clinical information to the parents other than what has already been shared. A multidisciplinary team conference may be helpful in the future but would take time to plan and would not deal with the immediate emotional needs of the parents.

This question illustrates the nurse characteristic of response to diversity.

**Reference:** Kenner, C.: Families in crisis. In Verklan, M.T., Walden, M. (Eds.): *Core Curriculum for Neonatal Intensive Care Nursing*, 4th ed. St. Louis, Saunders, 2010, pp. 354-355.

7. **(C)** The best action is to speak with the physician regarding the current sedation plan to control the physiologic parameters of tachycardia, agitation, and accompanying desaturation. Respiratory therapy staff would not be able to alter the current sedation order. Increasing oxygen administration during cares is a potential need, but only after sedation is maximized. The frequency of nursing care activities cannot always be decreased for a critically ill neonate.

This question illustrates the nurse characteristic of clinical judgment.

**Reference:** Askin, D.: Respiratory distress. In Verklan, M.T., Walden, M. (Eds.): *Core Curriculum for Neonatal Intensive Care Nursing*, 4th ed. St. Louis, Saunders, 2010, pp. 467-468.

8. **(D)** A team discharge conference is most likely to result in an optimal discharge plan. The social worker consultation is necessary, but other team members must be involved to provide the most comprehensive discharge plan, given the medical complexity of the case. Contacting a homeless shelter will not address the multitude of psychosocial factors in this situation.

Child protective services will be unable to assist with all aspects of the discharge plan.

This question illustrates the nurse characteristic of advocacy and moral agency.

**Reference:** Hummel, P.: Discharge planning and transition to home care. In Verklan, M.T., Walden, M. (Eds.): *Core Curriculum for Neonatal Intensive Care Nursing*, 4th ed. St. Louis, Saunders, 2010, pp. 385-387.

9. **(C)** Performing echocardiography to determine the type of congenital heart disease would be most important given the results of the hyperoxia test. With these initial blood gas results, it is not necessary to repeat the blood gas analysis before performing echocardiography. Prostaglandin therapy will be needed if a duct-dependent lesion is identified. The blood gas results do not indicate a need for intubation or mechanical ventilation.

This question illustrates the nurse characteristic of clinical judgment.

**Reference:** Sadowski, S.: Cardiovascular disorders. In Verklan, M.T., Walden, M. (Eds.): *Core Curriculum for Neonatal Intensive Care Nursing*, 4th ed. St. Louis, Saunders, 2010, pp. 551-552.

10. **(C)** Given the escalation of care, it would be most appropriate to have the mother speak directly with the neonatologist, who can discuss the mother's concerns and the forthcoming plan of care. The respiratory therapist would not be able to address the medical plan of care. The previous administration of surfactant has no impact on the current sepsis episode. A discussion of the clinical aspects of respiratory distress does not speak to the complications of infection.

This question illustrates the nurse characteristic of facilitator of learning.

**Reference:** Siegel, R., Gardner, S., Dickey, L.: Families in crisis: Theoretical and practical considerations. In Gardner, S.L., Carter, B.S., Enzman-Hines, M., et al. (Eds.): *Merenstein and Gardner's Handbook of Neonatal Intensive Care*, 7th ed. St. Louis, Mosby, pp. 878-879.

## I. CLINICAL JUDGMENT (80%)

A. Cardiovascular (10%)

1. Acute heart failure/pulmonary edema
2. Acute inflammatory disease (e.g., myocarditis, endocarditis, pericarditis)
3. Cardiac surgery
4. Cardiovascular pharmacology
5. Congenital heart defect/disease
6. Hemodynamic concepts
7. Pulmonary hypertension
8. Shock states (e.g., cardiogenic, hypovolemic/volume deficit)

B. Pulmonary (36%)

1. Acute respiratory failure, hypoxemia
2. Acute respiratory infections
3. Air-leak syndromes (e.g., spontaneous pneumo-thorax, bronch fistula, emphysema, PIE, pneumo-pericardium, pneumomediastinum)
4. Apnea of prematurity
5. Aspirations (e.g., aspiration pneumonia, meco-nium aspiration)
6. Chronic lung disease (e.g., bronchopulmonary dysplasia)
7. Congenital anomalies
8. Pulmonary hypertension in newborn
9. Respiratory distress syndrome
10. Respiratory pharmacology
11. Thoracic surgery (e.g., lung contusions, frac-tured ribs, hemothorax, pulmonary hemorrhage, lung reduction, pneumonectomy, lobectomy, tracheal surgery)
12. Transient tachypnea of the newborn
13. Ventilator management and ABG interpretation, mixed venous gases, CPAP, volutrauma and barotraumas

C. Endocrine (4%)

1. Acute hypoglycemia
2. Hormones and anatomy & physiology
3. Inborn errors of metabolism
4. Infant of diabetic mother

D. Hematology/Immunology (4%)

1. Anemia of prematurity
2. Hematology, blood products and plasma
3. Hyperbilirubinemia
4. Immunosuppression (e.g., Rh incompatibilities, ABO incompatibilities, hydrops fetalis)
5. Life-threatening coagulopathies (e.g., ITP, DIC) and non life-threatening coagulopathies

E. Neurology (6%)

1. Congenital neurological abnormalities (e.g., spina bifida, myelomeningocele, anencephaly, encephalocele)
2. Encephalopathy (e.g., hypoxic-ischemic, metabolic, edema, infectious)
3. Hydrocephalus
4. ICP monitoring
5. Intracranial hemorrhage/intraventricular hemorrhage
6. Neurologic infectious diseases (e.g., meningitis, congenital infections, viral infections, TORCH)
7. Seizure disorders

F. Gastrointestinal (7%)

1. Bowel infarction/obstruction/perforation (e.g., necrotizing enterocolitis, adhesions, shortgut)
2. Gastro-esophageal reflux
3. GI abnormalities at birth
4. Hepatic failure/coma

G. Renal (2%)

1. Acute renal failure (e.g., acute tubular necrosis, hypoxia)
2. Congenital renal-genitourinary abnormalities (e.g., polycystic kidneys, exstrophy of bladder, hydronephrosis)
3. Fluid balance concepts and renal anatomy & physiology
4. Life-threatening electrolyte imbalances (e.g., potassium, sodium, phosphorus, magnesium, calcium)

H. Multisystem (11%)

1. Asphyxia (e.g., neonatal-perinatal)
2. Life-threatening maternal-fetal complications (e.g., birth trauma and birth-related injuries, genetic disorders, maternal-fetal transfusion, abruptio placentae, placenta previa)
3. Low birth weight/prematurity
4. Septic shock/infectious diseases (e.g., congenital, viral, bacterial, line sepsis, nosocomial infections)
5. Toxic exposure (e.g., fetal exposure to drug/alcohol, drug withdrawal, anaphylaxis)

## II. PROFESSIONAL CARING AND ETHICAL PRACTICE (20%)

A. Advocacy/Moral Agency (2%)
B. Caring Practices (4%)
C. Collaboration (4%)
D. Systems Thinking (2%)
E. Response to Diversity (2%)
F. Clinical Inquiry (2%)
G. Facilitation of Learning (4%)